Please

ROSEI

CW00828923

FRONTIERS IN NUTRITIONAL SCIENCE

This series of books addresses a wide range of topics in nutritional science. The books are aimed at advanced undergraduate and graduate students, researchers, university teachers, policy-makers and nutrition and health professionals. They offer original syntheses of knowledge, providing a fresh perspective on key topics in nutritional science. Each title is written by a single author or by groups of authors who are acknowledged experts in their field. Titles include aspects of molecular, cellular and whole-body nutrition and cover humans and wild, captive and domesticated animals. Basic nutritional science, clinical nutrition and public health nutrition are each addressed by titles in the series.

Editor in Chief
P.C. Calder, University of Southampton, UK

Editorial Board
A. Bell, Cornell University, Ithaca, New York, USA
F. Kok, Wageningen University, The Netherlands
A. Lichtenstein, Tufts University, Massachusetts, USA
I. Ortigues-Marty, INRA, Thiex, France
P. Yaqoob, University of Reading, UK
K. Younger, Dublin Institute of Technology, Ireland

Titles available

1. *Nutrition and Immune Function*
   Edited by P.C. Calder, C.J. Field and H.S. Gill
2. *Fetal Nutrition and Adult Disease: Programming of Chronic Disease through Fetal Exposure to Undernutrition*
   Edited by S.C. Langley-Evans
3. *The Psychology of Food Choice*
   Edited by R. Shepherd and M. Raats

THE PSYCHOLOGY OF FOOD CHOICE

Edited by

Richard Shepherd and Monique Raats

Food, Consumer Behaviour and Health Research Centre
Department of Psychology
University of Surrey
Guildford, UK

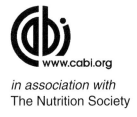

www.cabi.org

in association with
The Nutrition Society

CABI is a trading name of CAB International

CABI Head Office	CABI North American Office
Nosworthy Way	875 Massachusetts Avenue
Wallingford	7th Floor
Oxfordshire OX10 8DE	Cambridge, MA 02139
UK	USA

Tel: +44 (0)1491 832111
Fax: +44 (0)1491 833508
Email: cabi@cabi.org
Web site: www.cabi.org

Tel: +1 617 395 4056
Fax: +1 617 354 6875
Email: cabi-nao@cabi.org

A catalogue record for the hardcover edition of this book is available from the British Library, London, UK.

The Library of Congress has cataloged the hardcover edition as follows
The psychology of food choice / edited by Richard Shepherd and Monique Raats.
  p. cm.
    Includes bibliographical references and index.
    ISBN-13: 978-0-85199-032-3 (alk. paper)
    ISBN-10: 0-85199-032-0 (alk. paper)
    1. Food habits—Psychological aspects. I. Shepherd, R. (Richard)
II. Raats, Monique.
    [DNLM: 1. Food preferences—psychology. 2. Food Habits—psychology.
3. Emotions. 4. Age Factors. 5. Mass Media. QT 235 P974 2006]
TX357.S47 2006
394.1′2019—dc22

2005027934

ISBN-13: 978-0-85199-032-3 (hardback edition)
ISBN-13: 978-1-84593-723-2 (paperback edition)

First published 2006
Paperback edition 2010, reprinted 2011

Printed and bound in the UK by CPI Antony Rowe, Chippenham and Eastbourne.

Contents

Contributors

Armitage, Christopher J., *Department of Psychology, University of Sheffield, Sheffield S10 2TP, UK.*

Barnett, Julie, *School of Psychology, University of Surrey, Guildford GU2 7XH, UK.*

Bisogni, Carole A., *Division of Nutritional Sciences, Cornell University, Ithaca, NY 14853, USA.*

Bowen, Deborah J., *School of Public Health, University of Washington, Seattle, WA 98195-7660, USA and Fred Hutchinson Cancer Research Center, 1100 Fairview Ave N, M3-B232, Seattle, WA 98109-1024, USA.*

Brown, J. Lynne, *Department of Food Science, Penn State University, 205 A Borland, University Park, PA 16802, USA*

Caraher, Martin, *Department of Health Management and Food Policy, Institute of Health Sciences, City University, Goswell Place, Northampton Square, London EC1 0HB, UK.*

Clark, Christina, *School of Psychology, University of Surrey, Guildford GU2 7XH, UK.*

Conner, Mark, *Institute of Psychological Sciences, University of Leeds, Leeds LS2 9JT, UK.*

Devine, Carole M., *Division of Nutritional Sciences, Cornell University, Ithaca, NY 14853, USA.*

Gibson, E.L., *Clinical and Health Psychology Research Centre, School of Human and Life Sciences, Roehampton University, Whitelands College, Holybourne Avenue, London SW15 4JD, UK.*

Grunert, Klaus G., *MAPP – Centre for Research on Customer Relations in the Food Sector, Department of Marketing and Statistics, Aarhus School of Business, Haslegaardsvej 10, DK 8210 Aarhus V, Denmark.*

Harris, Peter, *Centre for Research in Social Attitudes, Psychology Department, University of Sheffield, Sheffield S10 2TP, UK.*

Higgs, Suzanne, *School of Psychology, University of Birmingham, Edgbaston, Birmingham B15 2TT, UK.*

Hilliard, Tracy, *School of Public Health, University of Washington, Seattle, WA 98195-7660, USA.*

Jastran, Margaret, *Division of Nutritional Sciences, Cornell University, Ithaca, NY 14853, USA.*

Landon, Jane, *National Heart Forum, Tavistock House South, Tavistock Square, London WC1H 9LG, UK.*

Lumbers, Margaret, *School of Management, University of Surrey, Guildford GU2 7XH, UK.*

McCartney, Glenda, *School of Psychology, Queen's University of Belfast, Belfast BT7 1NN, UK.*

Meiselman, Herbert L., *Natick Soldier Center, Natick, MA 01760-5020, USA.*

Miles, Susan, *School of Medicine, Health Policy and Practice, University of East Anglia, Norwich NR4 7TJ, UK.*

Muldoon, Orla, *School of Psychology, Queen's University of Belfast, Belfast BT7 1NN, UK.*

Pliner, Patricia, *Department of Psychology, University of Toronto at Mississauga, 3359 Mississauga Road, Mississauga, Ontario L5L 1C6, Canada.*

Raats, Monique, *Food, Consumer Behaviour and Health Research Centre, Department of Psychology, University of Surrey, Guildford GU2 7XH, UK.*

Reilly, Jacquie, *Public Health and Health Policy, University of Glasgow, 1 Lilybank Gardens, Glasgow G12 8RZ, UK.*

Rozin, Paul, *Department of Psychology, University of Pennsylvania, 3815 Walnut Street, Philadelphia, PA 19104-6196, USA.*

Salvy, Sarah-Jeanne, *Department of Psychology, University of Toronto at Mississauga, 3359 Mississauga Road, Mississauga, Ontario L5L 1C6, Canada.*

Scaife, Vicky, *School of Social Work and Psychosocial Sciences, University of East Anglia, Norwich NR4 7TJ, UK.*

Sheeran, Paschal, *Department of Psychology, University of Sheffield, Sheffield S10 2TP, UK.*

Shepherd, Richard, *Food, Consumer Behaviour and Health Research Centre, Department of Psychology, University of Surrey, Guildford GU2 7XH, UK.*

Sobal, Jeffery, *Division of Nutritional Sciences, Cornell University, Ithaca, NY 14853, USA.*

Trew, Karen, *School of Psychology, Queen's University of Belfast, Belfast BT7 1NN, UK.*

Wardle, Jane, *Health Behaviour Unit, Department of Epidemiology and Public Health, University College London, London WC1E 6BT, UK.*

Webb, Thomas L., *Department of Psychology, University of Sheffield, Sheffield S10 2TP, UK.*

Westerterp, Klaas R., *Department of Human Biology, Maastricht University, PO Box 616, 6200 MD Maastricht, The Netherlands.*

Yeomans, Martin R., *Department of Psychology, School of Life Sciences, University of Sussex, Falmer, Brighton BN1 9QG, UK.*

Preface

We all eat foods every day and in Western societies we are confronted with a vast array of different types of foods with different prices, offering different sensory experiences and of varying composition in terms of nutritional components. Although the proportion of income spent on food has declined, food nevertheless remains a major part of an ordinary person's expenditure and the various parts of the food industry including production, manufacturing, retail and catering represent a very significant part of the overall economy.

If we are interested in the nutrition of free-living people then we have to understand not only what factors influence people's choice of foods and how consumers make decisions in relation to the amounts of food eaten, but also the choice between different alternatives. Likewise, if we are interested in improving the nutritional status of individuals or populations then we need to understand what influences choice and how we might impact upon those choices. Since nutritional intake is a consequence of a complex set of behaviours, the behavioural sciences, including psychology, have a lot to offer in terms of furthering our understanding in this area.

The present book brings together insights from a number of sub-disciplines within psychology and also related disciplines, in terms of what they can tell us about the influences on human food choice. The book is organized in five main sections which cover: models of food choice; biological and learning influences on food choice; societal influences on food; food choices across the lifespan; and changing dietary behaviour.

One of the difficulties in this area is that because human food choice is influenced by so many potential factors, there is often a tendency to look at the impact of these factors in isolation rather than trying to arrive at some overall understanding of the interplay between different types of influences. The chapters in the first section present general overviews on how we might conceptualize the different types of influences on food choice and also bring these together in a more integrated framework.

The second section not only includes consideration of the underlying biological influences on food choice and the amounts of food consumed, but also adopts a learning approach to try to understand how people make choices about foods given that there are few in-built predispositions in humans to choose particular types of foods or sensory experiences. Most food choice is learned both during early childhood and also from experiences later in life. The chapters in this section explore the role of experience and learning and also related aspects of the relationship between mood and food choice and food cravings.

While there are clearly influences at the level of the individual, there are also wider societal influences on food choice and these ideas are explored in the third section of the book. Here such influences as the media, advertising and marketing of foods are considered, along with more general environmental impacts on eating.

The fourth section looks at food choices across the lifespan. Clearly the impact of different factors on food choice will vary as people move across the lifespan and the chapters in this section take as a starting point examination of some of these influences on people at different ages.

The final section deals with attempts at changing dietary behaviour. Dietary behaviour has important health consequences, being associated with, for example, cardiovascular diseases and various cancers and also the growing problems linked to overweight and obesity. One of the major interests in trying to understand food choice is often a desire to try to influence dietary behaviour and to improve the nutritional intake of individuals or populations. This final section explores dietary interventions and the application of psychological theories such as the stages of change theory, implementation intentions and the role which optimistic bias might play in affecting attempts at changing dietary behaviour.

Given the importance that food choice has in terms of nutritional consequences and also in terms of economics, social and cultural life and personal enjoyment, it is important to try and understand this particular type of human behaviour. The present volume seeks to explore some of the complexity of trying to understand human food choice and the ways in which our understanding might be improved in the future.

Richard Shepherd
Monique M. Raats
University of Surrey

1 A Conceptual Model of the Food Choice Process over the Life Course

JEFFERY SOBAL, CAROLE A. BISOGNI, CAROL M. DEVINE AND MARGARET JASTRAN

Division of Nutritional Sciences, Cornell University, Ithaca, NY 14853, USA

Introduction

Food choice involves the selection and consumption of foods and beverages, considering what, how, when, where and with whom people eat as well as other aspects of their food and eating behaviours. Food choices play an important role in symbolic, economic and social aspects of life by expressing preferences, identities and cultural meanings. Food choices are important because they create consumer demand for suppliers in the food system who produce, process and distribute food (Sobal *et al.*, 1998). Food choices also determine which nutrients and other substances enter the body and subsequently influence health, morbidity and mortality.

Because of their crucial biological, psychological, economic, social, cultural and epidemiological importance, many researchers and practitioners pay attention to food choices (e.g. Marshall, 1995; Meiselman and MacFie, 1996; Murcott, 1998). Three general approaches have been used to develop models of food choices (Sobal, 1997). First, existing models, frameworks and theories developed to explain other topics are applied to examine food choices, such as the theory of planned behaviour, health belief model, transtheoretical model, social cognitive theory, hedonic consumer choice model, etc. (e.g. Axelson and Brinberg, 1989; Lancaster, 1991, 1998; Baranowski *et al.*, 1999; Conner and Armitage, 2002). Second, new models to explain food choice have been deductively developed, where analysts create their own explanations about how food choices are made (e.g. Lucas, 1984; Krondl, 1990; Nestle *et al.*, 1998; Wetter *et al.*, 2001). Third, models of food choice have been inductively developed using qualitative research methods to produce emergent conceptualizations of how people think about and engage in food choices (e.g. Furst *et al.*, 1996; Palojoki, 1997).

This chapter focuses on an inductively developed and evolving model of the food choice process devised using in-depth qualitative interviews with adults in the USA that asked about how they constructed their food choices (Falk *et al.*, 1996;

Furst *et al.*, 1996; Connors *et al.*, 2001). The chapter considers this food choice process model's components, elaborations and applications. This model is compatible with a biopsychosocial perspective (Engel, 1980) in assuming that physiological, cognitive and sociocultural influences and processes are all involved together in making food choices. However, it emphasizes a constructionist approach (Berger and Luckmann, 1967; Spector and Kitsuse, 1987) in assuming that while sensory, biological, behavioural and social structural factors contribute to food choices, people actively consider, interpret and negotiate food choice possibilities and exercise their personal agency in perceiving, defining, conceptualizing, managing, presenting and enacting food choices. This model assumes that a key process in selecting foods is the construction of food choices based on cognitions and social negotiations. Overall, people are assumed to construct food choices in a variety of ways by actively selecting what, when, where, with whom and how to eat.

A Food Choice Process Model

The range of factors potentially involved in choosing foods is tremendously diverse and extensive. Many of the most important components of the construction of food choices are portrayed in the food choice process model presented in Fig. 1.1 (Falk *et al.*, 1996; Furst *et al.*, 1996; Connors *et al.*, 2001). This model seeks to be comprehensive and integrated by representing crucial parts of the process that people use in selecting foods and relationships between them, although the model is not exhaustive in explicitly listing all possible factors involved in making food choices. The components of the model also are not mutually exclusive of each other because they overlap and interact.

This food choice process model includes three major components that operate together when people construct food choices: the life course, influences and personal systems. In interviews about food choice, people often attribute current eating patterns to prior experiences, so the 'life course' is a key component of the model. As people describe food choices, they explain how various factors emerging from past experiences and current situations shape their eating, and these are labelled 'influences' in the model. The 'personal food system' for selecting foods is the process whereby people operationalize influences on food choices. The following sections present these components in greater detail and provide selected examples.

Life course

As people develop and change over time they are shaped by their environments and personally construct an individual life course that involves past and current food and eating experiences and situations as well as expectations about future possibilities. This suggests that food choices are dynamic and evolve over time. While developmental (e.g. growth, maturation and ageing) and life stage (e.g. childhood, adolescence, adulthood, later life) perspectives consider individual

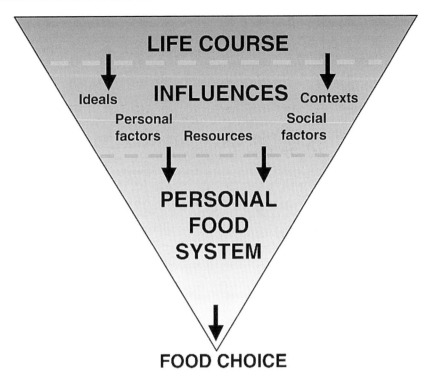

Fig. 1.1. A food choice process model. (Adapted from Falk *et al.*, 1996; Furst *et al.*, 1996; Connors *et al.*, 2001.)

growth over the lifespan, the more dynamic life course perspective provides additional insights by considering a person's agency in determining their own food choice trajectory, the accumulation of experiences over time, the anticipation of the future, and the importance of changes in contexts at specific points in time (Elder, 1985). A life course approach to food choice complements biological studies of early life programming and those that track dietary behaviour over time by including the changing social, behavioural and cultural contexts in which the individual eats. Key concepts developed in other work on the life course that also emerge in people's reports about how they construct food choices over time include trajectories, transitions, timing and contexts (Elder, 1985; Devine, 2005; Fig. 1.2).

  Trajectories are a central concept in life course thinking. Food choice trajectories include a person's 'persistent thoughts, feelings, strategies, and actions over the lifespan' (Devine *et al.*, 1998). Pathways in food choice behaviour and attitudes have been described over specific life course transitions such as bearing children (e.g. Devine *et al.*, 2000) and over longer periods in the lifespan such as mid-life (e.g. Edstrom and Devine, 2001). People develop food choice trajectories within specific situational and historical contexts that become persistent, exhibiting their own momentum and continuity (Devine *et al.*, 1998, 1999b). For example, a person may grow up with the family tradition of eating a salad at every evening meal and continue that trajectory for much or all of his or her life.

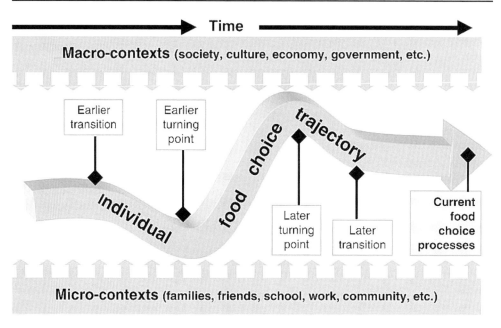

Fig. 1.2. A conceptual model of how food choice is shaped by contexts over time to form a food choice trajectory. (Adapted from Devine *et al.*, 1998.)

The food choice trajectories of lifelong salad eaters may differ, however, from those of salad eaters who only began that pattern as adults, and may lead to differential ability to persist in salad eating behaviour when life changes occur. Repeated food choices create momentum for making the same food selections in future circumstances. Food choice trajectories provide momentum leading to habitual food selections that can affect how individuals adjust to life course transitions such as ageing and changes in health (Paquette and Devine, 2000). People arrive at their current food choices within trajectories that are developed over the course of their lives, shaped by contexts they encounter and the past transitions they have made.

Transitions are shifts in a person's life that lead to changes or solidify the continuation of behaviours, including food choice patterns (Devine *et al.*, 1998, 1999a). Major life events such as entering or leaving school, changing employment, entering or leaving important personal relationships, migrating to a different area or culture, developing an illness and others represent transitions that may become turning points that have major impacts on food choices (Devine, 2005). These transitions and turning points change roles, resources, health or contexts in ways that perturb or disturb usual personal food systems and can lead to minor (in the case of transitions) or radical (in the case of turning points) reconstruction of food choice patterns that establish new personal food systems which begin different food choice trajectories.

Timing represents when a particular transition or turning point occurs in the life course of an individual, with the specific timing of an event influencing whether and how it may influence food choices. For example, many mothers adopt healthier food choices during pregnancy and child-rearing, but childbirth among young immature adolescents is 'off time' in the usual course of development of social roles and may not enhance the adoption of a healthier food choice trajectory (Devine *et al.*, 2000).

Contexts represent the environments within which life course changes occur, including social structure, economic conditions, historical eras and the changing physical environment (Devine, 2005). A person born at one period comes of age, lives through mid-life and becomes elderly within historically specific normative family patterns, employment and financial conditions, historical–cultural belief systems, patterns of food availability, eating standards, and epidemiological environments where particular diseases are or are not major risk factors. Thus a person growing up in the depression era of the 20th century developed different trajectories of food choices from those of their grandchildren growing up today. For example, people raising children early in the 20th century socialized their offspring in a different historical context of professional dietary advice than those currently teaching young people about food (Devine and Olson, 1991). Also, people growing up in an earlier historical era represent a cohort that is more concerned about wasting food than those in contemporary eras (Falk *et al.*, 1996).

In summary, a person's life course provides temporal individual and historical precursors and contexts for current food choices, with people developing personal food choice trajectories that are subject to change in relationship to particular life course transitions they experience at different periods in their lives. Each new food choice experience adds to a person's life course and shapes subsequent food choices. Investigation of changes in the food choice trajectories of groups of individuals provides an opportunity to examine the impact of social, economic and food system trends on food choices. A life course perspective provides a framework for considering a variety of individual and contextual influences on food choices.

Influences

A wide variety of influences operates to shape particular food choices. The food choice process model clusters these influences into five types: ideals, personal factors, resources, social factors and contexts (see Fig. 1.1). Each of these types of influences is embedded within and fluctuates over the life course of a person making food choices, interacts with all of the other influences, and is operationalized in the personal food system of the individual as they engage in specific eating practices. This section describes these five major categories of influences on food choices and provides selected examples.

Ideals are the standards people have learned through socialization and acculturation that they use to make food choices. Ideals represent normative gauges about what and how one should eat. Ideals are culturally learned through families and other institutions, and reflect the plans and expectations for food and eating. Cultural and sub-cultural norms establish which foods are acceptable and preferable for consumption among larger cultures and ethnic groups within cultures, and individuals consider those ideals in food selection (Sobal, 1998;

Devine *et al.*, 1999b). For many individuals, ideals about proper meals, appropriate manners and health are among the most crucial influences on their food choices. For example, Falk *et al.* (1996) found that the ideals about what a meal should be ('meat and potatoes') were held by older adults and constituted some of the most important factors driving their food choices.

Personal factors are characteristics of the individual that influence food choices. Personal factors include physiological factors (sensory, endocrinological, genetic, etc.), psychological or emotional characteristics (preferences, personalities, moods, phobias, etc.) and relational factors (identities, self-concept, etc.). These personal factors develop and are learned over time for each person and provide the basis for the unique and individualized construction of food choices. Dietary individualism, where people make different food choices from others, is based on the priority of personal factors over other influences (Bove *et al.*, 2003). For example, people establish personal food and eating identities (Jabs *et al.*, 1998a; Bisogni *et al.*, 2002) that represent their self-image as a specific type of eater and operate to shape their specific food selections. Some individuals experience food cravings and addictions that operate as personal factors in shaping food choices (Hetherington, 2001).

Resources are assets available to people for making food choices. Resources include tangible physical capital such as money, equipment, transportation and space; intangible human capital such as time, skills and knowledge; and intangible social capital such as help from others, advice and emotional support (e.g. Senauer *et al.*, 1991). Individuals construct food choices by being aware of the resources they can use in making food selections, often assessing food choice options by excluding those which are not possible given existing resources. In constructing food choices, most people consider some types of food choices 'out of bounds' because they do not have the money, time, facilities or cooking skills to choose them. For example, many low-income people manage food choices according to their changing financial situations as they experience greater or lesser food insecurity (Radimer *et al.*, 1992).

Social factors are relationships in which people are embedded that influence food choices. Roles, families, groups, networks, organizations, communities and other social units provide opportunities and obligations for constructing eating relationships and food choices. Most eating occurs in commensal groups, where individuals need to negotiate and manage their own food choices in conjunction with the food selections of others (Sobal and Nelson, 2003). Managing such eating relationships is a crucial and often contested part of the food choice process, and with whom someone eats often governs where, when, how and what they eat (Sobal, 2000). For example, spouses eat most of their meals together and negotiate joint food selections symmetrically (with both partners converging together) or asymmetrically (with one partner adopting the food choices of the other; Bove *et al.*, 2003).

Contexts are the broader environments within which people make food choices. Contexts include physical surroundings and behaviour settings, social institutions and policies, and seasonal and temporal climate. An important context within which people make food choices is the food and nutrition system (Sobal *et al.*, 1998), which determines which foods are available for individuals to choose from, how and where they are prepared, served and eaten, and the social meanings and functions with which they are imbued. The home and the workplace are two key contexts where food choices are made, with mutual 'spillover' occurring between those settings (Devine *et al.*, 2003). As people eat in an increasingly wider range of environments, the location-specific structural elements and social processes affecting food choices become ever more complex. Most contexts change, leading people to reconstruct their food choices, such as the seasonality of food availability or the historical evolution of mass media marketing, advertising and programming as a context for food information (Avery *et al.*, 1997).

In summary, influences on food choice include an extensive scope of biological, behavioural, psychological, cultural, economic, social, geographical, political, historical, environmental and other influences that are iteratively considered and reconsidered both simultaneously and sequentially in food choice decision-making in conscious and subconscious ways. The importance of particular factors may change over the life course and vary for particular situations. Influences provide input for the personal systems individuals develop for use in cognitively constructing specific food choices.

Personal food system

Personal food systems are the mental processes whereby people translate influences upon their food choices into how and what they eat in particular situations (Furst *et al.*, 1996; Connors *et al.*, 2001). Personal food systems represent ways that options, trade-offs and boundaries are constructed in the process of making food choices. Personal food systems include the processes of constructing food choice values, classifying foods and situations according to these values, negotiating these personally defined values in food choice settings, balancing competing values, and developing strategies for food selection and eating in different situations. These processes are presented in Fig. 1.3 and described in the following sections.

Food choice values represent a set of considerations important in constructing food choices (Falk *et al.*, 1996; Furst *et al.*, 1996; Connors *et al.*, 2001). These values involve personally developed interpretations and meanings related to food and eating as well as involving emotional affect and attachment (Smart and Bisogni, 2001). Food choice values are dynamic, changing over time as life course events and experiences shape food choice influences that may result in new or modified food choice values. Research finds that five types of values (taste, convenience, cost, health and managing relationships) consistently emerge as salient among many people, with other additional values also salient to some individuals and groups (Connors *et al.*, 2001).

Taste is a food choice value that represents the considerations that people develop related to their sensory perceptions in eating and drinking. People use the word 'taste' to describe many different characteristics of food and beverages that affect their food enjoyment and aversions, including appearance, odour, flavour, texture and other properties. Taste is a primary consideration for most people in nearly all food and drinking settings. It is important to recognize that

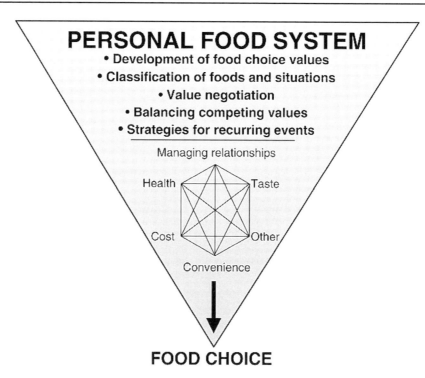

Fig. 1.3. Details of the personal food system. (Adapted from Connors *et al.*, 2001.)

individual taste preferences may change over time. Few people enthusiastically eat things that do not taste good to them, and thus taste is often used as a minimum criterion for whether or not a food or drink will be consumed. The importance of taste cannot be overstated, and the physiological, cultural, social, developmental and life stage aspects of taste have been topics of extensive study by other researchers (e.g. Rozin and Vollmecke, 1986; Meiselman and MacFie, 1996; Murcott, 1998).

Convenience is a value that refers to the time and effort considerations that people employ in constructing food choices. Convenience relates to the actual time, physical ability and the mental or physical involvement it takes for a person to acquire, prepare, consume and clean up after eating or drinking. Convenience is also a personal judgement about the opportunity cost of expending time and effort in relationship to the benefits from a particular food or drink (Gofton, 1995). Convenience to older adults often relates to transportation to acquire food or difficulty in opening a can or lifting a pot (Falk *et al.*, 1996). In contrast, time is frequently the primary meaning of convenience for students and people who are employed (Furst *et al.*, 1996; Connors *et al.*, 2001; Smart and Bisogni, 2001; Devine *et al.*, 2003). The consideration of convenience also varies according to cooking skills.

Cost is a value representing the monetary considerations that people construct related to food choices. Most food in contemporary post-industrial societies is purchased rather than self-produced, and the prices of buying food to eat at home or away from home are judged in food choices. The price of food related to someone's monetary resources is encompassed in this value, and this topic is an important and ongoing focus of food economists (Senauer *et al.*, 1991). However, the value of cost also includes the concept of 'worth'. People with unlimited disposable incomes may still be very sensitive to price increases because they do not feel that the product is 'worth it', whereas people with low incomes may still buy a food that is high in price because they believe that the food is essential to their well-being or satisfaction.

Health is a value that broadly represents food choice considerations constructed in relationship to physical well-being. Included in this value are considerations about immediate responses to food and drink such as digestive discomfort, allergic reactions, energy levels or athletic performance, as well as considerations about longer-term consequences such as growth, weight control, illness management or chronic disease prevention (Falk *et al.*, 1996; Furst *et al.*, 1996; Smart and Bisogni, 2001). Foods are often classified by the public as 'good' or 'bad' based on the meanings related to health and physical well-being. The definitions for health related to eating in the population vary considerably, including overall balance, nutrient balance, low fat, weight control, naturalness, disease management and disease prevention (Falk *et al.*, 2001).

Managing relationships is a value that represents how someone considers the interests and well-being of other people involved in a person's social world. When people provide food for others, share food with others or receive food from others, they typically consider the needs, preferences and feelings of those people related to what, how, when and where food is eaten. Personal needs and preferences are often compromised to build, maintain or repair relationships. Food is central to family harmony, and someone who adopts the role of the 'household food manager' is typically very attentive to the preferences, dislikes and patterns of eating of others (DeVault, 1990). For example, newly married couples must negotiate ways to make joint food choices (Bove *et al.*, 2003) and parent–child relationships contribute to constructing family food decisions (Birch, 1980). Being a host, guest or co-worker also shapes food choice situations where roles and relationships (e.g. politeness, organizational duties) are primary considerations in food choice (Devine *et al.*, 2003).

Other values that are considered in food choice include quality, variety, symbolism, ethics, safety and waste (Furst *et al.*, 1996; Jabs *et al.*, 1998b; Connors *et al.*, 2001). For some people, considerations related to these values are highly salient, whereas for other people they are considered only in certain circumstances. For example, religious beliefs, ethnic identity and environmental concerns are primary considerations in food choice for some people, whereas other people will be highly focused on their personally constructed expectations for 'quality' related to the way food is grown, stored, prepared or presented (Bisogni *et al.*, 1987).

Classification

When they think about eating, people categorize objects into foods and non-foods, and further classify foods according to their personally constructed food choice values (Furst *et al.*, 2000; Connors *et al.*, 2001; Falk *et al.*, 2001). People also classify food and eating situations, such as believing 'eating at home is healthy; eating out is not' (Connors *et al.*, 2001). Personally operational classification schemes for food and eating situations are embedded in classification schemes that are significant for one's close social environment (i.e. family or friends), which are embedded in classification schemes provided by the wider cultural environments (i.e. region or nation; Fig. 1.4). The concept of personally operational classification allows the same food to be viewed as 'healthy' or 'unhealthy' or as 'cheap' or 'expensive' by different people living in the same household. The concept of socially significant classifications acknowledges the shared categories (i.e. 'we both like', 'we make this food together') that two or more people develop for food and eating based on their eating relationships.

The classification of foods and eating situations is a way that people simplify food choices in a society where the food system is complex and many different ways of eating are possible and acceptable (Furst *et al.*, 2000; Connors *et al.*, 2001). People classify foods and eating situations according to multiple dimensions that they construct based on their food choice values. The study of consumers' perceptions of multidimensional food attributes is a focus of consumer research (e.g. Lancaster, 1991), and the inductively derived food choice process model emphasizes consumers' ways of constructing classifications.

Each particular food or eating situation may be seen as a bundle of different attributes that are bound together and must be considered simultaneously in

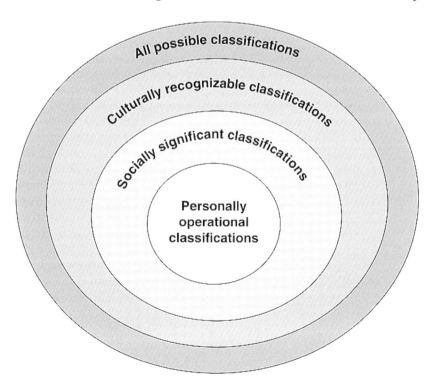

Fig. 1.4.   Multiple levels of food classifications. (Adapted from Furst *et al.*, 2000.)

making food choices (Lancaster, 1991). The characteristics of each specific food often represent conflicting values that require reconciliation in making food choices. For example, fresh broccoli may be seen by some household members as healthy and convenient but expensive and not tasty. These combined attributes of broccoli come together as one 'package' and must be evaluated as a composite whole in the process of considering broccoli as a possible food option.

Value negotiation is a key food choice process because only rarely can all food choice values be satisfied in a particular food and eating situation (Furst *et al.*, 1996). People prioritize values and weigh the options for how and what they will eat in a given setting. Prioritizing values into a hierarchy often occurs simultaneously as people rate foods according to their salient values and then order choice options according to their hierarchy for those values (Connors *et al.*, 2001). The priority of food choice values varies according to individual traits, personal states and situational contexts. Some values reinforce each other and lead to easier choices, whereas other values are in opposition and lead to difficult selections. Because value conflicts occur, people must often make choices that are 'trade-offs' between opposing values such as choosing a tasty or healthy snack or selecting between an inexpensive or convenient meal. For some individuals, certain values dominate all food choices and serve as limiting factors, such as a gourmand who consistently values taste and quality and would rather not eat in certain situations than compromise these values. Similarly, a person concerned about diabetes may base most food choices primarily on management of the disease.

Balancing is a process that people use to resolve many food choice value conflicts. People construct their own ways of ensuring that all of their salient values are met in food choices. Balancing occurs over personally defined frames of reference such as times (day, week, month), eating occasions, places or eating partners (Connors *et al.*, 2001). For example, some people eat healthy foods during the work week and indulge in less healthy foods on weekends. Other people vary the importance of health over months, restricting food choices at certain seasons of the year (Smart and Bisogni, 2001; Bisogni *et al.*, 2002). Others may limit the amount of money spent on food for everyday eating but not worry about cost on vacations or holidays. Still others may seek out spicy food when eating alone or with co-workers but accept eating bland food with their children (Bisogni *et al.*, 2002).

Strategies are the behavioural plans, routines and rules that people develop for how and what they eat in recurring situations (Falk *et al.*, 1996; Furst *et al.*, 1996; Connors *et al.*, 2001). Strategies simplify food choice by eliminating the cognitive effort and time required for deliberation about every food choice. Strategies emerge from initial conscious food choice decisions for a specific situation and eventually become less mindful when that situation occurs repeatedly. The strategies of a personal food system are congruent with the cognitive processes of developing schemas and scripts for different behavioural settings (Blake and Bisogni, 2003). Schemas are constructions of the personal assessment and meaning of a situation, and scripts represent the behavioural plan for that situation (Rumelhardt, 1984).

The strategies that people employ to expedite food choice in recurring situations can be characterized according to the nature of the heuristic being used for the strategy (Falk *et al.*, 1996, 2001; Connors *et al.*, 2001). Types of heuristics include: focusing on one value, routinization, elimination, limitation, substitution, addition and modification (Falk *et al.*, 1996, 2001; Connors *et al.*, 2001; Fig. 1.5). Focusing on only one value discounts other values as less relevant and defines a food choice setting in a very specific way so that values do not have to be negotiated. Routinization standardizes food choice decision-making processes or actual eating behaviours for a recurring situation into habits and automatic behaviours. Elimination excludes particular foods, food categories, eating locations or eating partners from all food choice options or makes exclusions for particular settings. Limitation restricts use of selected foods or ways of eating to simplify food choice decisions, but is more complex than elimination because it requires establishing acceptable levels and then monitoring adherence to those limits. Substitution replaces foods or ways of eating to accommodate conflicting values by supplanting one option with another that is more satisfactory. Addition selects particular foods or includes food components to satisfy specific values. Modification changes foods, their components or ways of eating to make them more acceptable.

Examples of these types of heuristics are reported in a study of college hockey players (Smart and Bisogni, 2001). The types of foods chosen by the players in the food choice events preceding a game or practice focused solely on 'health', defined by them as easily digestible food that made them feel 'explosive' on the ice. The pre-game meals consistently involved the same foods and

Strategy	Example
Focusing on one value (emphasize only cost, taste, health, relationships, convenience or another value)	Eat the cheapest food whenever possible
Routinization (standardize, systematize, ritualize)	Eat cereal every day for breakfast
Elimination (avoid, exclude, prohibit)	Never eat desserts
Limitation (restrict, regulate, reduce)	Drink only two cups of coffee each day
Substitution (replace, exchange, fill in)	Choose brown rice instead of white rice
Addition (augment, include, enhance)	Eat a salad with every evening meal
Modification (alter, adjust, transform)	Remove fat from meats and poultry

Fig. 1.5.   Selected strategies for simplifying food choices. (Adapted from Falk *et al.*, 1996.)

seating arrangements (routinization). Immediately after the competitive season, the players focused solely on another food choice value – taste – as they indulged in the higher-fat fast foods that they had desired but avoided in preceding months. Additional examples of the heuristics employed in food choice strategies come from studies of cardiac patients (Janas *et al.*, 1996; Falk *et al.*, 2001). Some cardiac patients managed personal food choice by abandoning former ways of eating and fully adopting the heart-healthy dietary recommendations that they permanently maintained (routinization). Other patients made less drastic dietary changes using some new foods (substitution) or recipes to reduce the fat in their typical diet (modification). Other approaches used by patients involved rejecting certain foods, food components or eating locations (elimination) to avoid food choice value conflicts.

Most people use multiple strategies for making food choices and the combinations of strategies that are used have been described as a repertoire (Falk *et al.*, 1996, 2001). While some people have developed and use one dominant strategy for their repertoire, others use multiple strategies simultaneously, sequentially or situationally to deal with varying food choice conditions (Janas *et al.*, 1996; Falk *et al.*, 2001). For example, one person may focus on convenience in all settings, whereas another person may focus on convenience during the work week but emphasize taste and quality on the weekend. Breakfast may be routinized for some people who also use a substitution heuristic for dinners. Individuals who have developed a variety of strategies that they can employ in various settings tend to be more adaptive eaters or food providers than those who have only a few strategies that they are not experienced with combining into different repertoires (Falk *et al.*, 1996).

The repertoires that someone uses for food choices are shaped by personal and social identities, and food choice repertoires also contribute to constructing identities (Bisogni *et al.*, 2002). For example, mothers described different food choice schemas for their personal eating and their roles in providing foods for their family (Blake and Bisogni, 2003). The predominant types of food choice schema for personal eating included dieter, health fanatic, picky eater, non-restrictive eater and inconsistent eater, and the major types of provider food schema included peacekeeper, healthy provider, struggler and partnership (Blake and Bisogni, 2003).

Strategies and repertoires for food choice are acquired over the life course by personally creating them or learning them from others. Strategies and repertoires are dynamic and responsive to changes in other food choice processes. For example, a new marriage or a new health condition is a life course transition that typically changes the influences of personal factors, resources, social contexts and food contexts (Janas *et al.*, 1993; Falk *et al.*, 2000, 2001; Bove *et al.*, 2003). For example, although someone's food choice values related to taste may remain the same, values related to managing relationships, costs and health may change in meaning and salience which results in new food classifications, new value negotiations and new ways of balancing food choices. In novel circumstances, food choices are typically reflective and mindful for a period of time while people try different ways of eating. When satisfactory ways of food choice emerge, they become automatized strategies for recurring food choice events.

In summary, the personal food system is the way that individuals construct food choices, considering values and employing other cognitive processes for selecting foods. Personal food systems may be particularly important to recognize in societies where many options for eating are available and few rules exist to guide how and what one eats (Fischler, 1988; Murcott, 1998). People construct primary food choice values (such as taste, convenience, cost, health and managing relationships), conceptually organize foods and eating situations according to these values, prioritize food choice values in specific situations, and negotiate values and balance ways of eating as needed and desired. Food choices in recurring situations are simplified by the construction of strategies that result in rules, routines and habits for decision making and food behaviours. Personal food systems are dynamic and evolving as they respond to new life course events and experiences as well as new food choice influences and situations that a person encounters.

Conclusion

The food choice process perspective presented here can be used as a framework or as a model (Sobal and Lee, 1997). A framework is a way to list and map disparate concepts into a more coherent whole, representing elements that are important to include and locating those elements with respect to each other. Thinking about the food choice process as including life course, influences and a personal system provides such a representation that incorporates and links a broad scope of factors involved in making food selections. A model is more integrated than a framework, making assumptions about mechanisms and processes operating together in a consistent theoretical manner. Thinking about food choice as a constructed activity where past experiences and contexts in the life course provide a basis for evaluating current influences and incorporating them into personal systems that lead to food selections permits specific modelling of the processes involved in how people choose foods.

Like all models, frameworks and theories, this food choice process model has several limitations. In an attempt to broadly consider multiple issues in making food choices, the model does not focus deeply on specific factors and does not explicitly consider some factors. The model was developed to examine individual food choices of consumers, and it needs to be further elaborated when applied to collective food choices of families and other multi-person units involving group decision making (Stratton and Bromley, 1999). The model was developed and has largely been applied in a post-industrial Western society in the late 20th and early 21st century and may require considerable adaptation, elaboration and extension to serve well in other cultures, places and historical eras. This model may not apply as well if multiple food options are not available, as in famines, subsistence cultures or settings where only a fixed menu is available, etc. (although the model is not irrelevant under those conditions). Also, the underlying constructionist assumptions of the food choice process model may be contested and challenged by thinking that takes other theoretical perspectives (e.g. Hacking, 1999).

This food choice process model has several applications in research settings. As a framework for considering the scope of factors involved in food choices, it is useful in identifying particular issues to examine, manipulate and consider as controls in analysis of food selections. For example, psychological analyses of cognitive food choice processes such as value negotiations may benefit from controlling for the influences described by the model and stratifying according to life course experiences. As a model of how people construct food choices, much future work needs to be done to elaborate processes and mechanisms, such as examining how influences such as resources specifically shape the operation of cost in value negotiations. The model also offers a broad map of potential factors involved in making food choices, and lets researchers who do focus on a particular biological, psychological, social, cultural, economic or other aspect of food choice locate their findings with respect to other factors involved in food choices.

This food choice process model can be applied in clinical, community and policy work (Bisogni, 2003; Bisogni *et al.*, 2003). Clinicians can use the model as a guide for assessing important factors involved in food choices of their clients, and as a guide for uncovering the personal food choice systems of the people with whom they work. Clinicians can use this food choice process model to work with clients to identify and dissect strategies and repertoires that habitually guide food choices, to understand clients' values as a way to identify what experiences are strongest in shaping current food choices, and to review these food choice processes as a first step in planning dietary changes. Community practitioners can use the model for identifying key influences of populations that can be modified, such as local cultural values or community food systems. Policy work can employ the model to consider how to leverage social and economic changes to improve healthy eating in populations and to target particular subgroups.

In summary, food choices can be conceptualized using existing, deductive and inductive models. The inductively developed food choice process model described here represents a broad, multifaceted, dynamic and integrated perspective for thinking about food choices, incorporating life course, influences and personal systems into a constructed system for choosing foods. Food choices are constructed using the thoughts, feelings and actions of individuals, with people creating their own systems for making food choices as they move through a life course. This food choice process model is not all-inclusive and may not meet the needs of every food choice analyst, but it may be useful to researchers and practitioners by providing a broad framework to use as a road-map for identifying and drawing attention to potential factors involved in food choices and as a more focused model representing the ways that people construct food choices.

Acknowledgements

The authors thank Georgie Fear, Karen Gunderson and Lisa Ranzenhoffer for helpful comments on the manuscript, and acknowledge support for this work from the United States Department of Agriculture (CSREES) and the Division of Nutritional Sciences at Cornell University.

References

Avery, R.J., Mathios, A., Shanahan, J. and Bisogni, C.A. (1997) Food and nutrition messages communicated through prime-time television. *Journal of Public Policy and Marketing* 16, 217–227.

Axelson, M.L. and Brinberg, D. (1989) *A Social–Psychological Perspective on Food-related Behavior*. Springer-Verlag, New York.

Baranowski, T., Cullen, K.W. and Baranowski, J. (1999) Psychosocial correlates of dietary intake: advancing dietary intervention. *Annual Review of Nutrition* 19, 17–40.

Berger, P.L. and Luckmann, T. (1967) *The Social Construction of Reality*. Anchor, New York.

Birch, L.L. (1980) The relationship between children's food preferences and those of their parents. *Journal of Nutrition Education* 12, 14–18.

Bisogni, C.A. (2003) *Communication about Food Choice: Tools for Professional Development*. Division of Nutritional Sciences, Cornell University, Ithaca, New York.

Bisogni, C.A., Ryan, G.J. and Regenstein, J.M. (1987) What is fish quality? Can we incorporate consumer perceptions? In: Kramer, D.E. and Liston, J. (eds) *Seafood Quality Determination*. Elsevier Science, Amsterdam, pp. 547–563.

Bisogni, C.A., Connors, M.M., Devine, C. and Sobal, J. (2002) Who we are and how we eat: a qualitative study of identities in food choice. *Journal of Nutrition Education and Behavior* 34, 128–139.

Bisogni, C.A., Sobal, J., Jastran, M. and Devine, C.M. (2003) *Creating Food Choice Dialogues*. Division of Nutritional Sciences, Cornell University, Ithaca, New York.

Blake, C. and Bisogni, C.A. (2003) Personal and family food choice schemas of rural women in upstate New York. *Journal of Nutrition Education* 35, 282–293.

Bove, C.F., Sobal, J. and Rauschenbach, B.S. (2003) Food choices among newly married couples: convergence, conflict, individualism, and projects. *Appetite* 40, 25–41.

Conner, M. and Armitage, C.J. (2002) *The Social Psychology of Food*. Open University Press, Buckingham, UK.

Connors, M.M., Bisogni, C.A., Sobal, J. and Devine, C. (2001) Managing values in personal food systems. *Appetite* 36, 189–200.

DeVault, M.L. (1990) *Feeding the Family: The Social Organization of Caring as Gendered Work*. University of Chicago Press, Chicago, Illinois.

Devine, C.M. (2005) A life course perspective: understanding food choices in time, social location, and history. *Journal of Nutrition Education and Behavior* 37, 121–128.

Devine, C.M. and Olson, C.M. (1991) Women's dietary prevention motives: life stage influences. *Journal of Nutrition Education* 23, 269–274.

Devine, C.M., Connors, M., Bisogni, C. and Sobal, J. (1998) Life course influences on fruit and vegetable trajectories: qualitative analysis of food choices. *Journal of Nutrition Education* 30, 361–370.

Devine, C.M., Sobal, J., Bisogni, C.A. and Connors, M. (1999a) Food choices in three ethnic groups: interactions of ideals, identities, and roles. *Journal of Nutrition Education* 31, 86–93.

Devine, C.M., Wolfe, W.S., Frongillo, E.A. and Bisogni, C.A. (1999b) Life-course events and experiences: association with fruit and vegetable consumption in 3 ethnic groups. *Journal of the American Dietetic Association* 99, 309–314.

Devine, C.M., Bove, C. and Olson, C. (2000) Continuity and change in women's weight orientations and lifestyle practices through pregnancy and the postpartum period: the influence of life course trajectories and transitional events. *Social Science & Medicine* 50, 567–582.

Devine, C.M., Connors, M., Sobal, J. and Bisogni, C.A. (2003) Sandwiching it in: spillover of work onto food choices and family roles in low- and moderate-income urban households. *Social Science & Medicine* 56, 617–630.

Edstrom, K.M. and Devine, C.M. (2001) Consistency in women's orientation to food and nutrition in midlife and older age: a 10-year qualitative follow-up. *Journal of Nutrition Education* 33, 215–223.

Elder, G. (1985) *Life Course Dynamics: Trajectories and Transitions 1968–1980.* Cornell University Press, Ithaca, New York.

Engel, G. (1980) The clinical application of the biopsychosocial model. *American Journal of Psychiatry* 137, 535–544.

Falk, L.W., Bisogni, C.A. and Sobal, J. (1996) Food choice processes of older adults. *Journal of Nutrition Education* 28, 257–265.

Falk, L.W., Bisogni, C.A. and Sobal, J. (2000) Diet change processes of participants in an intensive heart program. *Journal of Nutrition Education* 32, 240–250.

Falk, L.W., Sobal, J., Devine, C.M., Bisogni, C.M. and Connors, M. (2001) Managing healthy eating: definitions, classifications, and strategies. *Health Education & Behavior* 28, 425–439.

Fischler, C. (1988) Food, self, and identity. *Social Science Information* 27, 275–292.

Furst, T., Connors, M., Bisogni, C.A., Sobal, J. and Falk, L. (1996) Food choice: a conceptual model of the process. *Appetite* 26, 247–265.

Furst, T., Connors, M., Sobal, J., Bisogni, C.M. and Falk, L.M. (2000) Food classifications: levels and categories. *Ecology of Food and Nutrition* 39, 331–355.

Gofton, L. (1995) Convenience and the moral status of consumer practices. In: Marshall, D.W. (ed.) *Food Choice and the Consumer.* Blackie Academic, London, pp. 152–181.

Hacking, I. (1999) *The Social Construction of What?* Harvard University Press, Cambridge, Massachusetts.

Hetherington, M.M. (2001) *Food Cravings and Addiction.* Food Research Association, Leatherhead, UK.

Jabs, J.A., Sobal, J. and Devine, C.M. (1998a) Managing vegetarianism: identities, norms, and interactions. *Ecology of Food and Nutrition* 39, 375–394.

Jabs, J.A., Devine, C.M. and Sobal, J. (1998b) A model of the process of adopting vegetarian diets: health vegetarians and ethical vegetarians. *Journal of Nutrition Education* 30, 196–202.

Janas, B.G., Bisogni, C.A. and Campbell, C.C. (1993) A conceptual model for dietary change to lower serum cholesterol. *Journal of Nutrition Education* 25, 186–192.

Janas, B.G., Bisogni, C.A. and Sobal, J. (1996) Cardiac patients' mental representations of diet. *Journal of Nutrition Education* 28, 223–229.

Krondl, M. (1990) Conceptual models. In: Krasnego, N.A., Miller, G.D. and Simopoulos, A.P. (eds) *Diet and Behavior: Multidisciplinary Perspectives.* Springer Verlag, New York, pp. 5–16.

Lancaster, K.J. (1991) *Modern Consumer Theory.* Edward Elgar, Brookfield, Vermont.

Lancaster, K.J. (ed.) (1998) *Consumer Theory.* Edward Elgar, Northampton, Massachusetts.

Lucas, A.R. (1984) Psychosocial factors and food intake. In: White, P.L. and Selvey, N. (eds) *Malnutrition: Determinants and Consequences.* Alan R. Liss, New York, pp. 315–324.

Marshall, D. (ed.) (1995) *Food Choice and the Consumer.* Blackie Academic & Professional, New York.

Meiselman, H.L. and MacFie, H.J.H. (eds) (1996) *Food Choice, Acceptance and Consumption.* Blackie Academic & Professional, New York.

Murcott, A. (ed.) (1998) *The Nation's Diet: The Social Science of Food Choice*. Addison Wesley Longman, New York.

Nestle, M., Wing, R., Birch, L., DiSorgr, L., Drenowski, A., Middleton, S., Sigma-Grant, M., Sobal, J., Winston, M. and Economos, C. (1998) Behavioral and social influences on food choice. *Nutrition Reviews* 56, S50–S64.

Palojoki, P. (1997) *The Complexity of Food-related Activities in a Household Context: Study of Finnish Homemakers' Food Choices and Nutrition Knowledge*. Dissertation, Department of Teacher Education, University of Helsinki, Helsinki.

Paquette, M. and Devine, C.M. (2000) Dietary trajectories in the menopause transition among Québec women. *Journal of Nutrition Education* 32, 320–328.

Radimer, K.L., Olson, C.M., Greene, J.C., Campbell, C.C. and Habicht, J. (1992) Understanding hunger and developing indicators to assess it in women and children. *Journal of Nutrition Education* 24, S36–S45.

Rozin, P. and Vollmecke, T.A. (1986) Food likes and dislikes. *Annual Review of Nutrition* 6, 433–456.

Rumelhardt, D.E. (1984) Schema and the cognitive system. In: Wyers, R.S. and Siwl, T.K. (eds) *Handbook of Social Cognition*. Lawrence Erlbaum, Hillsdale, New Jersey, pp. 161–188.

Senauer, B., Asp, E. and Kinsey, J. (1991) *Food Trends and the Changing Consumer*. Eagan Press, St Paul, Minnesota.

Smart, L.R. and Bisogni, C.A. (2001) Personal food systems of college hockey players. *Appetite* 37, 57–70.

Sobal, J. (1997) Conceptualizing food choices. Presentation to the *Intercontinental Food Choice Conference*, Uppsala, Sweden.

Sobal, J. (1998) Cultural comparison research designs in food, eating, and nutrition. *Food Quality and Preference* 9, 385–392.

Sobal, J. (2000) Sociability and meals: facilitation, commensality, and interaction. In: Meiselman, H.L. (ed.) *Dimensions of the Meal: The Science, Culture, Business, and Art of Eating*. Aspen Publishers, Gaithersburg, Maryland, pp. 119–133.

Sobal, J. and Lee, S. (1997) Use of social science theories in community nutrition. *Korean Journal of Community Nutrition* 2, 671–679.

Sobal, J. and Nelson, M.K. (2003) Commensal eating patterns: a community study. *Appetite* 41, 181–190.

Sobal, J., Khan, L.K. and Bisogni, C.A. (1998) A conceptual model of the food and nutrition system. *Social Science & Medicine* 47, 853–863.

Specter, M. and Kitsuse, J.I. (1987) *Constructing Social Problems*. Aldine de Gruyter, Hawthorne, New York.

Stratton, P. and Bromley, K. (1999) Families' accounts of the causal processes in food choice. *Appetite* 33, 89–108.

Wetter, A.C., Goldberg, J.P., King, A.C., Sigman-Grant, M., Baer, R., Crayton, E., Devine, C., Drenowski, A., Dunn, A., Johnson, G., Pronk, N., Saelens, B., Snyder, D., Novelli, P., Walsh, K. and Warland, R. (2001) How and why do individuals make food and physical activity choices? *Nutrition Reviews* 59, S11–S20.

2

The Integration of Biological, Social, Cultural and Psychological Influences on Food Choice

PAUL ROZIN

Department of Psychology, University of Pennsylvania, 3815 Walnut Street, Philadelphia, PA 19104-6196, USA

Introduction

Almost everything influences food choice, at one time and place or another. Food is so important, and permeates human life in so many ways, that it engages and interacts with almost all of our activities: leisure, the arts, sex, work . . . everything but sleep . . . and there is nothing like a long sleep after a good meal.

Because of the richness and complexity of human food choice, many disciplines have something to say about it: biology, psychology, sociology, anthropology, economics, history and medicine, among others.

The plain fact is that the biggest determinant of what an individual eats is availability. One eats what is there, and more critically, one does not eat what is not there. This mundane fact should not discourage intellectual inquiry, because the determinants of what is available to any individual have biological, psychological, social, cultural and historical aspects.

One situation frequently focused upon by investigators, especially marketers, sensory testers and psychologists, has an individual facing a set of food choices. Under these conditions, we can say that psychological factors are probably pre-eminent, and that expectations about taste, convenience and health will predominate. The rich and complex interaction of expectations, beliefs and values can be modelled in this situation, as for example in the work of Richard Shepherd and his colleagues (Shepherd and Raats, 1996). As we focus more on availability, as opposed to the moment of choice, we are forced into considerations that take us well beyond psychology.

The 'moment' of food choice, for humans and other animals, is but a step in a series of behaviours organized for the quest for food. Typically, there is arousal by biological and cultural motives for nutrition (often described as hunger, in the former case, and 'mealtime' in the latter case). What follows, in the precultural environment, is the search for food, the detection of food or foods, the choice (or decision to accept or not), followed in some cases by capture of the food, then perhaps some preparation of the food, and finally its ingestion. For some species, especially food generalists, the stage of choice is particularly important. Food generalists such as humans, cockroaches and rats eat a wide range of foods, and encounter many different potential foods. 'To eat or not to eat' is a weighty decision, often made. The stakes are high: good food means life, and bad food may mean death. The risks are not just of consuming toxins, but of consuming nutritionally inadequate, unbalanced diets. For animals that eat a single type of food, like many carnivores and some herbivores, the choice situation is simplified. If it is the right size and alive, and capturable, the carnivore will go for it. There is no need to worry about toxins or imbalances: a live animal almost guarantees both safety and nutritional adequacy. For humans, cultural forces enhance the ambivalence of generalist eating. It is widely believed that 'you are what you eat'; that is, that people take on the properties of the foods they eat (Nemeroff and Rozin, 1989). These properties can be positive, such as strength, but also negative, such as animality.

Food and in particular, choosing and obtaining food, are as central to biological evolution as any activity. Furthermore, for the food generalist, there is usually no problem more difficult than finding nutritionally adequate foods, and avoiding toxins and imbalances. It is no accident that many animal groups are described in terms of their food habits: among the mammals (themselves named for their early milk drinking) there are Carnivora and Insectivora for example, and primates are often described in terms of their food habits: principally fruit or leaf eaters, for example.

Food choice assumes a central role in human evolution, with, according to most views, a shift from a primarily vegetarian diet to a more omnivorous diet with the movement from the forest to the savannah. And there is nothing more important in human cultural evolution than the twin advances of agriculture and animal domestication. As Diamond (1997) correctly notes, it is this major advance that makes most of the rest of the flowering of culture possible. It frees humans from day-to-day dependence on the vagaries of nature, and allows for the specialization of labour that leads to impressive technologies.

The quest for food plays a major role in the life of virtually all humans. For the less developed world, food probably accounts for 50% of total expenditures, in comparison to less than 25% for developed countries (Anon, 1990). But, of course, most human beings are in the former category. Among our daily activities, food-related behaviours are probably the third most time-consuming, following on sleep and work (Szalai, 1972).

Preadaptation and the Food Domain

Food would be complex enough for the reasons already stated. But for humans it is yet more complicated, because food has become integrated into many functions and activities that have nothing to do with nutrition. The process through which this has occurred is referred to as preadaption in biological evolution. As explained by Ernst Mayr (1960), preadaptation is the major source of innovation in evolution, and consists of the use of features already evolved to serve a particular function, to now serve a new function. In the process, the original function may be displaced, or there may be a sharing of function. Appropriately for a discussion of food, the human mouth is an excellent example. The mouth, its tongue and teeth, evolved for breathing and for processing of food. But when language arises in humans, it takes advantage of the preadapted food/breathing system, with oral cavity, teeth and tongue in the line of breathing. The teeth and tongue become an integral part of speech production, although they evolved for food functions.

In cultural evolution, preadaptation is even more important than it is in biological evolution. This is because, unlike in biological evolution, humans can conceive of a value for one system in another context, and make it happen. For example, fire is useful both to keep warm and to cook food. They can use a wheel in many ways. In the preadaptive history of food in human cultural evolution, food moves from its original function to assume many others (Fig. 2.1a).

Food becomes a social marker. It identifies one's group, as does a distinctive cuisine distinguish, say, Chinese from Indians. It also functions socially as the opportunity for family social interaction at meals, and for celebrations, such as marriages. In modern Western societies, it becomes a major arena for making

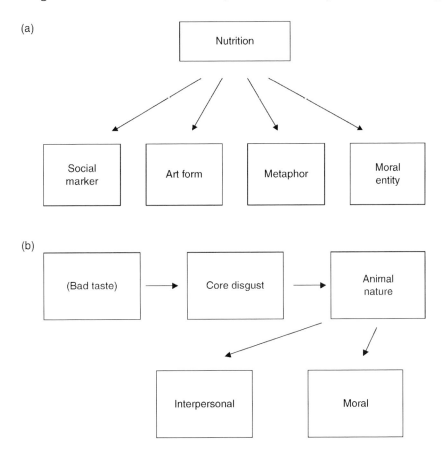

Fig. 2.1.   (a) Preadaptation and food; (b) preadaptation and disgust.

social contacts, dating or business deals. And it becomes an expression of affection and attachment, as in chocolate on Valentine's day and turkey on Thanksgiving. Sharing of food is a major sign of intimacy, cross-culturally. A purely nutritional perspective would be totally inadequate to capture these important uses of food.

Food also becomes a form of aesthetic satisfaction. The development of cuisine, and high cuisines in some cultures, represents an attempt to enrich life and produce aesthetic pleasure. There is no way in which nutrition requires fancy desserts, or the elaborate mixtures of spices in Indian cuisine. The social and aesthetic functions of food are so prevalent that a visitor from another planet might take some time to discover that food was 'essentially' about staying alive, about nutrition.

Food enters into our language, as part of communication, in yet another preadapted form. Food words are central parts of metaphors. Metaphors themselves are examples of preadaptation, where a term from one domain (in this case, food and nutrition) is used to describe another. So, when we say that someone is a sweet person, that we can't stomach a particular ideology, that we wish Rozin would get down to the meat of this paper (meat will be discussed later), we are using food for non-nutritional functions.

Finally (Fig. 2.1a), food plays a role in the moral world. The laws of kashrut in the Jewish religion and the various food transfer prohibitions between castes in Hindu India have to do not with nutrition, but with moral standing. The taking of the host in the Catholic Mass is a symbolic, moral use of food. In Hindu India, more than in the USA, food is an explicitly moral entity, described by Appadurai (1981) as a 'biomoral' substance. One can recreate the Hindu caste structure, based essentially on moral purity, by simply studying food transfer rules. In the USA, the moral function of food is more muted, although it is hard to escape noticing how cigarettes have become morally undesirable ingestants, and further, suggestions that high-calorie, sweet and fat foods have taken on a negative moral tinge (Stein and Nemeroff, 1995).

The spectacular elaboration of food and eating, and entry of food into all of the domains of life, is captured beautifully, for European civilization, by Leon Kass (1994) in his splendid book, *The Hungry Soul*. He describes the transformation, at one point, as from 'fressen to essen'. Eating on the spot and wolfing down food, as opposed to sitting at a table, eating with silverware, not taking bites of the food on another's plate and using the meal as a focus for conversation.

There is something special about food in this regard. While, in general, the development of culture is often associated with a de-emphasis of humans' biological functions (e.g. the general modesty about carrying out sexual and excretory functions), the biological function of gaining nutrition is typically accomplished in public, and often celebrated. Eating is the one biological function that has been both celebrated and transformed by culture. Human sex and excretion are much more like dog sex and excretion than is human eating like dog eating. Kass's story of the transformation of eating requires an integration of biological (nutritional and evolutionary), psychological, social, cultural and historical perspectives.

The cultural evolution of disgust, as studied by myself and my colleagues, April Fallon, Jonathan Haidt and Clark McCauley, illustrates the co-opting of a food function for a wide range of cultural purposes (Rozin and Fallon, 1987; Rozin *et al.*, 2000). The great majority of exemplars of disgust that we have elicited from Americans, Japanese and Asian Indians do not have to do with food. The varied involvements of the emotion of disgust in human life can be traced to a basic foundation emotion, which has to do with rejecting food (Fig. 2.1b). The prototype of disgust is the rejection of foods from the mouth based on a negative oral experience (taste, flavour, texture, temperature). In human cultural evolution, this response, which we can call the distaste response, transforms into a response that is basically about rejecting food because of its nature (ideational rejection), as opposed to its sensory properties. We call this 'core disgust', and it accounts for the principal food disgusts, such as responses in most cultures to specific spoiled foods, insects, animal wastes and other specific parts of animals. In our view, this type of disgust, which appears in children after the first few years of life, is what disgust is really about. Indeed, most adults do not label foods they do not like the taste of as disgusting. The original distaste system becomes disconnected from the disgust system.

The food-related core of disgust is evidenced in the following ways: (i) the word 'disgust', with similar derivations in some other languages, means bad taste; (ii) the facial expression of disgust, including a gape, is a gesture of oral rejection; and (iii) the physiological signature of disgust, nausea, is a symptom which specifically inhibits eating.

We hold that, in cultural evolution, this powerful rejection response has been co-opted by cultures to many things that are rejected by the culture. In the process of socialization, one can cause individuals to reject culturally undesirable entities by making them disgusting. According to our analysis, the major step in the cultural evolution has to do with disgust becoming attached to reminders of our animal nature, including aspects of sex, excretion, poor hygiene, indicators of our animal-like insides (blood, viscera) and, most interestingly, death, a property we share with animals. We note that the quintessential odour of disgust is the odour of decay or death.

We trace the cultural evolution of disgust (Fig. 2.1b) to two more domains of human life. Interpersonal disgust is about contact with other people, particularly people whom one does not like, or people from other groups. Finally, moral disgust has to do with attaching disgust to certain types of moral violations. These are usually what might be called violations of 'purity', best illustrated in Hindu India by disgust at contacts with less pure individuals or entities (associated with lower castes; see Miller, 1997, for an extended discussion of the invasion of the moral domain by disgust).

A central feature of core disgust is contagion: when a disgusting food touches otherwise acceptable foods, it renders them permanently inedible. This contagion property of disgust is carried along with disgust as it expands to a wider domain. Thus, individuals are disgusted by wearing clothing that had been worn by a person they consider immoral.

The trajectory described here for disgust, and that described for general food preadaptation by Kass (1994), illustrates the complex interactions of biological roots, individual psychology and culture in the shaping of the modern human mind and the physical and institutional world created by humans.

What is Food Choice?

The simplest manifestation of food choice is relative intake. Thus, we might note that the intake of rice is higher per capita in China than in the USA, but the intake of beef is higher in the USA. Food intake of particular foods is rather easy to obtain on a national basis, and is the focus of many economic analyses. It is motivated in part by preference and liking, but also, to a great degree, by availability, geographic and economic factors.

Preference has to do with a comparison of two of more foods, as part of a set from which a choice can be made. A prefers B to C means that when A is faced with a choice of B and C, under specified conditions, A prefers B. There are two important things to note about preference. First, although it influences intake, it is only one of many influences. Thus, Chinese might prefer beef to rice, but this would not be expressed in relative intake because of cultural, geographic and economic factors. Second, preference is related to liking, but does not stand for liking. One may prefer B to C, but like C better. For example, many Americans like ice cream more than salad, but will choose a salad because of concerns about weight and health.

Liking is the psychologically most interesting feature of food choice. It is most interesting because it motivates much food choice, and we do not really understand what gets people to like or dislike foods. It is easier to understand why health concerns or cost influence preference. So liking is a major determinant of preference, and preference is a major determinant of intake, but many other variables intervene.

The preference–liking distinction motivates a psychological taxonomy of foods, which in turn sets part of the agenda for understanding food choices. We can identify three basic motives for choosing or refusing potential foods: sensory properties (taste, flavour, smell, appearance), effects of ingestion (repletion, nausea, etc.) and ideational concerns (having to do with the nature or origin of a food; Rozin and Fallon, 1980). These three motives define four categories of food acceptance and rejection. With respect to rejections, distastes are motivated by sensory properties, and map rather clearly on to likings (examples might be hot pepper, black coffee or broccoli, depending on the individual). Dangers are motivated by concerns about the consequences of ingestion (examples for Americans include foods very high in fat or foods believed to contain toxins). Inappropriates are potential foods that just do not fit within the cultural definition of food (ideational rejection; examples include paper and sand). Finally, disgusts are multiply motivated rejections. They are primarily rejected because of their nature (ideational/inappropriate), but are also usually believed to be both harmful (dangers) and bad tasting (distastes). There is a corresponding division of accepted foods into those accepted because they are liked on sensory grounds (good tastes, e.g. candy), because they are thought to have positive consequences (beneficials, e.g. bread), because they are just classified as food (appropriates, e.g. turkey on Thanksgiving) and what we will call transvalued foods, the opposite of disgust, enhanced because of their nature or origin, and thought to be desirable on both sensory features and effects. Transvalued foods are much less common than their opposite, disgusting foods. Examples might be food prepared by or partaken by admired or loved others.

Finally, any food liking or preference is heavily dependent on context. Breakfast foods are preferred and liked only for breakfast; steak and whipped cream are both highly desirable to most people, but not mixed together. The importance and function of context have been explored and reviewed by a number of investigators, including Meiselman (1996) and Rozin and Tuorila (1993). Howard Schutz (1989), in considering this important feature of food choice, coins the apt term 'appropriateness' to describe it.

Perspectives on Human Food Choice

In this section, the disciplinary foci on food choice will be summarized across the four disciplines that have the most to say about food: biology, psychology, sociology and anthropology. Food selection in a broad perspective is treated in a number of edited volumes (Barker, 1982; Meiselman and MacFie, 1996; Meiselman, 2000).

Biological (physiological and evolutionary/adaptive) influences

Biological approaches to food choice take two forms. One focuses on physiological mechanisms, and its focus is explaining, at the moment, what is going on in the body and the brain when a food choice occurs. Most of this research is carried out with animals, particularly the domestic rat. The focus has been on the regulation of energy intake, but there is important information on food choice as well. The pioneer in this area is Curt Richter (1943). The case of sodium appetite is perhaps best investigated (Richter, 1956; Denton, 1982; Schulkin, 1991). The physiological approach has two aspects, metabolic and neural. That is, one aspect has to do with the processing of nutrients, and the metabolic events that become the stimuli for action, via communication of nutritional states to the nervous system. The second aspect focuses on the brain, and how and where information about metabolic state is integrated with information about the environment, other motives, etc., to lead to choice. This very important area, growing in relevance to human food choice with the recent development of non-invasive brain scanning techniques, will receive no more attention in this chapter (see relevant chapters in this book for further discussion of this perspective).

More central to the present review is the adaptive/evolutionary approach, which places an animal in its ecological niche, and in the context of its evolutionary history attempts to understand food choice, feeding strategies and the like. The critical frame for humans, in this respect, is as a food generalist (Rozin, 1976). As such, it is impossible to make adaptive decisions about the safety and nutritional quality of a potential food on just sensory properties. Hence, for the generalist, most knowledge about the food world must be acquired.

There are some biological predispositions that help the generalist to negotiate the world of literally thousands of potential foods and poisons. Most clear are
taste biases: innate biases to prefer sweet tastes (associated with fruit) and avoid
bitter (correlated with toxins; Steiner, 1979). As well, there seem to be innate aversions to very strong tastes, including salt or sour. There are early-onset fat preferences and irritant avoidances, which are also probably innate. As Bartoshuk
(1990) has noted, while the taste system has a number of innate links between
tastes and hedonic responses, the smell system is much more open-ended and
relies heavily on learning.

There is a complex of behaviours involving cautious sampling of new potential foods, a balance of neophobia and neophilia, most studied in rats.

There are specific learning mechanisms that facilitate the evaluation of
potential foods in terms of toxicity (taste aversion learning; Rozin and Kalat, 1971;
Garcia et al., 1974) and beneficial effects (Sclafani, 1999), allowing learning to
bridge the long delay between ingestion and the consequences of that ingestion
(illness or repletion). And there is the general tendency to come to like entities that
one experiences repeatedly (mere exposure; Zajonc, 1968). This can be enhanced
by social learning; at a minimum, increased exposure can be produced by the
food choices of local conspecifics (Galef, 1988).

Animals with specialized diets, such as koalas or anteaters, often have genetically prespecified means of detecting appropriate foods. With a very narrow
range of potential foods, such animals simply need one internal detection system
which indicates a need for energy (since all foods are essentially nutritionally
complete) and a sensory system for identifying that food (Rozin, 1976). Dietary
generalists have subsystems which operate like specialists. Thus, rats and humans
have a water system, which indicates a specific need for water, and some means
of detecting water or entities with high water content. A similar system exists, at
least in rats and some other animals, for salt (Richter, 1956; Denton, 1982;
Schulkin, 1991), and the hunger system provides guidance in the domain of
energy: hunger indicates the need for energy, and sweet and fat preferences help
to identify sources of calories.

None the less, the generalist, and in particular the human generalist, must
for the most part learn about what is good to eat, and what is not; and yet more
complicated, what combinations of foods are good, and what are not. The evo-
lutionary/adaptive approach to human food choice that has been described
looks at the behaviours that promote nutrition. Another approach, taken largely
by anthropologists, is an adaptationist programme which attempts to show that
traditional culinary practices are nutritionally adaptive. Marvin Harris (1985,
1987) and Solomon Katz (1982) are perhaps the strongest and most productive
advocates of this point of view. Examples include explaining the Mexican combination of beans and maize as together providing a satisfactory balance of amino
acids, the traditional leaching process that removes toxic cyanide from bitter
manioc, and the use of some spices and combination of spices which limit the
growth of bacteria (Billing and Sherman, 1998). These efforts are important and
interesting. They leave two questions (Rozin, P., 1982): (i) How much of traditional culinary practice can be accounted for by nutritional adaptations? (ii) How
were these processes discovered and institutionalized in cuisines?

Psychological influences

The experience with foods that any human has is largely determined by cultural traditions, since these determine what foods a person is exposed to. They constrain the operation of individual psychological factors, including genetic predispositions, parental influence and various other opportunities for learning. The mechanisms of acquisition of food preferences are reviewed in a few books, including Booth (1994) and Logue (2004), and edited books such as Meiselman and MacFie (1996) as well as in review articles (Rozin and Schulkin, 1990).

The developmental trajectory of humans in terms of food experience and preferences is striking. The initial 'food' of the fetus is blood, followed after birth by an exclusive milk diet and then the gradual introduction of adult foods. Weaning is, of course, a major event in this sequence.

Origin of preferences

Individuals *within a culture* vary widely in their food preferences. Many Americans like broccoli, lima beans and pork, and many do not. What is the source of this within-culture variation? The four most likely accounts are: genetics, early experience with parents, peer influences and other more general influences, such as the media. Of course, most of the latter are culture-wide influences, and hence cannot be easily invoked to explain within-culture differences. The most probable candidate is parental influences, because these encompass both genetic effects and early experience. Hence, it is quite surprising to discover that parent–child (with the children being young adults) correlations in food preferences are very low, in the range of 0 to 0.30, with a mean of about 0.15 (Rozin, 1991). Peers are another natural focus, although there is some evidence that peer influence may be smaller than expected (Rozin *et al.*, 2003). The origin of within-culture differences in preferences is, at this point in time, a mystery. There may be a substantial role for chance individual experiences. Also, results from marketing suggest that an important period for the development of preferences, specifically for genres of music, is between the ages of about 15 and 30 years (Holbrook and Schindler, 1989).

Acquisition of preferences

Psychologists have not paid much attention to the acquisition of preferences. We basically do not understand how food, music, pet or other preferences arise. There are three documented avenues to preference change.

1. *Mere exposure* (Zajonc, 1968). Generally, the more one is exposed to something, the more one likes it. Cultural traditions, family practices and peer preferences all influence the pattern of exposure an individual has. Mere exposure has been demonstrated as an influence on food preferences (Pliner, 1982).

2. *Evaluative conditioning*. Contingent pairing of tastes, appearances, etc. with biologically meaningful outcomes (e.g. sweet or bitter tastes) can cause acquired likes to occur by a Pavlovian mechanism (Rozin and Zellner, 1985), described, for the case of hedonics, as evaluative conditioning. The research group headed by Frank Baeyens in Belgium has carried out a major share of the work on this issue (de Houwer *et al.*, 2001). Taste aversion learning, in which specifically nausea following a novel taste rather reliably reduces the liking for that taste, is a quintessential example of evaluative conditioning.

3. *Social influence*. This is a vague but very important category. There is some evidence indicating that approval of admired others, experiencing the enjoyment of others on eating a particular food, and things of that sort can produce enhanced (or for the opposite case, decreased) liking. In her work on the development of food preferences, Leann Birch (reviewed in Birch *et al.*, 1996) has demonstrated some of these effects under controlled conditions. Baeyens and his colleagues (Baeyens *et al.*, 1996) have demonstrated evaluative conditioning, where the unconditioned stimulus is observation of a person consuming a drink (simultaneously consumed by the subject) and showing clear positive or negative facial expressions. Animal studies on food preferences suggest limited domains of social influence, often accomplished by mere exposure that results from social influence (Galef, 1988).

It is commonly believed by laypersons that a range of rewards and punishments is effective in shaping food preferences. There is no doubt that rewards and punishments can influence food intake, but it is not clear that they actually change liking. Some work by Leann Birch (reviewed in Birch *et al.*, 1996) casts doubt on the efficacy of instrumental rewards for changing liking.

Food choice in the moment

Acquisition aside, at a given moment humans face food choices, and a host of factors influence the selection. Among them are the physical arrangements of the foods, beliefs about the foods including their taste and health values, value systems (as with vegetarianism), knowledge about and experience with the particular foods available, and simple cost and convenience. Richard Shepherd and his colleagues (Shepherd and Raats, 1996) have modelled this situation with particular care and given a sense of the integration of factors, including the relation of attitudes and beliefs to actual choice. David Booth (1994) has also approached this problem from a number of perspectives.

Work by Daniel Kahneman and his colleagues (Kahneman *et al.*, 1997) has provided an important perspective on the moment of choice. These authors distinguish between anticipated, experienced and remembered pleasure. Faced with a choice about whether, for example, to buy a food product, an individual refers to his or her memories of past encounters with the choices (remembered pleasure), and considers his or her likely future hedonic trajectory with the product (anticipated pleasure). For example, if he/she buys a large box of X, will he/she continue to like it, grow in liking or decline in liking, with multiple experiences? In most choice situations except those in a food testing laboratory, an individual is not actually experiencing (tasting) the relevant choices. Kahneman and colleagues have shown two very important things, with research mostly from the domain of pain. First, valenced episodes are remembered quite differently from the way they are experienced. Duration of experience, a major determinant of the total pleasure received from an experience, is not recorded well in memory. Translating to the food domain, a few bites or a large number of bites of the same delicious food have very different effects on experienced pleasure, but are remembered as about equally pleasant (Rode *et al.*, unpublished). On the other hand, Kahneman has shown that people are poor at predicting their hedonic trajectories. Generally, they don't know whether repeated sampling of a given entity will increase or decrease their liking. Hence, in the purchase situation, individuals face distorted memories of past experiences with the foods in question, and poor abilities to predict their future reactions to the same foods.

CONTEXT. Understanding of any food choice must take into account both the surroundings (context) and the recent history of the person involved. Judgements are heavily influenced by the setting (décor, social situation; de Castro, 1990; Meiselman, 1996) and foods recently consumed (Rolls, 2000). (Contextual effects are reviewed in Rozin and Tuorila, 1993; Meiselman, 1996.)

Social influences (sociology)

The sociological approach to food choice is presented well in a few recent books (Murcott, 1983; Beardsworth and Keil, 1995; Maurer and Sobal, 1995). Sociologists have a particular interest in demographic variables as within-culture determinants of food choice. There are modest effects of age and gender on food preferences (for example, in the USA, meat avoidance is more common in women and, on account of greater weight concerns in women, preferences for low-calorie foods are higher in women). Gender, age and social status, while significant in accounting for food preference, do not account for very much variation (nor, as indicated above, do parents!).

Sociological concerns also deal with important influences on food choice and intake at the institutional level, such as in institutions and restaurants. The whole food system (Beardsworth and Keil, 1995; Maurer and Sobal, 1995), including the social organization of the growing of foods, delivery to markets and distribution of foods, has major influences on what is chosen.

And finally, one of the major influences on food choice is current fad movements, such as low-fat or 'lo-carb' or vegetarianism. These take their place, along with many other non-nutritional fads, in what appears to be a fundamental feature of human social organization.

Although this section is the shortest of the four on disciplinary influences on food, this reflects more on my own knowledge base than on its importance. The sociological perspective is vital in understanding food choice.

Cultural influences (anthropology)

In human food choice, culture is almost certainly the predominant influence. Consider the following. We have an unknown adult human being whose food preferences we wish to predict. We have only one question to ask before making our guesses. What is the most informative question? There is no doubt: it is 'What is your culture?' Individuals grow up embedded in a world highly determined by culture, which monitors the available foods and, indirectly, their costs, as well as general attitudes to food, the meaning of food and the way children should be socialized to food. Furthermore, of the social science disciplines relevant to the understanding of food (and this includes economics and history, as well as psychology and sociology), anthropology is the discipline that pays most attention to the role of food in daily life and the meaning of food. Concentrating as it does, through ethnographies, on the daily lives of people, it follows that food will play a central role (see de Garine, 1972 and Messer, 1984 for general discussion of cultural influences).

We can describe the complex of cultural traditions that bear directly on food as cuisine. Some of these traditions are about the particular foods one eats, the kinds of things that appear on the table from day to day, and are described in ethnically faithful cookbooks. Elisabeth Rozin (1982) has provided a framework within which to describe cuisine in this narrower sense, dividing into staple foods, flavouring ingredients and methods of preparation. Thus, Chinese cuisine is characterized by a rice base, with pork and other foods as common ingredients, flavourings centred on the 'flavour principle' of soy sauce, ginger root and rice wine, and the stir-fry technique. Mexican food, on the other hand, is built around maize and beans, with chilli pepper, tomato and lime as the repeating flavours, and with stewing as a basic technique.

There is much more to cuisine than the individual dishes. There is the meal (see Meiselman, 2000 for an excellent treatment of the meaning of the meal): what constitutes an appropriate meal, order of serving, and the like. And then there are table manners, the social organization of the meal, food and ritual, and the meaning of food in life and social intercourse. Food, preadaptively, often assumes symbolic roles. Because it involves shared substance, it is closely tied to the social world, functioning frequently as a homogenizing agent through sharing of food with individuals with whom one is close, and as a heterogenizing agent, as a way of distinguishing oneself from most others by not sharing food with them (Appadurai, 1981).

Among the Hua of Papua New Guinea (Meigs, 1984), food is believed to carry important vital essences. Among these are gender-specific essences. In order to protect young males, as they enter puberty, from feminization, the boys are kept in a separate house, are not allowed to consume any food touched in any way by fertile women (allowing contact with only prepubertal or postmenopausal women) and avoid consumption of any foods considered to contain feminine essence, which includes among other things fruits with soft, reddish interiors.

Focusing on the developed world, there are substantial cultural differences that affect not only the foods eaten, but also the role of food in life. For example, in comparison to Americans, the French eat smaller portions, take longer meals, consider food a more important part of life, worry less about the health effects of foods, organize their social life and celebrations around it, and are less receptive to the foods of other cultures ('ethnic foods'; Stearns, 1997; Rozin et al., 1999).

Five Examples of the Integration of Biological, Psychological and Cultural Factors

This particular book on food choice, and others that have preceded it, appropriately organizes food choice around issues such as origins, mechanisms and pathologies. Another orientation would be to use foods as a framework: vegetables, fruits, grains, dairy, meat and flavourings, for example. This is not how the field is organized, although food history is often so organized. One cannot organize a field simultaneously around foodstuffs and processes/influences. To help to redress this situation, and to illustrate the integration of forces in food choice, a brief discussion of five specific foods follows. The first three are components of the greatest food exchange in history: the mixture of foods and food traditions from the Western and Eastern hemispheres, consequent on the 'discovery' of the 'new' world by European explorers in the 15th–17th centuries. These and other examples are presented in somewhat more detail in Rozin, P. (1982) and by specific sources referred to in the discussion below.

Chocolate

Chocolate is one of the most popular foods in the Western world, and is the most craved food in the Western world. Its aroma and texture rank among the best of all foods. Chocolate comes from Mexico, and was introduced to Europe and the world by Cortez and the other early Spanish explorers (Coe and Coe, 1996). Raw chocolate was consumed by the ancient Aztecs in a bitter brew, seasoned with chilli pepper! It must have been very much an acquired taste. In the hands of the Europeans, a set of technologies were developed, involving drying and fermenting the beans, followed by grinding and extensive stirring under heat (conching), with the addition of sugar, vanilla (also a product of the Western hemisphere) and eventually milk. The result is the conversion of a bitter and gritty bean to a sweet and fat, luscious-tasting confection. The sweetness masks the bitterness. The aroma brought out by fermentation and other processes is irresistible. Of course, the critical addition of sugar depended on its availability, something that happened in the period prior to the European domestication of chocolate (Mintz, 1985). And most of the sugar came from plantations established by Europeans in the New World.

Chocolate is a perfect example of a culturally created super food. Its success is built on some human taste/texture predispositions: for sweet tastes and fatty textures (Drewnowski and Greenwood, 1983). Humans also seem to like foods that provide a dynamic sensory experience, changing in properties as they are consumed. The principal fat in chocolate is the only common fat that melts at body temperature. All of this is combined with the special, appealing aroma developed in processing. Chocolate also contains a number of pharmacologically active substances, including theobromine, caffeine and phenethylamine. These are all arousing substances. We still do not know their role in the popularity or craving for chocolate. What we do know is that chocolate is an example of culture capitalizing on some human food predispositions. It is expensive, and this may be part of the reason why it has not penetrated South America, Africa and

Asia to the degree that it has been accepted in Europe and North America. Economic and psychological factors, coupled by effective marketing, make it likely that chocolate will be a universal favourite in coming decades, particularly as the world moves towards Western tastes.

Chilli pepper

Chilli pepper is probably the world's most commonly consumed spice, other than garlic or salt (if one wishes to consider garlic and salt as spices; reviewed in Rozin, 1990). Chilli peppers come from the Americas, and were introduced to the Eastern hemisphere during the 15th–17th centuries. They now constitute basic flavourings in most of tropical Africa and Asia. It is hard to imagine Indian, Southwest Chinese, West African, Southeast Asian or Indonesian cuisines without chilli pepper. There is a flowering of varieties of chilli peppers, with different degrees of burn and different aromas, producing a range of mouth experiences that can be compared in some ways to the variety offered by cheese or wine.

The problem chilli pepper raises is that, on account of its oral irritant properties, it is innately aversive. It is, in an important sense, the opposite of sugar. In a still mysterious way, cultures have arranged to present chilli pepper as a flavouring in traditional foods, and choreographed gradual exposure to it in such a way that almost everyone in the relevant cultures is converted from a chilli hater to a chilli liker by the age of 6 years or so (Rozin, 1990). This is a case where culture has reversed an innate aversion; that is, opposed our biology. We do not yet know how this miracle occurs, but it is clear that the same burn that is negative initially becomes desirable through experience.

One of a number of accounts (all with insufficient evidence) for the production of chilli liking invokes the endorphin system. Endorphins are secreted in response to pain, and no doubt this happens on initial consumption of chilli pepper. The pain would normally stop further ingestion, but cultural pressures (such as, for children, eating what adults eat) keep it as an item of consumption for children. According to one model of addiction, opponent process theory, processes are set into operation on repeated exposure to pain which serve to neutralize the pain and perhaps, in some conditions, overcompensate for it. Thus, it is possible that excess endorphin secretion produces the pleasure that lovers of chilli pepper enjoy. This may or may not be a part of the acquisition mechanism; there are other possibilities (Rozin, 1990). But the important point about this example is that it illustrates a set of peculiar interactions among biology, psychology and culture. On the one hand, biological predispositions make chilli acceptance unlikely. On the other, in the face of repeated sampling, a biological (compensatory, homeostatic opponent) process is enlisted which, in this peculiar situation where an individual continues to administer pain to him- or herself, may reverse an aversion.

Maize

Maize comes from the Western hemisphere, specifically Mexico, along with chocolate and chilli pepper (and tomatoes, potatoes, squash, vanilla, manioc and groundnuts!). It entered Europe, and then spread around the world, in the same general manner as the other Western hemisphere products. Maize is a major source of energy, functioning as a staple food. It grows well in temperate climates, and is a highly efficient crop in terms of energy yield per hectare. Like all other vegetable foods, it does not contain sufficient amounts of all nutrients to be able to support mammals as their only food.

Maize functions as a staple food in Mexico and many other parts of the Americas. Katz (1982) has described in some detail how it has fitted into an adapted, nutritionally adequate cuisine. In Mexico, it is consumed along with beans, which have a complementary distribution of some critical amino acids; together they constitute a satisfactory array of essential amino acids. The tortilla is the major form in which maize is consumed in Mexico. Katz and his colleagues have shown how the traditional technique for making tortillas, which includes boiling the maize in an alkali solution, improves the nutritional quality of maize in a number of ways. These improvements are important, but none has rapid and dramatic effects, and it is not clear how they were discovered and maintained. Interestingly, when asked why they boil maize in alkali, Mexican women display no knowledge of the nutritional advantage, but point to a more palpable aspect of the tortilla technology (Rozin, P., 1982). The alkali softens the maize husks, and makes it easier to roll out a smooth tortilla. Katz's adaptive evolutionary account of tortilla technology raises interesting psychological problems as to how individuals discovered and retained the technique.

Maize had much less of an impact on the Eastern hemisphere than many other foods from the Americas: chilli peppers, chocolate, tomatoes, potatoes, manioc and groundnuts to name a few. In spite of its ability to grow well in Europe, it never became a human staple. But indirectly, it had a major effect on European eating because it became a principal source of animal feed.

It is not clear why maize was not readily accepted as a human food. One account is of particular interest, because it highlights the importance of unique and chance events in culinary history, and hence in food choice. Mexicans consume maize, a rather mealy and not particularly sweet staple, in the form of tortillas. Tortillas may well be tastier to most humans than maize itself, and are more nutritive as well. The tortilla-making technology is somewhat involved, and it is probable that none of the men in Cortez's expedition or other expeditions ever learned how to make them. Mexican men rarely do. So maize and maize seed were brought back to Europe but not the critical technology that made it more palatable and nutritious (Katz, 1982). Had there been a single Spanish woman on the expeditions to the New World, the tortilla technology might have been transferred back to Europe, with perhaps much more adoption of maize as a staple in Europe and beyond (the beyond being accomplished by later European colonization of Africa and Asia).

Milk

Milk is the special and unique food of baby mammals. As a food, it is as biological/predetermined as one could imagine. It is essentially a complete food.

The problem is that weaning from milk must occur, to allow a young mammal to find ways to obtain nutrition from the environment and free the mother for other activities, including having more offspring. Milk is a food only available to baby mammals.

Enter the domestication of animals, and the development of dairying traditions. Milk and milk products are now available to adult humans. But milk is specifically adapted as a food for the very young. Its substantial and energetically important carbohydrate component is in the form of lactose, a sugar that exists only in milk. Appropriately, the gut enzyme lactase, found only in mammals, breaks lactose down into two utilizable monosaccharides, glucose and galactose. But lactase is deprogrammed at about the time of weaning, so that, prior to dairying, no human adults could digest milk sugar. The result is what are called lactose-intolerant adults: the undigested lactose becomes a food for hindgut bacteria, with gas pains in the hindgut, diarrhoea and poor absorption of gut contents. Not fatal, but painful and inefficient.

So humans created a new adult food that they were biologically unprepared to deal with. As established largely by the work of Frederick Simoons (reviewed in Simoons, 1982), two solutions emerged that permitted the appropriation of milk, a very rich food, for adults.

1. *The cultural response.* Milk is an excellent food if one can digest lactose. The cultural solution is to digest lactose outside the body, and then drink the milk or milk product. Through a process of *culturing* (appropriately named), the milk is exposed to bacteria that break the lactose down to its two utilizable monosaccharides, glucose and galactose. In this form, with minimal levels of lactose, milk is a superb food for mammals. Cheese and yoghurt are two of the most ubiquitous outcomes of microbial digestion of lactose in milk.

2. *The biological response.* In one of relatively few clear demonstrations of how cultural forces have changed the human genome, the origin of dairying is connected with a genetic change that blocks the deprogramming of lactase at about the time of weaning. This single dominant gene mutation had obvious adaptive value, and through a process not yet documented became the dominant gene among the dairying cultures of northern Europe and among a few dairying groups in Africa. The rest of the world remained predominantly lactose-intolerant.

The problem of milk as an adult food was handled in two opposite ways. But there are still some important biocultural problems about milk as a human food. It is notable that milk and milk products are absent from China, home to one of the greatest and widely consumed cuisines in the world. The Chinese are known for their culinary ingenuity, having produced such complex products as soy sauce and tofu. Surely, they could have discovered that even leaving milk around for a few days would make it an acceptable food? This was discovered by many other cultures. The answer may well be that the rejection of dairy products by the Chinese had a sociocultural base. Milk and fermented milk products were basic foods for the Mongols, who conquered and ruled China. It may have been negative reactions to the Mongols that motivated the Chinese not to incorporate milk or milk products into their cuisine.

Yet another problem posed by milk, and a problem with a more biological account, has to do with weaning. It is an extraordinary and rare problem, in the animal world, to initially have a highly nutritive and exclusive food, and then be forced not only to wean from it, but for it to never be available again. What is to prevent young mammals from vainly seeking a beloved but unavailable food? There are apparently a number of biological adaptations to make this process easier (Rozin and Pelchat, 1988). Lactose intolerance develops at about the time of weaning. It is preprogrammed and not the result of declining milk intake. As a consequence, the late nursing mammal starts to experience the negative symptoms of lactose intolerance late in weaning, a contingency that would surely discourage milk ingestion. In addition, milk sugar, lactose, is much less sweet than most other sugars and its two monosaccharide components. Perhaps the low sweetness is there to detract from what is so positioned to be a super food. And, on the cultural side, weaning is often accomplished gradually, accompanied by introduction of other palatable foods, and, in many cases, by explicit discouragement of nursing by placement of bitter or irritant substances on the nipple.

The story of milk, biological, psychological and cultural, is particularly important, and particularly interactive. How could it not be? The universal first food remains at the centre of cuisine in some cultures, and disappears completely in others.

Meat

Like milk, meat plays a very important role in human evolutionary history and in human diets around the world. It is the quintessential complete food; since the nutrient requirements of most vertebrates are about the same, they essentially form packages of complete nutrients for other vertebrates. Meat can legitimately be claimed to be the most favoured and the most tabooed food across the culinary landscape (Simoons, 1961; Tambiah, 1969). It is the quintessentially ambivalent food for human beings, and this is the core of its great psychological interest. In many parts of the world, individuals or cultural groups are vegetarian. There is a dedication to a meat-free diet which is not paralleled by a dedication to a vegetable product-free diet; that is, there are few if any 'meatatarians'. While meat, particularly beef and chicken, is a favourite food among Americans, the most offensive foods for Americans are also of animal origin, indeed just move inches from a beef steak or chicken breast and we have kidneys, skin and guts, which are strongly repulsive to most Americans. Why?

Meat involves eating another living animal. By the 'you are what you eat' principle, this could involve taking on these animal's properties. And one of these properties is being *like* an animal, a core theme eliciting the emotion of disgust.

More than any other food, meat is associated with some things that are basically human. Hunting of larger animals, and adaptations to do it, provided one of the major motives for fundamental changes in humans as they evolved. Larger animal foods are a major factor promoting food sharing and social eating occasions. A hunter or particular family happens upon much more food than it can consume before it goes bad. This is rarely true for vegetable foods. On the other hand, the killing that necessarily goes with eating meat is cause for both appeal (as in hunting) and concern. Among foods, meat is the focus of moral concerns. It plays a central role in moral concerns in some cultures, as Hindu India, and among dedicated groups of vegetarians within meat-eating cultures (see Twigg, 1983; see also Fiddes, 1991, for discussions of the meaning of meat).

Conclusion

The message of this chapter is that food and food choice can only be understood by a mixture of biological, psychological, social and cultural perspectives, all taken within a historical context. Culinary history is a major part of human history: directly, as it affects an important part of life, and indirectly, as it motivates other activities, such as the exploration and colonization of the Americas. Strong social movements, often describable as 'fads', characterize the history of foods, especially in more affluent countries. The story of food in America over the last 200 years, as told by historians such as Levenstein (1988, 1993) and Whorton (1982), is a complex mixture of religion, morality and other social forces, harnessed to a developing and powerful food industry, and more recently, major concerns about body image and health. The politics of food (Nestle, 2002), such as agreement on and dissemination of dietary standards and the food pyramid, and trust in institutions (Frewer and Salter, 2003), now has much to do with food choice. We are just beginning to understand all of this.

References

Anon. (1990) *The Economist Book of Vital World Statistics* (Introduction by Paul Samuelson). Random House, New York.

Appadurai, A. (1981) Gastro-politics in Hindu South Asia. *American Ethnologist* 8, 494–511.

Baeyens, F., Kaes, B., Eelen, P. and Silverans, P. (1996) Observational evaluative conditioning of an embedded stimulus element. *European Journal of Social Psychology* 26, 15–28.

Barker, L.M. (ed.) (1982) *The Psychobiology of Human Food Selection*. AVI, Westport, Connecticut.

Bartoshuk, L.M. (1990) Distinctions between taste and smell relevant to the role of experience. In: Capaldi, E.D. and Powley, T.L. (eds) *Taste, Experience and Feeding*. American Psychological Association, Washington, DC, pp. 62–72.

Beardsworth, A. and Keil, T. (1995) *Sociology on the Menu*. Routledge, London.

Billing, J. and Sherman, P.W. (1998) Antimicrobial functions of spices: why some like it hot. *The Quarterly Review of Biology* 73, 3–49.

Birch, L.L., Fisher, J.O. and Grimm-Thomas, K. (1996) The development of children's eating habits. In: Meiselman, H.L. and MacFie, H.J.H. (eds) *Food Choice, Acceptance and Consumption*. Blackie Academic & Professional, London, pp. 161–206.

Booth, D.A. (1994) *Psychology of Nutrition*. Taylor and Francis, London.

Coe, S.D. and Coe, M.D. (1996) *The True History of Chocolate*. Thames and Hudson, London.

De Castro, J.M. (1990) Social facilitation of duration and size but not rate of the sponta-neous meal intake of humans. *Physiology and Behavior* 47, 1129–1135.

De Garine, I. (1972) The socio-cultural aspects of nutrition. *Ecology of Food and Nutrition* 1, 143–163.

De Houwer, J., Thomas, S. and Baeyens, F. (2001) Associative learning of likes and dislikes: a review of 25 years of research on human evaluative conditioning. *Psychological Bulletin* 127, 853–869.

Denton, D. (1982) *The Hunger for Salt.* Springer-Verlag, Berlin.

Diamond, J. (1997) *Guns, Germs, and Steel. The Fates of Human Societies.* W.W. Norton, New York.

Drewnowski, A. and Greenwood, M.R.C. (1983) Cream and sugar: human preferences for high-fat foods. *Physiology & Behavior* 30, 629–633.

Fiddes, N. (1991) *Meat. A Natural Symbol.* Routledge, London.

Frewer, L.J. and Salter, B. (2003) The changing governance of biotechnology: the politics of public trust in the agri-food sector. *Applied Biotechnology, Food Science and Policy* 1, 199–211.

Galef, B.G. Jr (1988) Communication of information concerning distant diets in a social central-place foraging species: *Rattus norvegicus.* In: Zentall, T. and Galef, B.G. Jr (eds) *Social Learning: A Comparative Approach.* Lawrence Erlbaum, Hillsdale, New Jersey, pp. 119–140.

Garcia, J., Hankins, W.G. and Rusiniak, K.W. (1974) Behavioral regulation of the milieu interne in man and rat. *Science* 185, 824–831.

Harris, M. (1985) *Good to Eat: Riddles of Food and Culture.* Simon and Schuster, New York.

Harris, M. (1987) Foodways: historical overview and theoretical prolegomenon. In: Harris, M. and Ross, E.B. (eds) *Food and Evolution: Toward a Theory of Human Food Habits.* Temple University Press, Philadelphia, Pennsylvania, pp. 57–90.

Holbrook, M. and Schindler, R.M. (1989) Some exploratory findings on the development of musical tastes. *The Journal of Consumer Research* 16, 119–124.

Kahneman, D., Wakker, P.P. and Sarin, R. (1997) Back to Bentham? Explorations of experienced utility. *The Quarterly Journal of Economics* 112, 375–405.

Kass, L. (1994) *The Hungry Soul.* The Free Press, New York.

Katz, S.H. (1982) Food, behavior and biocultural evolution. In: Barker, L.M. (ed.) *The Psychobiology of Human Food Selection.* AVI, Westport, Connecticut, pp. 171–188.

Levenstein, H. (1988) *Revolution at the Table. The Transformation of the American Diet.* Oxford University Press, New York.

Levenstein, H. (1993) *Paradox of Plenty. A Social History of Eating in Modern America* Oxford University Press, New York.

Logue, A.W. (2004) *The Psychology of Eating and Drinking,* 3rd edn. Brunner-Routledge, New York.

Maurer, D. and Sobal, J. (eds) (1995) *Eating Agendas. Food and Nutrition as Social Problems.* Aldine de Gruyter, Hawthorne, New York.

Mayr, E. (1960) The emergence of evolutionary novelties. In: Tax, S. (ed.) *Evolution after Darwin.* Vol. 1. *The Evolution of Life.* University of Chicago Press, Chicago, Illinois, pp. 349–380.

Meigs, A.S. (1984) *Food, Sex, and Pollution: A New Guinea Religion.* Rutgers University Press, New Brunswick, New Jersey.

Meiselman, H.L. (1996) The contextual basis for food acceptance, food choice, and food intake: the food, the situation, and the individual. In: Meiselman, H.L. and

MacFie, H.L.H. (eds) *Food Choice, Acceptance and Consumption*. Blackie Academic & Professional, London, pp. 239–263.

Meiselman, H.L. (ed.) (2000) *Dimensions of the Meal. The Science, Culture, Business and Art of Eating*. Aspen Publishers, Gaithersburg, Maryland.

Meiselman, H.L. and MacFie, H.L.H. (eds) (1996) *Food Choice, Acceptance and Consumption*. Blackie Academic & Professional, London.

Messer, E. (1984) Anthropological perspectives on diet. *Annual Review of Anthropology* 13, 205–249.

Miller, W.I. (1997) *The Anatomy of Disgust*. Harvard University Press, Cambridge, Massachusetts.

Mintz, S.W. (1985) *Sweetness and Power*. Viking, New York.

Murcott, A. (ed.) (1983) *The Sociology of Food and Eating*. Gower, London.

Nemeroff, C. and Rozin, P. (1989) 'You are what you eat': applying the demand-free 'impressions' technique to an unacknowledged belief. *Ethos. The Journal of Psychological Anthropology* 17, 50–69.

Nestle, M. (2002) *Food Politics*. University of California Press, Berkeley, California.

Pliner, P. (1982) The effects of mere exposure on liking for edible substances. *Appetite* 3, 283–290.

Richter, C.P. (1943) Total self regulatory functions in animals and human beings. *Harvey Lecture Series* 38, 63–103.

Richter, C.P. (1956) Salt appetite of mammals: its dependence on instinct and metabolism. In: *L'Instinct dans le Comportement des Animaux et de l'Homme*. Masson, Paris, pp. 577–629.

Rode, E., Rozin, P. and Durlach, P. (unpublished) Experienced and remembered pleasure for meals: duration neglect but minimal peak-end effects. Submitted to *Appetite*.

Rolls, B.J. (2000) Sensory specific satiety and variety in the meal. In: Meiselman, H. (ed.) *Dimensions of the Meal: The Science, Culture, Business, and Art of Eating*. Aspen Publishers, Gaithersburg, Maryland, pp. 107–116.

Rozin, E. (1982) The structure of cuisine. In: Barker, L.M. (ed.) *The Psychobiology of Human Food Selection*. AVI, Westport, Connecticut, pp. 189–203.

Rozin, P. (1976) The selection of foods by rats, humans, and other animals. In: Rosenblatt, J., Hinde, R.A., Beer, C. and Shaw, E. (eds) *Advances in the Study of Behavior*, Vol. 6. Academic Press, New York, pp. 21–76.

Rozin, P. (1982) Human food selection: the interaction of biology, culture and individual experience. In: Barker, L.M. (ed.) *The Psychobiology of Human Food Selection*. AVI, Westport, Connecticut, pp. 225–254.

Rozin, P. (1990) Getting to like the burn of chili pepper: biological, psychological and cultural perspectives. In: Green, B.G., Mason, J.R. and Kare, M.R. (eds) *Chemical Senses*. Vol. 2. *Irritation*. Marcel Dekker, New York, pp. 231–269.

Rozin, P. (1991) Family resemblance in food and other domains: the family paradox and the role of parental congruence. *Appetite* 16, 93–102.

Rozin, P. and Fallon, A.E. (1980) Psychological categorization of foods and non-foods: a preliminary taxonomy of food rejections. *Appetite* 1, 193–201.

Rozin, P. and Fallon, A.E. (1987) A perspective on disgust. *Psychological Review* 94, 23–41.

Rozin, P. and Kalat, J.W. (1971) Specific hungers and poison avoidance as adaptive specializations of learning. *Psychological Review* 78, 459–486.

Rozin, P. and Pelchat, M.L. (1988) Memories of mammaries: adaptations to weaning from milk in mammals. In: Epstein, A.N. and Morrison, A. (eds) *Advances in Psychobiology*, Vol. 13. Academic Press, New York, pp. 1–29.

Rozin, P. and Schulkin, J. (1990) Food selection. In: Stricker, E.M. (ed.) *Handbook of Behavioral Neurobiology*. Vol. 10. *Food and Water Intake*. Plenum, New York, pp. 297–328.

Rozin, P. and Tuorila, H. (1993) Simultaneous and temporal contextual influences on food choice. *Food Quality and Preference* 4, 11–20.

Rozin, P. and Zellner, D.A. (1985) The role of Pavlovian conditioning in the acquisition of food likes and dislikes. *Annals of the New York Academy of Sciences* 443, 189–202.

Rozin, P., Fischler, C., Imada, S., Sarubin, A. and Wrzesniewski, A. (1999) Attitudes to food and the role of food in life: comparisons of Flemish Belgium, France, Japan and the United States. *Appetite* 33, 163–180.

Rozin, P., Haidt, J. and McCauley, C.R. (2000) Disgust. In: Lewis, M. and Haviland, J. (eds) *Handbook of Emotions*, 2nd edn. Guilford, New York, pp. 637–653.

Rozin, P., Riklis, J. and Margolis, L. (2003) Mutual exposure or close peer relationships do not seem to foster increased similarity in food, music or television program preferences. *Appetite* 42, 41–48.

Schulkin, J. (1991) *Sodium Hunger. The Search for a Salty Taste*. Cambridge University Press, Cambridge, UK.

Schutz, H.G. (1989) Beyond preference: appropriateness as a measure of contextual acceptance of food. In: Thomson, D.M.H. (ed.) *Food Acceptability*. Elsevier Applied Science, Essex, UK, pp. 115–134.

Sclafani, A. (1999) Macronutrient-conditioned flavor preferences. In: Berthoud, H.-R. and Seeley, R.J. (eds) *Neural Control of Macronutrient Selection*. CRC Press, Boca Raton, Florida, pp. 93–106.

Shepherd, R. and Raats, M.M. (1996) Attitudes and beliefs in food habits. In: Meiselman, H.L. and MacFie, H.L.H. (eds) *Food Choice, Acceptance and Consumption*. Blackie Academic & Professional, London, pp. 346–364.

Simoons, F.J. (1961) *Eat Not this Flesh: Food Avoidances in the Old World*. University of Wisconsin Press, Madison, Wisconsin.

Simoons, F.J. (1982) Geography and genetics as factors in the psychobiology of human food selection. In: Barker, L.M. (ed.) *The Psychobiology of Human Food Selection*. AVI, Westport, Connecticut, pp. 205–224.

Stearns, P.N. (1997) *Fat History. Bodies and Beauty in the Modern West*. New York University Press, New York.

Stein, R.L. and Nemeroff, C.J. (1995) Moral overtones of food: judgments of others based on what they eat. *Personality and Social Psychology Bulletin* 21, 480–490.

Steiner, J.E. (1979) Human facial expressions in response to taste and smell stimulation. In: Reese, H.W. and Lipsitt, L.P. (eds) *Advances in Child Development and Behavior*, Vol. 13. Academic Press, New York, pp. 257–295.

Szalai, A. (ed.) (1972) *The Use of Time. Daily Activities of Urban and Suburban Populations in Twelve Countries*. Mouton, The Hague, The Netherlands.

Tambiah, S.J. (1969) Animals are good to think and good to prohibit. *Ethnology* 8, 423–459.

Twigg, J. (1983) Vegetarianism and the meanings of meat. In: Murcott, A. (ed.) *The Sociology of Food and Eating. Essays on the Sociological Significance of Food*. Gower, London, pp. 18–30.

Whorton, J.C. (1982) *Crusaders for Fitness*. Princeton University Press, Princeton, New Jersey.

Zajonc, R.B. (1968) Attitudinal effects of mere exposure. *Journal of Personality and Social Psychology* 9, 1–27.

This page intentionally left blank

3 Social Psychological Models of Food Choice

MARK CONNER[1] AND CHRISTOPHER J. ARMITAGE[2]

[1]Institute of Psychological Sciences, University of Leeds, Leeds LS2 9JT, UK;
[2]Department of Psychology, University of Sheffield, Sheffield S10 2TP, UK

Introduction

The study of food choice focuses on the question 'Why do individuals eat the foods they do?' At first blush, this may seem a rather simple question, but the answer is often complex. After all, an individual does not have to be hungry, he/she does not *always* choose the most preferred option, and some influences may not be open to introspection. The complexity associated with this kind of research is reflected in the range of key contributions made in this field by pharmacologists, physiologists, geneticists, economists and sociologists, as well as psychologists, and means that a scientific analysis of food choice must be able to account for the underlying physiological mechanisms such as innate preference, nutrient-specific appetites and learned food aversions. However, we would argue that social psychological research provides the best explanation of food choice (Conner and Armitage, 2002), as evidenced by the fact that the impact of physiology on food choice is mediated by social influences, such as the decision-making processes studied by social psychologists (e.g. Bagiella *et al.*, 1991; Teff and Engelman, 1996; Birch, 1999). For example, in their review of physiological mechanisms of food choice, Rogers and Blundell (1990) concluded: 'Often, food choice will be guided by an individual's conscious appraisal of the likely after-effects of consuming a particular food' (p. 35) and that 'social factors may be particularly important in influencing the development of preferences for foods' (p. 38).

Social Psychological Approaches to Food Choice

The evidence would therefore suggest that although physiological processes are fundamental to understanding food choice, their impact on behaviour is likely to be mediated by social psychological variables. The implication is that social psychological variables such as attitudes (e.g. Teff and Engelman, 1996) or an 'individual's conscious appraisal of the likely after-effects of consuming a particular food' (Rogers and Blundell, 1990, p. 35) will provide insight into more proximal determinants of food choice. Perhaps more importantly, these more proximal determinants of food choice may be more directly amenable to change and could exert a more powerful influence on food choice than physiological processes. This chapter focuses on social psychological research into food choice and models of how social psychological variables influence choice.

In common with other branches of psychology, social psychological research into food choice has its roots in animal research on learning theory. Through systematic study of animal behaviour, both Herrnstein's (1961, 1970) matching law and optimal foraging theory (e.g. Broughton, 1994) have been developed as normative models of food choice. Whilst these models have been successfully applied to some human food choice behaviours, it is the exclusively human models of behavioural decision making (as applied to food choice) that have particularly concerned social psychologists.

Expectancy–value theory

Expectancy–value (EV) theory (e.g. Peak, 1955; Fishbein, 1967a) is a general model of human decision making that has been widely applied to understanding food choice. Comparable with the matching law and optimal foraging theory, EV theory is based on the assumption that individuals are motivated to maximize the chances of desirable outcomes occurring and minimize the chances of undesirable outcomes occurring. Given a choice between two objects, individuals choose the one associated with the most desirable outcome (i.e. the one *evaluated* most positively). This global evaluation (*attitude*) is derived from the perceived likelihood that the object possesses a number of key attributes (e.g. outcomes associated with purchasing a product), weighted by the evaluation of those outcomes.

Perhaps the most influential advocate of EV theory in social psychology has been Martin Fishbein. In his summative model of attitudes, Fishbein (1967a, 1967b) argued that individuals may possess a large number of beliefs about a particular object, although only a subset of these are likely to be salient at any one time (see also Ajzen, 1996; Ajzen and Fishbein, 2000). Thus, attitudes towards objects (e.g. behaviours, products) are determined by *salient* underlying beliefs computed by multiplying (weighting) the perceived likelihood of salient outcomes occurring with the value attached to those particular outcomes. The formal equation is:

$$\text{Attitude} = \sum_{i=1}^{n} b_i e_i$$

where b refers to the outcome belief and e refers to the evaluation of that belief, which when multiplied together are referred to as behavioural beliefs. i represents a particular attribute and n represents the number of attributes salient at any one time. The salient beliefs are then summed to produce an overall evaluation, or attitude. By way of an example, in choosing between cheese A and cheese B, a consumer might judge the likelihood of the cheeses having a strong flavour, a long shelf-life and being a recognized brand. These judgements would then be weighted by the evaluation of each of these attributes (e.g. is strong flavour good or bad? Is the shelf-life good or bad? Is the brand good or bad?) and summed to provide an overall evaluation. If the consumer values strongly flavoured cheese with a short shelf-life and a recognized brand name and perceives that cheese A is more likely to possess these qualities than cheese B, she or he is more likely to choose cheese A. By the same token, if the attitude object is a behaviour (e.g. eating five portions of fruit and vegetables per day), the individual might rate the likelihood and evaluation that (for example) eating 5-a-day will reduce the risk of heart disease, will be tasty, will reduce weight. Again, the sum of these beliefs will provide an overall attitude towards eating 5-a-day which will be compared with not eating 5-a-day. The course of action evaluated most positively is the one most likely to be pursued. At this point, it should be noted that this approach to attitude formation is regarded as a representation, rather than a realistic description of the processes involved, as Ajzen and Fishbein (2000) state: 'In actuality, although the investigator does perform these computations, people are not assumed to do so. We merely propose that attitude formation may be *modeled* in this fashion' (pp. 7–8).

As we have already pointed out, there are a number of possible outcomes associated with consuming particular foods (e.g. putting on weight, whether it will satisfy hunger, feeling ill), but it is the outcomes that are *salient* at the time that are held to be important (Fishbein and Ajzen, 1975). Perceptions of these outcomes result partly from our interaction with foods, but also from socially transmitted information. These include beliefs about which foods are healthy and unhealthy, which foods are generally acceptable and which are not. Thus whilst some food choices are clearly based upon experience with food (e.g. taste aversions), other choices are based upon the cultural meaning of food (e.g. the concern in Western culture with not eating too much is clearly linked to the current culturally ideal slim body shape for both men and women; Grogan, 1999).

Although the EV model is one of general behavioural decision making, it provides insight into the psychological processes influencing human food choice decisions. A number of studies have investigated this. For example, Towler and Shepherd (1992) interviewed 34 people about the outcomes they associated with eating four food groups associated with excessive fat intake: meat, meat products, dairy products and fried foods. Salient outcomes about each of the food groups were elicited, three of which were identical across the food groups ('. . . is healthy', '. . . is high in fat', '. . . tastes good'). Other beliefs included 'expense' (meat and meat products), 'protein' (meat and dairy products) and 'convenience' (meat products and fried foods). Towler and Shepherd (1992) tested the ability of these beliefs to predict attitudes towards these food groups in a sample of 240 individuals. Findings indicated that 'taste' and 'health' were important determinants of attitudes towards each food group, while 'fat' was predictive of only dairy products and fried foods. In addition, 'expense' and 'vitamins' were predictive of attitudes towards meat, and 'vitamins' was predictive of attitudes towards dairy products. Towler and Shepherd's (1992) study provided evidence to support the utility of the EV approach to understanding attitudes: different behavioural beliefs underpinned attitudes to specific food groups.

Similar research has utilized the EV model to examine attitudes to whole diets. For example, eating a low-fat diet is a key UK government health target: given the serious health risks from excessive fat intake, it is recommended that individuals consume no more than 35% of their food energy from fat in the diet (Department of Health, 1992). EV theory predicts that an individual's overall attitude to eating a low-fat diet will be determined by the salient outcomes associated with that behaviour. In a study conducted by Armitage and Conner (1999a), eight salient outcomes were identified through pilot interviews, of which four were predictive of attitudes towards eating a low-fat diet ('. . . makes me feel good about myself', '. . . reduces my enjoyment of food', '. . . helps to maintain a lower weight', '. . . eating fat makes me feel guilty'). Interestingly, health outcomes (e.g. '. . . reduces my risk of coronary heart disease') were unrelated to attitudes. The implication is that appeals designed to change dietary intake via targeting health might be relatively ineffective, compared with those targeting weight loss and taste of low-fat alternatives.

Research by van der Pligt and de Vries (1998) suggests that the importance placed on beliefs is significant. Reasoning that more important beliefs are likely to be more salient, they asked individuals to nominate the three beliefs that they regarded as most important. The results are striking: the three most important beliefs were strongly correlated ($r = 0.63$) with overall attitude, in contrast with the correlation between the 12 less important beliefs and attitude ($r = 0.15$). Although van der Pligt and de Vries's (1998) study examined attitudes towards smoking, the inclusion of measures of belief importance might well enhance the predictive validity of the EV model (for a review of alternative approaches, see van der Pligt et al., 2000).

The research by Towler and Shepherd (1992) and Armitage and Conner (1999a) demonstrates the utility of the EV model for predicting food choice attitudes. However, while it is clearly important to study the decision-making processes underpinning attitudes towards food, the real power of this approach lies in the ability of attitudes to predict actual food choice. The following section focuses on research that has investigated the proposed relationship between attitudes and behaviour.

The attitude–behaviour relationship

The social psychological study of attitudes has been one of the core areas of the discipline for decades (Allport, 1935). This concept has spawned a considerable amount of work in social psychology and has been defined in various ways (for reviews see Eagly and Chaiken, 1993; Ajzen, 2001). For example, Eagly and Chaiken (1993) define an attitude as 'a psychological tendency that is expressed by evaluating a particular entity with some degree of favor or disfavor' and state that evaluative responding may be 'overt or covert, cognitive, affective, or behavioral' (p. 1). As we have already noted, overt attitudes towards food have been shown to mediate the effects of biology on behaviour.

Commensurate with the amount of research attention directed at the attitude–behaviour relationship in general, many studies have examined this in conjunction with food choice. Indeed, Conner (Meta-analysis of the attitude–behaviour relationship in food choice, unpublished raw data, School of Psychology, University of Leeds, UK) conducted a meta-analysis of 143 tests of the relationship between food choice attitudes and behaviour, and found that correlations were in the moderate ($0.21 < r < 0.40$) to large ($0.41 < r < 0.60$) range. This is directly comparable to the mean size of the attitude–behaviour relationship ($0.30 < r < 0.49$) across all behaviours (e.g. Kim and Hunter, 1993; Kraus, 1995). These data have often been taken as providing strong support for the idea that attitudes are a strong correlate of food-related behaviours. However, these data hide the fact that the average frequency-weighted correlation between attitudes and behaviour was 0.35. Whilst this figure equates with explaining more than 12% of the variance in behaviour, clearly the correspondence between attitudes and behaviour is less than perfect. There have been two dominant approaches towards explaining this lack of correspondence. The first approach has examined variables that affect the *relationship* between attitudes and behaviour (i.e. moderating factors), most notably imprecise measurement. The second approach has explored possible *mediating variables*, or the idea that the influence of attitudes on behaviour is actually indirect, filtered through some other variable.

Measurement issues and the attitude–behaviour relationship

Fishbein and Ajzen's (1975) principle of correspondence stems from the finding that attitudes are most predictive of behaviour when the two measures are congruent with respect to action (e.g. eating), target (e.g. an apple), time (e.g. this afternoon) and context (e.g. during a meeting). Thus, the principle of correspondence states that in order to maximize the relationship between attitude and behaviour, one must measure both components with similar levels of specificity. For the example provided above, an individual's attitude might be measured using an item such as:

My eating an apple during this afternoon's meeting would be . . .

Negative   –3   –2   –1   0   +1   +2   +3   Positive

and her/his behaviour should be measured at a similar level of specificity (e.g. did I eat an apple during my meeting this afternoon?). Clearly, this level of specificity is likely to maximize the relationship between attitudes and behaviour (for a review see Ajzen and Fishbein, 1977), but is unlikely to provide useful information about more general behaviour. However, the principle of correspondence allows for the prediction of more general behaviours by emphasizing the fact that it is the *correspondence* between measures that is important, rather than the level of specificity. In short, general attitudes should be more predictive of a general measure of behaviour than will a specific attitude. For example, a healthy eating attitude could be measured by responses to the following item:

My eating a healthy diet in the next 12 months would be . . .

Negative   –3   –2   –1   0   +1   +2   +3   Positive

A year-long assessment of dietary intake in the same individual would provide a measure of behaviour at a suitable level of correspondence, and one might expect a reasonable attitude–behaviour correlation across individuals. In fact, Conner's (unpublished data) meta-analysis for food and attitudes confirmed this, demonstrating that measures showing good levels of correspondence in relation to action and target produced stronger attitude–behaviour correlations ($r = 0.40$) than measures with relatively poor correspondence ($r = 0.33$).

Indirect effects of attitudes on behaviour

A second strand of Fishbein and Ajzen's (1975) work suggests an *indirect* link between attitudes and behaviour, proposing behavioural intention as a mediating variable. Behavioural intention is defined as the motivation required to perform a particular behaviour: the more one intends to perform a behaviour, the more likely will be its performance. Explicit within these conceptualizations is the causal link between salient (behavioural) beliefs, attitudes, intention and behaviour, respectively. Support for this view is reported by the meta-analysis of Conner (unpublished data), who found that the overall frequency-weighted correlation between attitudes and behaviour was significantly weaker than either the attitude–intention ($r = 0.46$) or the intention–behaviour relationship ($r = 0.43$). The implication is that the indirect impact of attitudes on behaviour via intentions is greater (0.20) than the direct effect (0.15). This is partial support for behavioural intentions as mediators of the attitude–behaviour relationship in relation to food choice. More direct evidence is provided by studies into the theories of reasoned action and planned behaviour, which include measures of attitude and behavioural intention within a broader theoretical framework.

The theory of reasoned action

The behavioural beliefs, attitude, intention and behaviour model forms the basis of Fishbein and Ajzen's (1975) theory of reasoned action (TRA; see also Ajzen and Fishbein, 1980). In addition, the TRA proposes a second determinant of intention: subjective norms. Subjective norms are defined as perceptions of general social pressure to perform or not to perform a given behaviour. Underlying subjective norms are normative beliefs: the perceived social pressure from salient referents weighted by an individual's motivation to comply with those referents. For example, one might perceive social pressure from one's parents to eat cabbage, but this social pressure will only be influential to the extent that one is motivated to comply with one's parents. Congruent with behavioural beliefs, salient normative beliefs are held to determine subjective norms. A schematic representation of the TRA is presented in Fig. 3.1.

Several quantitative and narrative reviews have provided support for use of the TRA in the prediction of a number of behaviours (e.g. Sheppard *et al.*, 1988; Van den Putte, 20 years of the theory of reasoned action of Fishbein and Ajzen: a meta-analysis, unpublished data, University of Amsterdam, The Netherlands). More specifically, the model has been used to predict both specific and more

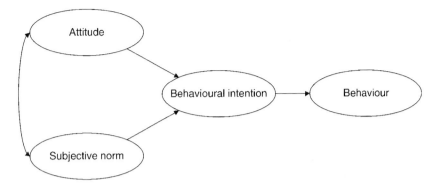

Fig. 3.1. Schematic representation of the theory of reasoned action.

general food choices. For example, Saunders and Rahilly (1990) used the TRA to predict reducing fat and sugar consumption in students who were either majoring in health studies or not majoring in health studies. Taking the sample as a whole, both attitude and subjective norm were predictive of intentions, accounting for 41% of the variance. Interestingly, when the sample was divided into health majors and non-health majors, attitudes were the dominant predictors of the intentions of health majors, whereas subjective norms were the dominant predictors of non-health majors. The implication is that the health majors were more knowledgeable about the outcomes associated with reducing fat and sugar intake, making their decision to eat healthily less open to the influence of social pressure.

In another study, Anderson and Shepherd (1989) examined the ability of the TRA to predict 'healthier eating' in a sample of 95 women attending ante- and postnatal clinics. Again, the predictive validity of the model was supported, with attitude and subjective norm together accounting for 28% of the variance in intentions. However, in this case, only attitude was a significant predictor: subjective norm did not exert a significant effect on the decisions of these women. Thus a number of applications of the TRA to food choice have provided support for the model. However, in spite of all the supporting evidence, Ajzen (1998) himself concedes, 'The theory of reasoned action was developed explicitly to deal with purely volitional behaviors' (p. 127); in other words, simple behaviours, where successful performance of the behaviour required only the formation of an intention. The implication was that behaviours were solely dependent on personal agency (i.e. the formation of an intention), and that control over behaviour (e.g. personal resources or environmental determinants of behaviour) was relatively unimportant.

The theory of planned behaviour

Ajzen (1988) proposed 'a conceptual framework that addresses the problem of incomplete volitional control' (p. 132) which would address the limitations of

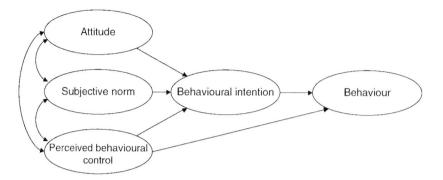

Fig. 3.2. Schematic representation of the theory of planned behaviour.

the TRA: the theory of planned behaviour (TPB; Ajzen, 1988, 1991). The TPB (see Fig. 3.2) extended the TRA by including a measure of perceived behavioural control (PBC) as a determinant of both intentions and behaviour. The inclusion of PBC as a predictor of behaviour is based on the rationale that: holding intention constant, greater perceived control will increase the likelihood that enactment of the behaviour will be successful. Further, to the extent that perceived control reflects actual control, PBC will directly influence behaviour. PBC therefore acts as both a proxy measure of actual control and a measure of confidence in one's ability. Within the TPB, PBC is posited as a third determinant of intention: the easier a behaviour is, the more likely one will be to intend to perform it. Congruent with the other belief components, salient control beliefs determine these global perceptions of control. Control beliefs are the perceived frequency of occurrence of facilitating or inhibiting factors multiplied by the perceived power of those factors to inhibit/facilitate the behaviour in question.

Applications of the theory of planned behaviour to food choice

A series of narrative and quantitative reviews (e.g. Ajzen, 1991; Conner and Sparks, 1996; Godin and Kok, 1996; Conner and Armitage, 1998; Armitage and Conner, 2001; Armitage and Christian, 2003; B. van den Putte, University of Amsterdam, 1991, unpublished manuscript) have shown the efficacy of the TPB in predicting behaviour in general. Sparks (1994) has reviewed applications of the TPB to food choice, which demonstrates that the PBC component makes a significant contribution to the predictive power of the TRA, providing support for the TPB.

More specifically, there have been several applications of the TPB to predict food choice intentions, from the use of gene technology in food production (e.g. Sparks *et al.*, 1995) to fat intake (e.g. Nguyen *et al.*, 1996). For example, Cox *et al.* (1998) found that the TPB accounted for between 33% and 47% of the variance in intentions to increase fruit and vegetable consumption, with attitude being the dominant predictor, followed by subjective norm and perceived behavioural control. Comparably, Nguyen *et al.* (1996) found that attitude, subjective norm and perceived behavioural control independently contributed to the prediction of the intention to eat fatty foods. The final model accounted for 51% of the variance in intention.

Several studies have examined the more pertinent relationship of the TPB to food choice behaviour. For example, comparable with the work reviewed above, Povey et al. (2000) found that the TPB explained 57% of the variance in intentions to eat five daily portions of fruit and vegetables. Importantly, Povey et al. (2000) assessed actual behaviour a month later, finding that the TPB accounted for 32% of the variance in actual fruit and vegetable consumption. Similarly, Armitage and Conner (1999a) conducted a study that asked participants about their attitudes and intentions towards eating a low-fat diet. These participants were contacted again after a month and asked whether or not they had eaten a low-fat diet in the intervening period. Analyses of these responses revealed that the TPB accounted for 39% of the variance in behaviour. However, unlike fruit and vegetable consumption, where it is possible to count portions with at least some level of accuracy, it is harder for people to assess how much fat they have actually eaten in the past month. So, in addition participants completed a food frequency questionnaire to obtain a more objective measure of behaviour (Cade and Margetts, 1988). Interestingly, this measure was only modestly correlated ($r = 0.37$) with the self-perception measure, providing support for the idea that people find it hard to accurately judge the fat content of their own diets. Consistent with this, the TPB was only able to account for 18% of the variance in behaviour using this more objective measure of behaviour.

Consistent with Conner's (unpublished data) review of the attitude–behaviour relationships within food choice research, it is clear that the TPB accounts for considerably more of the variance in specific dietary behaviours than more global dietary behaviours. Povey et al. (2000) showed that the TPB accounted for 32% of the variance in fruit and vegetable consumption, compared with 18% variance explained in Armitage and Conner's (1999a) low-fat diet study. This effect may be attributable to the fact that specific actions are easier to predict because the number of ways of achieving them is, by definition, limited (for a review see Baranowski et al., 1999). In contrast, more general classes of behaviours (or goals) such as eating a low-fat diet might be achieved in a number of different ways and it is likely that a range of other factors will be important in addition to the general attitude (or goal attitude). By the same token, eating a low-fat diet is more complex than eating five portions of fruit and vegetables per day because there are more component behaviours (e.g. identifying high-fat foods, locating low-fat alternatives, purchasing appropriate foods, etc.). The implication is that more complex models are required for more complicated behaviours and that, for a goal such as eating a low-fat diet, one needs to assess a range of attitudes rather than simply a global attitude to eating a low-fat diet.

Additional variables within the theory of planned behaviour

Notwithstanding the differences in the behaviours studied by Povey et al. (2000) and Armitage and Conner (1999a), it is clear that the TPB was less than perfect at predicting food choice. One clear goal for researchers has been to increase the proportion of variance explained in intentions and behaviour. A number of approaches have been adopted, most notably the inclusion of variables in addition to attitude, subjective norm and PBC. The inclusion of these additional variables is regarded as an effective way of accounting for more variance in intentions and behaviour. Two variables in particular have attracted the attention of social psychologists in relation to food choice: self-identity and perceived need.

Sparks (2000) regards *self-identity* as being 'synonymous with self-perception or self-concept' and that it 'refers to the relatively enduring characteristics that people ascribe to themselves' (p. 35). Self-identity is held to exert motivational significance insofar as individuals seek to perform behaviours that maintain their sense of self. In food choice, one might be more likely to eat healthily if one sees oneself as 'health-conscious' and to eat environmentally friendly foods if one is a 'green consumer'. A number of empirical investigations have supported the independent predictive power of self-identity. For example, Sparks and Shepherd (1992) found that self-identification as a 'green consumer' significantly contributed to the prediction of intentions to consume organically grown vegetables, over and above the effects of TPB variables. Related work has demonstrated effects in relation to eating a low-fat diet (Sparks and Guthrie, 1998; Armitage and Conner, 1999a) and eating a healthy diet (Armitage and Conner, 1999b). Thus, the way in which one sees oneself exerts significant influence on the motivation to choose certain foods.

There are two explanations of the self-identity–intention relationship. First, Charng *et al.* (1988) argue that whilst models such as the TRA/TPB are predictive of people's behaviour initially, over time people are more motivated by their need to retain their sense of self, rather than by their attitudes or by perceived social pressure. Thus, Charng *et al.* (1988) argue that repeated performance of behaviour develops one's self-concept. Applying this to the Sparks and Shepherd (1992) study on green consumerism, the implication is that to the extent that the behaviour is repeated over time, one's intention to purchase organic foods will be driven solely by self-identity. The second explanation for the self-identity–intention relationship argues that individuals are motivated to communicate their values and identity to others (c.f. Katz, 1960; Shavitt, 1990). To extend this view to the Sparks and Shepherd (1992) paper, this implies that choosing organic food is a communicative act, designed to express one's credentials as a 'green consumer'. To date, it is unclear which provides the better account of the self-identity–intention relationship.

Paisley and Sparks (1998) have demonstrated that *perceived need* is an important predictor of intentions to eat healthily. These authors argue that whilst the TPB includes measures of individuals' overall evaluations, there is no assessment of whether individuals see themselves as needing to (for example) eat a low-fat diet. Paisley and Sparks (1998) have shown that perceived need adds significantly to the prediction of behavioural intentions, over and above the effects of TPB variables. More recently, Povey *et al.* (2000) reported that perceived need added 11% and 6% to variance explained in intentions with respect to eating five portions of fruit and vegetables per day and eating a low-fat diet, respectively. However, given that perceived need is so closely related to behavioural intention ($r = 0.67$ and 0.73, respectively; Povey *et al.*, 2000), it is unclear whether the construct truly adds anything distinct to the TPB. Given that behavioural intention is regarded as a summary of the motivation required to engage in a particular behaviour, it is possible that perceived need might more usefully be incorporated in measures of intention. One way to address this issue would be to experimentally manipulate perceived need and so attempt to dissociate it from effects on behavioural intention.

More generally, in spite of the contributions made by self-identity and perceived need, the true value of their contribution is open to question. First, it is notable that each of these variables exerts its influence on actual food choice *indirectly*, via behavioural intentions. As discussed above, this approach can provide only a partial account of actual food choice: the challenge is to identify variables that exert direct influence on behaviour. Second, Conner and Armitage's (1998) meta-analysis indicated that, on average, self-identity explained only 1% unique variance in intention. Whilst meta-analytic data on perceived need are not currently available, it is clear that the variable contributes less to the prediction of intention than the components of the TPB. Third, the majority of studies that have tested the role of additional variables within the TPB have only investigated additive effects. That is, researchers typically statistically control for the effects of TPB variables before seeing whether the additional variable of choice explains significant additional variance. Very few studies have investigated interactive or moderator (see Baron and Kenny, 1986) effects of additional variables, which might equally add to our understanding of food choice. For example, it is possible that self-identity might moderate the attitude–intention relationship such that the attitudes of high identifiers are more predictive of intentions than are those of individuals who do not identify themselves as (for example) green consumers. The potential contribution of this approach was demonstrated in a study of voting behaviour: Granberg and Holmberg (1990) demonstrated that the intentions of high identifiers were more predictive of behaviour than were the intentions of low identifiers.

Some food choice studies *have* tested moderator effects, although the focus has been upon investigating the *properties* of TPB variables rather than on variables that might add to the prediction of intention/behaviour. One property that has recently been investigated is that of temporal stability, or the idea that (for example) the attitudes of some individuals may be more stable over time and hence more predictive of intention and behaviour. In fact, this is one of the early assumptions of models like the TPB (e.g. Fishbein and Ajzen, 1975) and given that many studies assess TPB variables and behaviour several months apart, controlling for the (in)stability of components means that extraneous influences such as mass media campaigns, spontaneous changes in attitudes, or exposure to uncontrolled health promotion materials can be accounted for. For example, Conner *et al.* (2000) found that more stable intentions were more predictive of eating a low-fat diet 3 months later. More recently, Conner *et al.* (2003) extended these findings by testing the predictive validity of the TPB across a 6-year time period. Consistent with Conner *et al.* (2000), Conner *et al.* (2003) found that stable intentions were more predictive of an objective measure of healthy eating taken 6 years later than were unstable intentions. Stability is therefore one property that enhances the predictive power of behavioural intentions. Moreover, similar stability effects have been reported with respect to the influence of perceived behavioural control on behaviour (see Conner *et al.*, 2000).

The second property of TPB variables that has been investigated has been that of attitude strength, and stronger attitudes have been shown to be more predictive of intentions (e.g. Sparks *et al.*, 1992). More recently, a number of social psychologists have considered the possibility that attitudes might be multidimensional. As we have already noted in our discussion of the EV model, attitudes towards objects are generally held to be summaries of decision-making processes. The implication is that individuals 'decide' whether or not they are positively or negatively disposed towards an attitude object and that this changes only if the underlying beliefs change. This unidimensional view of attitudes has been the dominant approach in social psychology (see Eagly and Chaiken, 1993).

Recently, however, it has been recognized that attitudes may be multidimensional. Thus, rather than arguing that attitudes are simply positive or negative, individuals can be simultaneously positive and negative towards an attitude object. For example, an individual's attitude towards the consumption of junk food may be positive because they like the taste of it, while simultaneously being negative because of the high fat content. This bidimensional view of attitudes is known as attitudinal ambivalence (see Thompson *et al.*, 1995; Olsen, 1999; Conner and Sparks, 2001). The idea of attitudinal ambivalence with respect to food choice is particularly appealing, given that food choice has long been associated with ambivalence (Beardsworth, 1995) and competing motives (see Herrnstein, 1970; Mischel *et al.*, 1989). For example, Sparks *et al.* (2001) note that, 'people may have mixed feelings about consuming animal products because the sensory appeal of such products may be accompanied by moral concerns with animal welfare issues' (p. 56). Similarly, the positive evaluations associated with the taste of cream cakes may be experienced simultaneously with negative evaluations concerning weight gain.

As well as capturing potentially conflicting influences on food choice, the consequences of ambivalent attitudes are also important. Given that more ambivalent attitudes capture both positive and negative evaluations of objects, they are likely to be less extreme than less ambivalent (or univalent) attitudes. In other words, they are likely to be weaker than univalent attitudes (see Thompson *et al.*, 1995). Of particular relevance to the present discussion, attitudinal ambivalence is likely to moderate the relationship between attitudes and intention/behaviour, such that stronger (i.e. less ambivalent) attitudes are more predictive. A number of recent studies have explored this possibility. For example, Sparks *et al.* (2001) examined ambivalence with respect to eating meat and chocolate and found that greater ambivalence was associated with weaker attitude–intention relationships. Similarly, Povey *et al.* (2001) examined the determinants of eating meat, vegetarian and vegan diets; in each case more ambivalent attitudes were associated with weaker attitude–intention correlations. Thus, Sparks *et al.* (2001) and Povey *et al.* (2001) have found that attitudinal ambivalence undermines the relationship between attitudes and intentions.

Armitage and Conner (2000, Study 1) replicated these findings in the context of eating a low-fat diet. In addition, they also found that attitudinal ambivalence moderated the attitude–behaviour relationship such that less ambivalent attitudes were more predictive of behaviour 3 months later. The latter finding is of particular note because it is an example of a study that has simultaneously measured both attitude and intention and found a direct effect of attitude. The implication is that the strong, univalent attitudes by-passed intentions to predict behaviour directly, unmediated by intentions. In a second study, Armitage and Conner (2000) designed an intervention to change attitudes. The intervention materials were based on the work of Fishbein and Ajzen (1975) and were designed to change beliefs about salient outcomes and the evaluation of those outcomes (see also Ajzen and Fishbein, 1980). Examining differences between more- and less-ambivalent individuals, Armitage and Conner (2000) found that individuals high in ambivalence were more easily persuaded. Again, this suggests that ambivalent attitudes are weak and therefore more susceptible to a persuasive communication. Thus, research into attitudinal ambivalence suggests that attitudes can predict behaviour directly, but they need to be of a certain strength. In addition, attempts to persuade individuals to change their diet might need to take the strength of attitudes into account.

To date, research on attitudinal ambivalence has focused almost exclusively on what we term *global* ambivalence, or general positive and negative evaluations of behaviour. However, when thinking about evaluative conflict with respect to food choice, the conflict between heart and head – or *affect* and *cognition* – is also relevant (c.f. Rosenberg and Hovland, 1960). Thus, foods can elicit both emotional and cognitive reactions, and attitudinal ambivalence might usefully be extended to incorporate simultaneous affective and cognitive evaluations. For example, a chocolate cake might be simultaneously perceived as enjoyable (positive, affective), beneficial (positive, cognitive), harmful (negative, cognitive) or unpleasant (negative, affective). Given that cognitive outcomes (e.g. health risks, not wasting food) are likely to be more long-term than affective outcomes (e.g. pleasure, guilt), it is perhaps unsurprising that health risks are often not predictive of food choice attitudes (e.g. Armitage and Conner, 1999a).

Conclusions

This chapter has focused on EV models and the TPB in particular as the dominant social psychological models applied to food choice (see Conner and Armitage, 2002). Such models have provided valuable insights into the determinants of food choice. More importantly, the identified factors appear to both mediate the impact of other influences on food choice (e.g. physiological, sociodemographic) and be potentially modifiable. This latter aspect is particularly important in relation to developing interventions to change health behaviours. Finally, we should note that the present focus on the TPB is not to deny the value of other social psychological models. Indeed, we would note the value of implementation intentions (Sheeran *et al.*, 2005) and stage models (Sutton, 2005) to further our understanding of food choice (see later chapters in this volume). In addition, other models such as protection motivation theory (Maddux and Rogers, 1983; Norman *et al.*, 2005) and social cognitive theory (Bandura, 1982, 2001; Luszczynska and

Schwarzer, 2005) may also represent useful additional models in relation to food choice, but have as yet not been sufficiently widely applied to evaluate.

References

Ajzen, I. (1988) *Attitudes, Personality and Behavior.* Open University Press, Milton Keynes, UK.

Ajzen, I. (1991) The theory of planned behavior. *Organizational Behavior and Human Decision Processes* 50, 179–211.

Ajzen, I. (1996) The directive influence of attitudes on behavior. In: Gollwitzer, P. and Bargh, J.A. (eds) *Psychology of Action.* Guilford, New York, pp. 385–403.

Ajzen, I. (1998) Models of human social behavior and their application to health psychology. *Psychology & Health* 13, 735–739.

Ajzen, I. (2001) Nature and operation of attitudes. *Annual Review of Psychology* 52, 27–58.

Ajzen, I. and Fishbein, M. (1977) Attitude–behavior relations: a theoretical analysis and review of empirical research. *Psychological Bulletin* 84, 888–918.

Ajzen, I. and Fishbein, M. (1980) *Understanding Attitudes and Predicting Social Behavior.* Prentice-Hall, Englewood Cliffs, New Jersey.

Ajzen, I. and Fishbein, M. (2000) Attitudes and the attitude–behavior relation: reasoned and automatic processes. *European Review of Social Psychology* 11, 1–33.

Allport, G.W. (1935) Attitudes. In: Murchison, C. (ed.) *Handbook of Social Psychology.* Clark University Press, Worcester, Massachusetts, pp. 798–844.

Anderson, A.S. and Shepherd, R. (1989) Beliefs and attitudes toward 'healthier eating' among women attending maternity hospital. *Journal of Nutrition Education* 21, 208–213.

Armitage, C.J. and Christian, J. (eds) (2003) Special issue: On the theory of planned behaviour. *Current Psychology* 22, 187–280.

Armitage, C.J. and Conner, M. (1999a) Distinguishing perceptions of control from self-efficacy: predicting consumption of a low-fat diet using the theory of planned behavior. *Journal of Applied Social Psychology* 29, 72–90.

Armitage, C.J. and Conner, M. (1999b) Predictive validity of the theory of planned behaviour: the role of questionnaire format and social desirability. *Journal of Community and Applied Social Psychology* 9, 261–272.

Armitage, C.J. and Conner, M. (2000) Attitudinal ambivalence: a test of three key hypotheses. *Personality and Social Psychology Bulletin* 26, 1421–1432.

Armitage, C.J. and Conner, M. (2001) Efficacy of the theory of planned behaviour: a meta-analytic review. *British Journal of Social Psychology* 40, 471–499.

Bagiella, E., Cairella, M., del Ben, M. and Godi, R. (1991) Changes in attitude toward food by obese patients treated with placebo and serotoninergic agents. *Current Therapeutic Research* 50, 205–210.

Bandura, A. (1982) Self-efficacy mechanism in human agency. *American Psychologist* 37, 122–147.

Bandura, A. (2001) Social cognitive theory: an agentic perspective. *Annual Review of Psychology* 52, 1–26.

Baranowski, T., Cullen, K.W. and Baranowski, J. (1999) Psychosocial correlates of dietary intake: advancing dietary intervention. *Annual Review of Nutrition* 19, 17–40.

Baron, R.M. and Kenny, D.A. (1986) The moderator–mediator variable distinction in social psychological research: conceptual, strategic, and statistical considerations. *Journal of Personality and Social Psychology* 51, 1173–1182.

Beardsworth, A. (1995) The management of food ambivalence: erosion or reconstruction? In: Maurer, D. and Sobal, J. (eds) *Eating Agendas: Food and Nutrition as Social Problems*. De Gruyter, New York, pp. 38–42.

Birch, L.L. (1999) Development of food preferences. *Annual Review of Nutrition* 19, 41–62.

Broughton, J.M. (1994) Declines in mammalian foraging efficiency during the Late Holocene, San Francisco Bay, California. *Journal of Anthropological Archaeology* 13, 371–401.

Cade, J.E. and Margetts, B.M. (1988) Nutrient sources in the English diet: quantitative data from three English towns. *International Journal of Epidemiology* 17, 844–848.

Charng, H.-W., Piliavin, J.A. and Callero, P. (1988) Role identity and reasoned action in the prediction of repeated behavior. *Social Psychology Quarterly* 51, 303–317.

Conner, M. and Armitage, C.J. (1998) Extending the theory of planned behavior: a review and avenues for further research. *Journal of Applied Social Psychology* 28, 1429–1464.

Conner, M. and Armitage, C.J. (2002) *The Social Psychology of Food*. Open University Press, Buckingham, UK.

Conner, M. and Sparks, P. (1996) The theory of planned behaviour and health behaviours. In: Conner, M. and Norman, P. (eds) *Predicting Health Behaviour*. Open University Press, Buckingham, UK, pp. 121–162.

Conner, M. and Sparks, P. (2001) Ambivalence and attitudes. *European Review of Social Psychology* 12, 37–70.

Conner, M., Sheeran, P., Norman, P. and Armitage, C.J. (2000) Temporal stability as a moderator of relationships in the theory of planned behaviour. *British Journal of Social Psychology* 39, 469–493.

Conner, M., Povey, R., Sparks, P., James, R. and Shepherd, R. (2003) Moderating role of attitudinal ambivalence within the theory of planned behaviour. *British Journal of Social Psychology* 42, 75–94.

Cox, D.N., Anderson, A.S., Lean, M.E.J. and Mela, D.J. (1998) UK consumer attitudes, beliefs and barriers to increasing fruit and vegetable consumption. *Public Health Nutrition* 1, 61–68.

Department of Health (1992) *The Health of the Nation: A Strategy for Health in England*. HMSO, London.

Eagly, A.H. and Chaiken, S. (1993) *The Psychology of Attitudes*. Harcourt Brace Jovanovich, Fort Worth, Texas/Philadelphia, Pennsylvania.

Fishbein, M. (1967a) A behavior theory approach to the relations between beliefs about an object and the attitude toward the object. In: Fishbein, M. (ed.) *Readings in Attitude Theory and Measurement*. Wiley, New York, pp. 389–400.

Fishbein, M. (1967b) Attitude and the prediction of behavior. In: Fishbein, M. (ed.) *Readings in Attitude Theory and Measurement*. Wiley, New York, pp. 477–492.

Fishbein, M. and Ajzen, I. (1975) *Belief, Attitude, Intention, and Behavior*. Wiley, New York.

Godin, G. and Kok, G. (1996) The theory of planned behavior: a review of its applications to health-related behaviors. *American Journal of Health Promotion* 11, 87–98.

Granberg, D. and Holmberg, S. (1990) The intention–behavior relationship among US and Swedish voters. *Social Psychology Quarterly* 53, 44–54.

Grogan, S. (1999) *Body Image: Understanding Body Dissatisfaction in Men, Women and Children*. Routledge, London.

Herrnstein, R.J. (1961) Relative and absolute strength of response as a function of frequency of reinforcement. *Journal of the Experimental Analysis of Behavior* 4, 267–272.

Herrnstein, R.J. (1970) On the law of effect. *Journal of the Experimental Analysis of Behavior* 13, 243–266.

Katz, D. (1960) The functional approach to the study of attitudes. *Public Opinion Quarterly* 24, 163–204.

Kim, M.-S. and Hunter, J.E. (1993) Attitude–behavior relations: a meta-analysis of attitudinal relevance and topic. *Journal of Communication* 43, 101–142.

Kraus, S.J. (1995) Attitudes and the prediction of behavior – a meta-analysis of the empirical literature. *Personality and Social Psychology Bulletin* 21, 58–75.

Luszczynska, A. and Schwarzer, R. (2005) Social cognitive theory. In: Conner, M. and Norman, P. (eds) *Predicting Health Behaviour: Research and Practice with Social Cognition Models*, 2nd edn. Open University Press, Maidenhead, UK, pp. 127–169.

Maddux, J.E. and Rogers, R.W. (1983) Protection motivation and self-efficacy: a revised theory of fear appeals and attitude change. *Journal of Experimental Social Psychology* 19, 469–479.

Mischel, W., Shoda, Y. and Rodriguez, M.L. (1989) Delay of gratification in children. *Science* 244, 933–938.

Nguyen, M.N., Otis, J. and Potvin, L. (1996) Determinants of intention to adopt a low-fat diet in men 30 to 60 years old: implications for heart health promotions. *American Journal of Health Promotion* 10, 201–207.

Norman, P., Boer, A. and Seydel, A. (2005) Protection motivation theory. In: Conner, M. and Norman, P. (eds) *Predicting Health Behaviour: Research and Practice with Social Cognition Models*, 2nd edn. Open University Press, Maidenhead, UK, pp. 81–126.

Olsen, S.O. (1999) Strength and conflicting valence in the measurement of food attitudes and preferences. *Food Quality and Preference* 10, 483–494.

Paisley, C.M. and Sparks, P. (1998) Expectations of reducing fat intake: the role of perceived need within the theory of planned behaviour. *Psychology & Health* 13, 341–353.

Peak, H. (1955) Attitude and motivation. In: Jones, M.R. (ed.) *Nebraska Symposium on Motivation*, Vol. 3. University of Nebraska Press, Lincoln, Nebraska, pp. 149–188.

Povey, R., Conner, M., Sparks, P., James, R. and Shepherd, R. (2000) Application of the theory of planned behaviour to two dietary behaviours: roles of perceived control and self-efficacy. *British Journal of Health Psychology* 5, 121–139.

Povey, R., Wellens, B. and Conner, M. (2001) Attitudes towards following meat, vegetarian and vegan diets: an examination of the role of ambivalence. *Appetite* 37, 15–26.

Rogers, P.J. and Blundell, J.E. (1990) Psychobiological bases of food choice. *The British Nutrition Foundation Nutrition Bulletin* 15, 31–40.

Rosenberg, M.J. and Hovland, C.I. (1960) Cognitive, affective, and behavioral components of attitudes. In: Hovland, C.I. and Rosenberg, M.J. (eds) *Attitude Organization and Change: An Analysis of Consistency Among Attitude Components*. Yale University Press, New Haven, Connecticut, pp. 1–14.

Saunders, R.P. and Rahilly, S.A. (1990) Influences on intention to reduce dietary intake of fat and sugar. *Journal of Nutrition Education* 22, 169–176.

Shavitt, S. (1990) The role of attitude objects in attitude functions. *Journal of Experimental Social Psychology* 26, 124–148.

Sheeran, P., Milne, S., Webb, T.L. and Gollwitzer, P.M. (2005) Implementation intentions and health behaviours. In: Conner, M. and Norman, P. (eds) *Predicting Health Behaviour: Research and Practice with Social Cognition Models*, 2nd edn. Open University Press, Maidenhead, UK, pp. 276–323.

Sheppard, B.H., Hartwick, J. and Warshaw, P.R. (1988) The theory of reasoned action: a meta-analysis of past research with recommendations for modifications and future research. *Journal of Consumer Research* 15, 325–343.

Sparks, P. (1994) Attitudes towards food: applying, assessing and extending the 'theory of planned behaviour'. In: Rutter, D.R. and Quine, L. (eds) *Social Psychology and Health: European Perspectives*. Avebury Press, Aldershot, UK, pp. 25–46.

Sparks, P. (2000) Subjective expected utility-based attitude–behavior models: the utility of self-identity. In: Terry, D.J. and Hogg, M.A. (eds) *Attitudes, Behavior and Social Context: The Role of Norms and Group Membership*. Lawrence Erlbaum, London, pp. 31–46.

Sparks, P. and Guthrie, C.A. (1998) Self-identity and the theory of planned behavior: a useful addition or unhelpful artifice? *Journal of Applied Social Psychology* 28, 1394–1411.

Sparks, P. and Shepherd, R. (1992) Self-identity and the theory of planned behavior – assessing the role of identification with green consumerism. *Social Psychology Quarterly* 55, 388–399.

Sparks, P., Hedderley, P. and Shepherd, R. (1992) An investigation into the relationship between perceived control, attitude variability and the consumption of two common foods. *European Journal of Social Psychology* 22, 55–71.

Sparks, P., Shepherd, R. and Frewer, L.J. (1995) Assessing and structuring attitudes toward the use of gene technology in food production: the role of perceived ethical obligation. *Basic and Applied Social Psychology* 16, 267–285.

Sparks, P., Conner, M., James, R., Shepherd, R. and Povey, R. (2001) Ambivalence about health-related behaviours: an exploration in the domain of food choice. *British Journal of Health Psychology* 6, 53–68.

Sutton, S.R. (2005) Stage theories of health behaviours. In: Conner, M. and Norman, P. (eds) *Predicting Health Behaviour: Research and Practice with Social Cognition Models*, 2nd edn. Open University Press, Maidenhead, UK, pp. 223–275.

Teff, K.L. and Engelman, K. (1996) Palatability and dietary restraint: effect on cephalic phase insulin release in women. *Physiology & Behavior* 60, 567–573.

Thompson, M.M., Zanna, M.P. and Griffin, D.W. (1995) Let's not be indifferent about (attitudinal) ambivalence. In: Petty, R.E. and Krosnick, J.A. (eds) *Attitude Strength: Antecedents and Consequences*. Lawrence Erlbaum Associates, Mahwah, New Jersey, pp. 361–386.

Towler, G. and Shepherd, R. (1992) Application of Fishbein and Ajzen's expectancy–value model to understanding fat intake. *Appetite* 18, 15–27.

Van der Pligt, J. and de Vries, N.K. (1998) Belief importance in expectancy–value models of attitudes. *Journal of Applied Social Psychology* 28, 1339–1354.

Van der Pligt, J., de Vries, N.K., Manstead, A.S.R. and van Harreveld, F. (2000) The importance of being selective: weighing the role of attribute importance in attitudinal judgment. *Advances in Experimental Social Psychology* 32, 135–200.

This page intentionally left blank

4 Biological Influences on Energy Intake

KLAAS R. WESTERTERP

Department of Human Biology, Maastricht University, PO Box 616, 6200 MD Maastricht, The Netherlands

Introduction

Adult humans maintain a balance between their energy intake and energy expenditure. The energy store of their bodies does not fluctuate much, as the constancy of body weight and body composition shows. Food energy is consumed in the form of carbohydrate, protein, fat and alcohol, together forming the macronutrients of the diet. The regulation of food intake is a multifactor system. Studies on the measurement of food intake in daily life have to rely on self-reporting with consequences for their validity. In the present chapter, biological influences on food intake are presented in a case-oriented approach. The cases are: reported food intake as a measure of energy intake; regulation of body weight primarily through intake; regulation of intake as a multifactorial system; the alcohol paradox; why does carbohydrate make fat; why is protein not fattening; and one is as fat as one eats.

Reported Food Intake as a Measure of Energy Intake

The measurement of habitual food consumption in man is one of the hardest tasks in energy balance studies. The two basic problems are the accurate determination of a subject's customary food intake, and the conversion of this information to nutrient and energy intakes. Any technique used to measure food intake should not be so intensely applied as to interfere with the subject's dietary habits and thus alter the parameter being measured. The next problem is for how long food intake should be measured before the information can be said to be a true reflection of habitual food intake, i.e. the food an individual normally consumes to provide the energy and nutrient requirements for his regular everyday activities. Basiotis *et al.* (1987) calculated that the minimum time interval to measure habitual energy intake was 31 days for the individual level and 3 days for the group level. For accurate estimation of separate nutrients such as fat, the number of days required is 6 for a measurement at group level and about 65 for a measurement at individual level. The focus in the following is on methods to measure food intake at the individual level, i.e. dietary record and dietary recall. The food record method requires subjects to record types and amounts of all foods consumed over a given time interval. The foods are weighed or recorded in household measures like cups and spoons. The latter information is translated to weight or volume by measuring the actual 'tools' used or adopting standard values from reference tables. Dietary recalls use the subjects' report of intake over the previous 24 h period (24 h recall) or the report of customary intake over the previous week up to the past year(s) (diet history); the same methods are then used to quantify the reported intake from information on portion size.

Nowadays there are a number of reference methods to verify the results of dietary assessment. Reference methods include urine nitrogen, total energy expenditure, resting metabolic rate and physical activity, and total water loss. The most widespread reference method is total energy expenditure as assessed by the doubly labelled water method. It is the most accurate method for the validation of reported energy intake by subjects in free-living situations. Hill and Davies (2001) reviewed studies using doubly labelled water in conjunction with self-reported energy intake. Considering data included in that review plus in one study published afterwards (Lanigan *et al.*, 2001), most studies showed a lower value for reported energy intake than for measured total energy expenditure. Women did not show more or less under-reporting than men. Values for normal-weight subjects were mostly in the range of 0–25% with a grand average of 16% (Fig. 4.1). Values for obese subjects were more in the 25 to 50% range with a grand average of 41%, i.e. generally twice as high as in normal-weight subjects (Fig. 4.2). An important point was that in studies where a person other than the subject was responsible for recording dietary intake, such as parents of young children, reported intake generally was not lower than measured expenditure. A typical example is a study in children and adolescents with severe disabilities. The recorded intake of the children, by the caregivers who also fed the children, was about 50% higher than measured energy expenditure (Stallings *et al.*, 1996). Studies with depleted nursing home patients also reported an overestimation of the habitual food intake (Johnson *et al.*, 1993; Kayser-Jones *et al.*, 1998). The increased awareness by the nurses during the food-recording period resulted in a higher figure than real intake. In studies where a 'neutral observer' recorded intake, there was no difference between recorded intake and doubly labelled water-assessed energy expenditure (Sjödin *et al.*, 1994; Hise *et al.*, 2002).

Recent studies analysing misreporting of habitual food intake and its consequences for the study of dietary intake are now considered. Under-reporting of habitual intake can be explained by under-recording and undereating. Some studies have discriminated between the two errors mentioned, by comparing reported food intake and water intake with energy expenditure and water loss. When subjects record food intake they record simultaneously water intake. In healthy individuals, water balance is preserved and is therefore an independent indicator for under-recording. The recording precision of water intake is

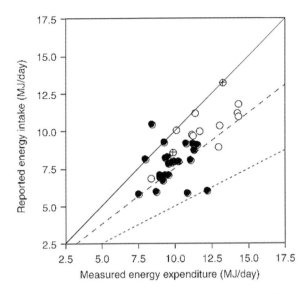

Fig. 4.1. Reported energy intake plotted against energy expenditure as measured with doubly labelled water from studies on normal-weight (body mass index 20–25 kg/m²) adult subjects (○, women, *n* = 482; ●, men, *n* = 226; ⊕, gender mixed, *n* = 46). The lines denote no under-reporting (—), 25% under-reporting (– – –) and 50% under-reporting (- - -).

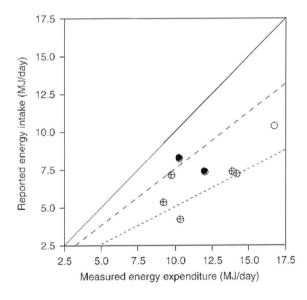

Fig. 4.2. Reported energy intake plotted against energy expenditure as measured with doubly labelled water from studies on obese subjects (○, women, *n* = 17; ●, men, *n* = 30; ⊕, gender mixed, *n* = 85). The lines denote no under-reporting (—), 25% under-reporting (– – –) and 50% under-reporting (- - -).

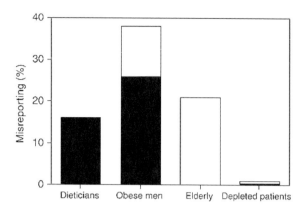

Fig. 4.3.   Percentage of misreporting, divided into misrecording (▫) and a change in diet (■), as observed in lean women, obese men, elderly men and women, and depleted patients. Data are presented as [(measured energy expenditure – recorded energy intake)/measured energy expenditure] × 100 (%).

assumed to be representative for total food recording, as most foodstuffs contain water. Undereating during food recording is monitored by measurement of body mass. Body mass changes over a food-recording period are compared with normal body mass fluctuations. Figure 4.3 shows the percentage of misreporting, divided into misrecording and a change in diet as observed in lean women (Goris and Westerterp, 1999), obese men (Goris et al., 2000), elderly men and women (Goris et al., 2001) and depleted patients (Goris et al., 2003). Both the obese men and lean women ate less while recording food intake, but probably for different reasons. The lean women ate less because weighing and recording food intake was perceived as a great burden, which might also count for the obese men. However, the obese men used the recording period also as an opportunity to start dieting. The recording error observed in the obese men and the elderly men and women was probably due to underestimation of food portion sizes and to not recording all foods consumed. Only the depleted patients reported their food intake accurately and they did not change their diet while recording food intake.

Many studies on dietary intake show figures for total energy intake much lower than figures for total energy expenditure reported in comparable subject groups. A correction for energy intake is not a possibility to solve the problem of misreporting of food intake as intake of macronutrients might be misreported selectively. Under-reporting of food intake does not result from a systematic underestimation of portion sizes for all food items but seems to concern specific food items which are generally considered 'bad for health' (Lissner et al., 1998). The relationship between nutrient intake and health parameters can be overestimated or hidden as a consequence of selective under-reporting (Greenwald et al., 1997). One example is the relationship between fat intake and obesity entitled 'the American paradox'. In the US adult population the prevalence of overweight has increased since 1976 by 31% and at the same time reported energy intake and percentage of energy from fat have decreased. This might be due to a lower physical activity and a higher consumption of

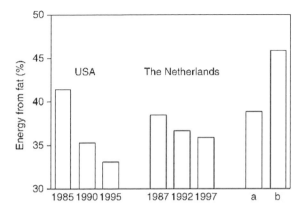

Fig. 4.4.   Percentage of energy from fat as measured in national food consumption studies in the USA in 1985, 1990 and 1995; in The Netherlands in 1987, 1992 and 1997; and in obese men, uncorrected (a) and corrected for under-reporting (b). (From Goris *et al.*, 2000.)

low-energy foods but under-reporting has also increased since 1976 (Heitmann *et al.*, 2000). Combining the results of studies showing selective under-reporting of fat intake, the reported decrease in energy and fat intake in the USA seems to be doubtful (Kennedy *et al.*, 1999; Goris *et al.*, 2000; Tomoyasu *et al.*, 2000). Campaigns aimed at lowering fat intake might not be as successful as is concluded from the results of national food consumption measurements showing a decline in reported fat intakes over several years. Figure 4.4 shows reported percentage of energy from fat of national food consumption studies in The Netherlands and the USA and the percentage of energy from fat reported by obese men, corrected and uncorrected for under-reporting (Goris *et al.*, 2000).

Thus, there is not yet a method for the accurate determination of dietary intake. Physical and psychological characteristics of study participants play an important role in the observed reporting bias (Hill and Davies, 2001; Trabulsi and Schoeller, 2001). The degree of misreporting might increase with repeated dietary assessment in the same subjects, confounding the results of intervention studies (Goris *et al.*, 2001). A potential solution is to confront subjects with earlier results of food reporting. In a group of motivated women this method of confrontation improved the food reporting of a second time (Goris and Westerterp, 2000). Whatever method is used, it remains very difficult to get accurate data from food reporting at the individual level (Lanigan *et al.*, 2001). Consequently, when studying biological influences on energy intake, data on reported food intake have to be interpreted with care.

Regulation of Body Weight Primarily through Intake

An adult human maintains a balance between energy intake and energy expenditure. This can be achieved either by the control of intake or the expenditure of energy. Humans do not balance energy intake and energy expenditure on a daily basis, whereas smaller animals do. Apparently humans can afford to rely on their body reserves while smaller species sooner show signs of energy shortage such as lowered body temperature and reduced physical activity. Smaller species have a higher energy expenditure on a kg body mass basis plus a relatively smaller body energy reserve. Thus a mouse does not survive a period of 3 days without food while a normal adult survives more than 30 days.

Of course, humans maintain a perfect energy balance in the long term as shown by a constant body weight in adult life. Energy intake correlates highly with energy expenditure on a weekly basis. Discrepancies on a daily basis between intake and expenditure are especially large when days with high energy expenditure are alternated with quieter intervals. Military cadets did not show an increase in energy intake on days with higher energy expenditure when they joined a drill competition. The corresponding increase in energy intake came about 2 days afterwards (Edholm et al., 1955). A more recent review based on 69 subjects from six energy balance studies also ended with the conclusion that there is no precise short-term control mechanism. Humans can change their energy intake by a factor of at least 3 for adapting it to the expenditure of energy. Under sedentary living conditions the energy balance is maintained at about 1.5 times basal metabolic rate, while during sustained exercise levels of 4.5 times basal metabolic rate are reached (Westerterp, 2001).

The possibility that humans adapt their expenditure to the energy intake is often called into question. It is even stated sometimes that the control of energy expenditure is contrary to what body weight would require in view of hyperactivity in anorectics and hypoactivity in obesity. However, a decrease in energy intake has consequences for energy expenditure. Body weight does not remain at equilibrium as during ad libitum conditions and this causes a drop in energy expenditure. Some metabolic savings will result from the mere fact that one handles and digests less food. Over and above these 'automatic' consequences of a lowered energy intake for energy expenditure, there is a 'real' adaptation of energy expenditure to a decreasing energy intake. The underfed subject spends less energy on a given function (e.g. protein turnover, or muscular effort for a given behaviour) than would do a conspecific of the same weight and body composition eating ad libitum. Evolution has provided the individual with a special capability of eking out its provisions in order to increase the chance that it may tide over temporary food scarcity, a condition common in many places in history and even nowadays in several parts of the world. On the other hand, this is a 'problem' for many well-fed people in the Western world these days. Many of them struggle to maintain a 'normal' body weight. Most of them are finding themselves overweight or manifestly overweight. They want to spend more energy, even on an energy-restricted diet, to get rid of body mass mainly in the form of body fat.

Energy expenditure in overfeeding has been studied in several laboratories, mainly to increase the understanding of the causes and consequences of obesity. Lean people are persuaded to gain weight to increase the understanding of 'spontaneous' obesity. From classical overfeeding studies it can be concluded that most of the energy added to a maintenance diet is stored. Norgan and

Durnin (1980) fed subjects with a mean energy expenditure of 11.4 MJ/day a diet supplying 17.5 MJ/day for 42 days, i.e. the added energy over 42 days was on average 256 MJ and the energy gain was on average 144 MJ or 56%. Webb and Annis (1983) fed subjects with a mean energy expenditure of 9.2 MJ/day a diet supplying 13.2 MJ/day for 30 days, i.e. the added energy over 30 days was on average 120 MJ and the energy gain was on average 76 MJ or 63%.

There is very little information on the consequences of a decrease in energy expenditure for energy intake and the resulting energy balance. It is often suggested that we eat according to our needs to maintain energy balance, only to prevent a negative energy balance. In evolution, there has nevertheless been selection against or even selection in favour of mechanisms to promote a positive energy balance. Thus, there might be no adaptive mechanism to reduce energy intake after a decrease in energy expenditure.

Everybody knows people gain weight after a decrease in energy expenditure through a reduction in physical activity. Common examples are athletes quitting training or people quitting manual work. A more complicated example is weight gain in people stopping smoking. Traditionally, the weight gain after the cessation of smoking is ascribed to an increase in energy intake. However, there are indications that smokers do have higher energy expenditure than non-smokers. Stopping smoking would thus mean a decrease of the energy expenditure, explaining why people gain weight even when energy intake remains the same. Unfortunately, there are no systematic studies on energy intake and energy balance in subjects before and after a reduction of energy expenditure.

The consequences of an increase in energy expenditure for energy intake and energy balance have been measured by raising the physical activity. Novice athletes starting a training programme manage to maintain energy balance (Westerterp *et al.*, 1992). Reported energy intake did not show significant changes. However, measured total energy expenditure increased to a value on average 21 ± 10% higher than before the start of the training. Body mass did not show much change, indicating that subjects were in energy balance. The discrepancy between the observed increase in energy expenditure without a significant increase in intake clearly is an artefact. It is another example of the difficulties of measuring food consumption. The conclusion must be that it is possible to maintain energy balance after an increase in energy expenditure by an increase in energy intake. Usually, there is at least initially a negative energy balance and in the long term an increased level of physical activity affects body composition.

Regulation of Intake as a Multifactorial System

The alcohol paradox

Nation-wide epidemiological studies show a paradoxical association between alcohol intake and body weight. While alcohol energy is additive to the normal diet, there is no positive correlation with body weight. Alcohol is a significant component of the diet in many countries. Per capita alcohol consumption is about 3–9% of daily energy intake. Alcohol seems to supplement rather than displace food-derived energy (Rose *et al.*, 1995). Studies on the effects of alcohol consumption on food consumption have led to the conclusion that alcohol consumption is associated with minimal compensatory down-regulation of energy intake from other foods (Poppitt and Prentice, 1996). Even increased energy intake after an aperitif, due to decreased control caused by lightheadedness, is not compensated for (Westerterp-Plantenga and Verwegen, 1999).

The lack of a relationship between the apparent alcohol energy surplus and body mass index in epidemiological studies has led to the suggestion that alcohol energy has a low biological efficiency. However, ethanol is readily absorbed and is principally eliminated by metabolism in the liver, urinary losses being about 0.3% of the dose. Since ethanol is not stored in the body, it must be oxidized preferentially to other fuels. Thus, alcohol ingestion results in a short-term reduction of fat oxidation. Controlled feeding studies have shown that ethanol is utilized with the same efficiency as other nutrients like carbohydrate (Rumpler *et al.*, 1996).

In the controlled studies mentioned above, the life-style of the subjects was not taken into account. We assessed habitual physical activity and habitual alcohol intake in the daily environment, hypothesizing that the addition of alcohol to energy intake might be offset by higher physical activity-induced energy expenditure (Westerterp *et al.*, 2004). Between subjects, there was a positive association between the level of habitual physical activity and alcohol intake ($r = 0.41$, $P < 0.01$). Subjects with higher alcohol intake had a higher activity level. On days with and days without alcohol consumption there was no difference in physical activity within subjects. In conclusion, we showed evidence for the lack of increasing body weight through additional energy intake from alcohol in that subjects who are habitually more active have higher alcohol consumption.

Why does carbohydrate make fat?

All macronutrients, alcohol, carbohydrate, protein and fat, are fattening when consumed in excess of daily requirement. However, there is a hierarchy in macronutrient oxidation with the sequence alcohol, protein, carbohydrate and fat. When the sum of the energy in alcohol, protein and carbohydrate intake is higher than daily energy requirement, a surplus of energy intake is stored by direct storage of dietary fat. In a situation where energy intake is lower than energy expenditure, normally fat stores permit covering the energy deficit by fat mobilization. Thus, an effect of a macronutrient on energy balance is through an effect on energy intake.

Carbohydrate-sweetened beverages such as soft drinks are thought to increase the risk of over-consumption resulting in excess body fat. When humans ingest energy-containing beverages such as soft drinks, energy compensation is less precise than when solid foods are ingested (DiMeglio and Mattes, 2000). Raben *et al.* (2002) investigated the effect of long-term supplementation with drinks and foods containing sucrose or artificial sweeteners on *ad libitum* food intake and body weight. Subjects who were given supplemental drinks and foods containing sucrose experienced increases in energy intake, body weight and fat mass. This was not observed in a similar group of subjects given similar drinks and foods containing artificial sweeteners. The increase in energy intake was mostly as beverages.

Epidemiological data show that the development of obesity in the USA has a temporal relationship to the consumption of beverages sweetened with high-fructose corn syrup (Bray *et al.*, 2004). The metabolism of fructose favours *de novo* lipogenesis. In the USA, the intake of high-fructose corn syrup with sweetened beverages increased from about zero in 1970 to 75 g/day per person in 1985 with a further increase to nearly 100 g/day per person in the year 2000. The parallel with the trend in the prevalence of obesity is striking. Indeed, there is a study showing that the consumption of beverages sweetened with high-fructose corn syrup is linked with increased energy intake and weight gain (Ludwig *et al.*, 2001).

Why is protein not fattening?

Protein as a nutrient is of primary importance for the amino acid supply of the body, especially the amino acids the body cannot make, known as essential amino acids. Protein requirement to maintain protein equilibrium is commonly estimated at 0.8 g/kg body weight. The figure of 0.8 g/kg body weight translates into about 10% of energy intake in a situation where intake covers energy expenditure. Diets with higher protein content are used as low-energy diets for weight loss. In the following, the focus is on the function of protein in a weight maintenance diet.

The main effect of protein on energy balance is thought to be related to protein-induced thermogenesis. Theoretically, based on the amount of ATP required for the initial steps of metabolism and storage, the diet-induced thermogenesis (DIT) is different for each nutrient. Reported DIT values for separate nutrients are 0–3% for fat, 5–10% for carbohydrate and 20–30% for protein (Tappy, 1996). In healthy subjects with a mixed diet, DIT represents about 10% of the total amount of energy ingested over 24 h. When a subject is in energy balance, where intake equals expenditure, DIT is 10% of daily energy expenditure.

High-protein/high-carbohydrate diets result in a higher satiety score after the meal, as well as over 24 h, than a high-fat diet (Westerterp-Plantenga *et al.*, 1999). The observed DIT-related satiety might be ascribed to the high protein rather than the high carbohydrate content of the diet. Postprandial thermogenesis was increased 100% on a high-protein/low-fat diet versus a high-carbohydrate/low-fat diet in healthy subjects (Johnston *et al.*, 2002). The DIT increases body temperature, which may be translated into satiety feelings. High-protein diets are favoured for weight maintenance and also after weight loss, by favouring maintenance or regain of fat-free mass, by reducing energy efficiency through a higher thermogenesis and by reducing intake through an increased satiety (Westerterp-Plantenga, 2003). Thus, protein plays a key role in body weight regulation.

One is as fat as one eats

The shift in the composition of the diet to a higher contribution of fats in Western countries has often been quoted as the reason for the increasing incidence of overweight, i.e. of a positive energy balance. There is experimental evidence that a change to a diet containing more fat leads to an increase in body weight. Combining this with the fact that obese people tend to eat foods containing more fat, leads to the conclusion that overweight can be prevented by reducing the fat content of the diet. The mechanism for the effect of the fat content of the diet on energy balance is not yet fully known. Theoretically there are two possibilities: a diet containing more fat reduces energy expenditure or increases energy intake.

Evidence for the first statement, a diet containing more fat reduces energy expenditure, is lacking. The second statement, a diet containing more fat increases energy intake, seems to be more realistic. Fat is often used to increase the palatability of food and fat is the nutrient with the highest energy density, more than twice that of carbohydrate and protein. Despite the potential of fat to increase energy intake because of a high palatability and energy density, direct evidence is weak. Many studies conclude that the influence of fat on energy balance is independent of energy intake. However, the conclusion was based on epidemiological observations and not the result of intervention studies.

In one study, the effect of dietary fat on energy balance was assessed with a dietary intervention (Westerterp et al., 1996). The study was part of a multi-centre study on the long-term health effects of realistic consumption of reduced-fat products. In a 6-month parallel study, free-living non-obese volunteers received either reduced-fat or full-fat products and body composition was measured before and after 6 months. Simultaneous measurements of energy and macronutrient intakes allowed analysis of the effect of dietary fat on body fat under normal living conditions.

A total of 220 subjects completed the intervention. Twenty-one subjects, 12 women and nine men, gave up for various reasons including disappointment on being assigned to the full-fat group. They did not differ in entry characteristics from those who completed the study. The diet intervention caused on average a change in fat intake and body fat mass in subjects of the reduced-fat group of -5 ± 29 g/day ($P < 0.05$) and -0.1 ± 2.1 kg (not significant), respectively, and of $+23 \pm 31$ g/day ($P < 0.0001$) and $+0.5 \pm 2.3$ kg ($P < 0.05$) in subjects of the full-fat group. Figure 4.5 shows the change in body mass for a subgroup of subjects where measurements covered a full year from June to June, including the diet intervention from August to February. The change in fat content of the diet was positively related to a change in energy intake, the latter explaining 5% of the variation in the change in body fat mass. Subjects changing the fat content of the diet showed a consequent change in body fat mass only when energy intake changed as well.

It is often suggested that the influence of fat on energy balance is independent of energy intake. The study clearly showed that the fat content of the diet had an effect on body fat as a function of the effect of dietary fat on energy intake. Subjects changing the fat content of the diet showed a consequent change in body fat mass only when energy intake changed as well. When subjects, without

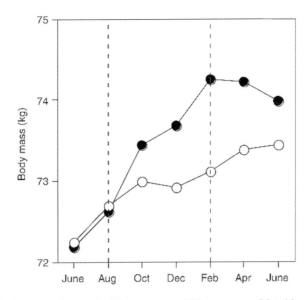

Fig. 4.5. Body mass change in 36 women and 33 men, age 36 ± 11 years (range 19–55 years) and body mass index 24 ± 2 kg/m² (range 21–30 kg/m²), equally distributed over a group consuming reduced-fat products (○) and a group consuming full-fat products (●) from August to February.

the intention to reduce energy intake, limit fat intake by switching from *ad libitum* consumption of full-fat products to reduced-fat products, body weight gain is prevented (Fig. 4.5). Thus, consumption of reduced-fat products is effective for weight maintenance. However, *ad libitum* consumption of reduced-fat products is not effective for the induction of weight loss in overweight or obese subjects.

Discussion

The regulation of body weight is thought to be primarily through energy intake. However, it is impossible to measure energy intake with sufficient accuracy to get confirmation of this point. Acheson *et al.* (1980) evaluated three methods of determining individual food intake: dietary record, dietary recall and the double portion technique with bomb calorimetry. Twelve subjects, all males spending a year on an Antarctic base, participated in the study. The period of investigation on different individuals varied between 6 and 12 months. The tedious job of weighing and recording of food intake and collecting of duplicate food samples requires a high degree of motivation but, in the confined area of a resident base camp, the subject is easier to encourage. During the study, the food intake of each subject was determined for at least 1 week of each month. During that week the subjects weighed and recorded all food consumed. Once during this week the subjects were asked to write down everything they could remember eating during the previous 24 h. The dietary record method and the use of food composition tables underestimated energy intake by a mean of 7% compared with analysis of duplicate meals by bomb calorimetry. Errors of over 20% were found in energy intake determined with dietary recall. In 62 out of 68 occasions the recall underestimated the real food consumption. The authors suggested that the discrepancy might have been smaller if the subjects had been interviewed by a skilled and persistent interviewer. Errors of over 20% are unacceptable in an energy balance study. A way to improve the recall procedure is the cross-check. A trained interviewer asks about the food eaten in the recent past and cross-checks this information against data on food purchases. With a skilled interviewer and a cooperative subject one assumes the standard deviation of the estimate to be 10% but the error is probably greater. The best an interviewer can do is to find out what people think they eat and this is often far from reality. Garrow (1981) concludes that, however intensively the eating habits of people may be studied, it is impossible to predict their energy intake over a period of a week or longer with accuracy much better than 10%.

For the study of food intake regulation in relation to the maintenance of energy balance, an accuracy of 10% is far beyond the requirements. This can be illustrated with a realistic example from daily life. Somebody adopts the habit of drinking daily one glass of beer. The question is whether the beer consumption displaces or supplements daily energy intake, assuming daily energy expenditure remains the same. The energy value of one glass of beer is 370 kJ. Over a year, the energy value adds up to 135 MJ or 4.5 kg body weight, assuming an energy equivalent of 30 MJ/kg body mass. This is a theoretical maximum. In practice, part of the supplemented energy is needed for diet-induced energy expenditure and, when the remaining energy is stored, the resulting increase in body weight results in an increase in energy expenditure for maintenance and body movement, even when the amount of body movement remains the same. Thus, the daily drinking of one glass of beer results over 1 year in an energy excess of 75 MJ or 2.5 kg body weight (Westerterp et al., 1995). The 75 MJ is only 2% of the total energy intake for an average subject with an energy turnover of 10 MJ/day, while the resulting increase in body weight is higher than is observed for an adult in the general population. The value of 2% is already five times lower than the maximum accuracy we can reach with measurements of food intake. Thus, we cannot study the effect of alcohol consumption on body weight with measurements of energy intake in daily life conditions.

Similarly, all reports on the explanation of the increased prevalence of obesity, in the USA and in many other countries, from data on reported energy intake remain speculative. An example is the paper 'Obesity in Britain: gluttony or sloth?' (Prentice and Jebb, 1995). The authors observe increasing obesity in the face of decreasing food intake and conclude that levels of energy expenditure have declined faster than energy intake, leading to an over-consumption of energy relative to a greatly reduced requirement. Since then, many studies have shown under-reporting of energy intake, especially in the obese. Thus, the secular trend in obesity might go together with an increase in under-reporting of energy intake, obscuring a relationship between 'real' energy intake and obesity.

Contrary to the suggestion of Prentice and Jebb (1995), that modern inactive life-styles are at least as important as diet in the aetiology of obesity and possibly represent the dominant factor, excessive energy intake is a more plausible explanation. Man is a discontinuous eater and a continuous metabolizer. A typical human eats three to four times a day to cover total daily energy expenditure. Thus, daily energy intake takes 30 to 60 min for 24 h energy expenditure, a behaviour selected for during evolution in an environment with a high predation pressure. Nowadays, food is often readily available and can be consumed in a safe environment. Thus, the normal eating rate at four to five times the expenditure rate during high-intensity exercise results in a high risk for overeating.

Currently, there is a trend for low-carbohydrate foods in the 'battle' against obesity. Whatever diet is consumed, it is not the diet composition but total energy intake that counts. Every 'diet rule' restricts the diet choice with a potential limiting effect on energy intake. Additional effects are, as described, through energy density and DIT. The apparent success of low-carbohydrate foods in the prevention of overweight can be linked to a reduction of food intake by the deliberate limitation of food choice and by a higher thermogenesis-induced satiety when the reduction of carbohydrate intake results in an increase in protein intake.

References

Acheson, K.J., Campbell, I.T., Edholm, O.G., Miller, D.S. and Stock, M.J. (1980) The measurement of food and energy intake in man – an evaluation of some techniques. *American Journal of Clinical Nutrition* 33, 1147–1154.

Basiotis, P.P., Welsh S.O., Cronin, F.J., Kelsay, J.L. and Mertz, W. (1987) Number of days of food intake records required to estimate individual and group nutrient intakes with defined confidence. *Journal of Nutrition* 117, 1638–1641.

Bray, G.A., Nielsen, S.J. and Popkin, B.M. (2004) Consumption of high-fructose corn syrup in beverages may play a role in the epidemic of obesity. *American Journal of Clinical Nutrition* 79, 537–543.

DiMeglio, D.P. and Mattes, R.D. (2000) Liquid versus solid carbohydrate: effects on food intake and body weight. *International Journal of Obesity and Related Metabolic Disorders* 24, 179–187.

Edholm, O.G., Fletcher, J.G., Widdowson, E.M. and McCance, R.A. (1955) The energy expenditure and food intake of individual men. *British Journal of Nutrition* 9, 286–300.

Garrow, J.S. (1981) *Treat Obesity Seriously, A Clinical Manual.* Churchill Livingstone, Edinburgh.

Goris, A.H.C. and Westerterp, K.R. (1999) Underreporting of habitual food intake is explained by undereating in highly motivated lean women. *Journal of Nutrition* 129, 878–882.

Goris, A.H.C. and Westerterp, K.R. (2000) Improved reporting of habitual food intake after confrontation with earlier results on food reporting. *British Journal of Nutrition* 83, 363–369.

Goris, A.H.C., Westerterp-Plantenga, M.S. and Westerterp, K.R. (2000) Undereating and underrecording of habitual food intake in obese men: selective underreporting of fat intake. *American Journal of Clinical Nutrition* 71,130–134.

Goris, A.H.C., Meijer, E.P. and Westerterp, K.R. (2001) Repeated measurement of habitual food intake increases under-reporting and induces selective under-reporting. *British Journal of Nutrition* 85, 629–634.

Goris, A.H.C., Vermeeren, M.A.P., Wouters, E.F.M., Schols, A.M.W.J. and Westerterp, K.R. (2003) Energy balance in depleted ambulatory patients with chronic obstructive pulmonary disease; the effect of physical activity and oral nutritional supplementation. *British Journal of Nutrition* 89, 725–729.

Greenwald, P., Sherwood, K. and McDonald, S.S. (1997) Fat, caloric intake, and obesity: lifestyle risk factors for breast cancer. *Journal of the American Dietetic Association* 97, S24–S30.

Heitmann, B., Lissner, L. and Osler, M. (2000) Do we eat less fat, or just report so? *International Journal of Obesity and Related Metabolic Disorders* 24, 435–442.

Hill, R.J. and Davies, P.S.W. (2001) The validity of self-reported energy intake as determined using the doubly labelled water technique. *British Journal of Nutrition* 85, 415–430.

Hise, M.E., Sullivan, D.K., Jacobsen, D.J., Johnson, S.L. and Donnelly, J.E. (2002) Validation of energy intake measurements determined from observer-recorded food records and recall methods compared with doubly labeled water method in overweight and obese individuals. *American Journal of Clinical Nutrition* 75, 263–267.

Johnson, L.E., Dooley, P.A. and Gleick, J.B. (1993) Oral nutritional supplement use in elderly nursing home patients. *Journal of the American Geriatrics Society* 41, 947–952.

Johnston, C.S., Day, C.S. and Swan, P.D. (2002) Postprandial thermogenesis is increase 100% on a high-protein, low-fat diet versus a high-carbohydrate, low-fat diet in healthy, young women. *Journal of the American College of Nutrition* 21, 55–61.

Kayser-Jones, J., Schell, E.S., Porter, C., Barbaccia, J.C., Steinbach, C., Bird, W.F., Redford, M. and Pengilly, K. (1998) A prospective study of the use of liquid oral dietary supplements in nursing homes. *Journal of the American Geriatrics Society* 46, 1378–1386.

Kennedy, E.T., Bowman, S.A. and Powell, R. (1999) Dietary-fat intake in the US population. *Journal of the American College of Nutrition* 18, 207–212.

Lanigan, J.A., Wells, J.C.K., Lawson, M.S. and Lucas, A. (2001) Validation of food diary method for assessment of dietary energy and macronutrient intake in infants and children aged 6–24 months. *European Journal of Clinical Nutrition* 55, 124–129.

Lissner, L., Heitmann, B.L. and Lindroos, A.K. (1998) Measuring intake in free-living human subjects: a question of bias. *Proceedings of the Nutrition Society* 57, 333–339.

Ludwig, D.S., Peterson, K.E. and Gortmaker, S.L. (2001) Relation between consumption of sugar-sweetened drinks and childhood obesity: a prospective observational analysis. *Lancet* 357, 505–508.

Norgan, N.G. and Durnin, J.V.G.A. (1980) The effect of 6 weeks of overfeeding on the body weight, body composition, and energy metabolism of young men. *American Journal of Clinical Nutrition* 33, 978–988.

Poppitt, A.D. and Prentice, A.M. (1996) Energy density and its role in the control of food intake: evidence from metabolic and community studies. *Appetite* 26, 153–174.

Prentice, A.M. and Jebb, S.A. (1995) Obesity in Britain: gluttony or sloth? *British Medical Journal* 311, 437–439.

Raben, A., Vasilaras, T.H., Moller, A.C. and Astrup, A. (2002) Sucrose compared with artificial sweeteners: different effects on *ad libitum* food intake and body weight after 10 wk of supplementation in overweight subjects. *American Journal of Clinical Nutrition* 76, 721–729.

Rose, D., Murphy, S.P., Hudes, M. and Viteri, F.E. (1995) Food energy remains constant with increasing alcohol intake. *Journal of the American Dietetic Association* 95, 698–700.

Rumpler, W.V., Rhodes, D.G., Baer, D.J., Conway, J.M. and Seale, J.L. (1996) Energy value of moderate alcohol consumption by humans. *American Journal of Clinical Nutrition* 64, 108–114.

Sjödin, A.M., Andersson, A.B., Högberg, J.M. and Westerterp, K.R. (1994) Energy balance in cross country skiers: a study using doubly labeled water and dietary record. *Medicine and Science in Sports and Exercise* 26, 720–724.

Stallings, V., Zemel, B., Davies, J., Cronk, C. and Charney, E. (1996) Energy expenditure of children and adolescents with severe disabilities: a cerebral palsy model. *American Journal of Clinical Nutrition* 64, 627–634.

Tappy, L. (1996) Thermic effect of food and sympathetic nervous system activity in humans. *Reproduction, Nutrition, Development* 36, 391–397.

Tomoyasu, N., Toth, M. and Poehlman, E. (2000) Misreporting of total energy intake in older African Americans. *International Journal of Obesity and Related Metabolic Disorders* 24, 20–26.

Trabulsi, J. and Schoeller, D.A. (2001) Evaluation of dietary assessment instruments against doubly labeled water, a biomarker of habitual energy intake. *American Journal of Physiology, Endocrinology and Metabolism* 281, E891–E899.

Webb, P. and Annis, J.F. (1983) Adaptation to overeating in lean and overweight men and women. *Human Nutrition: Clinical Nutrition* 37C, 117–131.

Westerterp, K.R. (2001) Limits to sustainable human metabolic rate. *Journal of Experimental Biology* 204, 3183–3187.

Westerterp, K.R., Meijer, G.A.L., Janssen, E.M.E., Saris, W.H.M. and Ten Hoor, F. (1992) Long term effect of physical activity on energy balance and body composition. *British Journal of Nutrition* 68, 21–30.

Westerterp, K.R., Donkers, J., Fredrix, E.W.H.M. and Boekhoudt, P. (1995) Energy intake, physical activity and body weight; a simulation model. *British Journal of Nutrition* 73, 337–347.

Westerterp, K.R., Verboeket-van de Venne, W.P.H.G., Westerterp-Plantenga, M.S., Velthuis-te Wierik, E.J.M., De Graaf, C. and Weststrate, J.A. (1996) Dietary fat and body fat: an intervention study. *International Journal of Obesity and Related Metabolic Disorders* 20, 1022–1026.

Westerterp, K.R., Meijer, E.P., Goris, A.H.C. and Kester, A.D.M. (2004) Alcohol energy intake and physical activity in older adults. *British Journal of Nutrition* 91, 149–152.

Westerterp-Plantenga, M.S. (2003) The significance of protein in food intake and body weight regulation. *Current Opinion in Clinical Nutrition and Metabolic Care* 6, 635–638.

Westerterp-Plantenga, M.S. and Verwegen, C.R.T. (1999) The appetizing effect of an alcohol aperitif in overweight normal weight humans. *American Journal of Clinical Nutrition* 69, 205–212.

Westerterp-Plantenga, M.S., Rolland, V., Wilson, S.A.J. and Westerterp, K.R. (1999) Satiety related to 24 h diet-induced thermogenesis during high protein/carbohydrate vs high fat diets measured in a respiration chamber. *European Journal of Clinical Nutrition* 53, 495–502.

This page intentionally left blank

5   Food Neophobia in Humans

PATRICIA PLINER AND SARAH-JEANNE SALVY

Department of Psychology, University of Toronto at Mississauga, 3359 Mississauga Road, Mississauga, Ontario L5L 1C6, Canada

Introduction

Food neophobia, a reluctance to ingest novel foods, is a characteristic of omnivorous animals, including humans. Such organisms, exposed to the hazards of an environment in which many food sources may be toxic, approach novel foods with caution, eschewing them in favour of familiar foods whenever possible. It has been suggested that food neophobia is a conservative force, operating to keep the organism's feeding behaviour 'locked in on a safe track' by preventing its taste preferences from straying from familiar foods known to be harmless (Schulze and Watson, 1995, p. 230).

Bases for rejection of foods

Rozin and Fallon's (1980; Fallon and Rozin, 1983) taxonomy of the bases for rejection of foods provides a useful starting point for the discussion of the rejection of novel foods by humans. These researchers have proposed that in humans there are three main bases for rejection of a food: (i) dislike of its sensory characteristics; (ii) danger, a fear of negative consequences of eating it; and (iii) disgust, arising from the idea of the food's nature or origin. While Rozin and Fallon focused on familiar foods, there is evidence for the relevance of each of these factors as a basis for rejection of novel foods as well.

In the case of dislike, Pliner *et al.* (1993) found that participants expected novel foods to be less palatable than familiar ones, and beliefs about their palatability predicted willingness to taste them. Danger, as a motivation for rejecting a novel food, is related to 'learned safety', one of the classic notions in the literature on food selection in animals (Kalat and Rozin, 1973). According to this idea, only after a number of very limited exposures to a novel food in the absence of negative consequences does the animal learn the food is safe and ingest significant quantities of it. Pliner *et al.* (1993) found that participants rated novel foods presented to them in the laboratory as slightly more dangerous than their familiar counterparts, and these ratings of dangerousness predicted willingness to taste them. Rozin *et al.* (1993) suggested that disgust might serve to counter individuals' tendencies to approach novel foods, after finding a negative correlation between their Disgust Scale (Haidt *et al.*, 1994) and the Sensation Seeking Scale (Zuckerman, 1979), which assesses preferences for novel and exciting stimuli. Similarly, Pliner (unpublished data) found a strong positive correlation between scores on the Food Neophobia Scale, a measure of the trait of food neophobia, and the Disgust Scale.

Factors affecting food neophobia

While humans generally reject novel foods, there are large situational differences in the extent to which such neophobic behaviour occurs. We describe these shortly. In addition, there are also large individual differences in the extent of food neophobia. Thus, it is sometimes useful to characterize food neophobia as a personality trait, a continuum along which people can be located in terms of their stable propensity to approach or avoid novel foods. In this chapter we will sometimes be discussing food neophobia as a behaviour involving rejection of a novel food or foods in a particular situation; at other times we will be referring to food neophobia as a personality characteristic involving a relative preference for familiar over novel foods that is stable over time and consistent across situations.

Measuring food neophobia

In keeping with the distinction between food neophobic behaviour displayed at a particular time in a particular situation and the trait of food neophobia, we describe measures of both – the former in this section and the latter in a later section of the chapter. In a typical study assessing neophobic behaviour, participants see an array of foods, some novel and some familiar, and are asked to indicate their degree of willingness to taste each later in the session, with the clear implication that their responses will determine which foods they will actually taste. Neophobia is defined in terms of the average willingness to taste the novel foods, usually divided by the average willingness to taste the familiar foods, so as to take into account willingness to accept any food at all at that time and in that situation. Low scores on this 'behaviouroid' measure are indicative of high neophobia. Some investigators have defined behavioural neophobia as reported 'willingness to eat more of' a particular novel food or in terms of ratings of liking for the taste, odour or even appearance of a novel food.

Situational Factors Affecting Food Neophobia

Information

Indirect information about taste and beneficiality

Rozin (1988) has argued that foods that are accepted are usually those that (are expected to) taste good and those that are seen to be beneficial. It will be noted that these characteristics of food describe the opposites of two of the bases for rejection described earlier – namely dislike and danger. It might, therefore, be expected that any situational factor that induces the expectation of their opposite poles – good taste or beneficial consequences – might reduce neophobia. In several studies, participants have been presented with information intended to promote these expectations, finding that good taste information does increase willingness (Tuorila *et al.*, 1994; Pelchat and Pliner, 1995; McFarlane and Pliner, 1997; Martins *et al.*, 1997). For example, students in one of Pelchat and Pliner's (1995) studies encountered a novel food in a cafeteria line; for some, the food was accompanied by a sign reading '9 out of 10 students said "tastes great!"' The latter were more likely to sample a portion of the food than were appropriate controls. The evidence concerning the efficacy of inducing anticipation of beneficial consequences as a means for eliminating rejection of novel foods is more complicated. Pelchat and Pliner (1995) included a condition in which the novel food was accompanied by a sign saying 'a good source of iron' and found no increase in the proportion of students accepting the food. Indeed, two studies found that beneficial consequences information actually decreased the likelihood of trying novel foods (Woodward, 1945; Koster *et al.*, 1987). However, information about the beneficial consequences of a food does seem to increase willingness to eat a novel food for individuals for whom this information is important or relevant (McFarlane and Pliner, 1997) or in a context where the new food is believed to be readily available (Martins *et al.*, 1997). To complicate matters further, whereas providing information seems effective for some kinds of foods, it appears to be relatively ineffective for reducing rejections mediated by strong emotional reactions such as disgust. Martins *et al.* (1997) found that neither taste information nor beneficial consequences information increased participants' willingness to taste novel animal foods.

Direct information about taste and beneficiality

Another means of providing information about a novel food relies on the individual's own experience. Here we refer to the literature on the 'mere exposure' effect (Zajonc, 1968). Birch and her colleagues (Birch and Marlin, 1982; Birch *et al.*, 1987) gave young children varying amounts of exposure to novel cheeses or fruits. After the exposure phase, the children were shown all possible pairs of foods and asked to choose the one they wanted to 'eat more of' or 'liked the best'. There was a positive effect of number of exposures on choice and liking. These results are typically interpreted in terms of 'learned safety'; with repeated exposures individuals learn that the food is 'safe' and does not produce negative gastrointestinal consequences. Other investigators, testing both infant and adult participants, have obtained similar results (Pliner, 1982; Zellner et al., 1983; Birch et al., 1998).

Generalization of direct information

Aside from the safety argument described above, individuals anticipate that novel foods will have an unpleasant taste. Exposure to palatable novel foods might help them realize that their negative expectations regarding novel foods are unfounded. That is, positive experiences with novel foods might generalize to other novel foods and decrease neophobia in a more general and enduring manner. Sullivan and Birch (1990) found that exposure affected children's preferences only for the specific food items exposed. However, a similar study by Pliner et al. (1993) obtained very different results. After an exposure phase in which they tasted either a set of good-tasting novel foods or a similar set of familiar foods, adult participants chose from a set of different foods, both familiar and novel, which ones they would taste later. Participants pre-exposed to good-tasting novel foods chose more novel items than did the familiar-food controls. In a subsequent study, Loewen and Pliner (1999) provided 7- to 9-year-old and 10- to 12-year-old children with taste exposure to good-tasting familiar, good-tasting novel or bad-tasting novel foods. For older children, exposure to the novel–good foods increased willingness to taste a different set of novel foods in comparison to the familiar–good control, while exposure to the novel–bad foods had no effect. For younger children, exposure to both novel–good and novel–bad foods decreased willingness to taste novel foods. Thus, to some extent, creating positive experiences with novel tastes seems to generalize to willingness to taste other novel foods.

Social influence

In several studies, social influence had strong effects on acceptance of and liking for foods; the children in these studies followed the lead of a 'model', liking and choosing the same foods (Duncker, 1938; Marinho, 1940; Birch, 1980a). These findings raise the question of whether social influence would also affect reactions to novel foods; specifically, if exposure to a model who accepts novel foods would increase an observer's acceptance of such foods. In a study by Harper and Sanders (1975), children were more likely to accept a novel food if they saw their mothers eat it first. Hendy (2002) examined the effect of trained peer models on pre-school children's willingness to accept novel foods, finding that only the girls were effective models. Hendy and Raudenbush (2000) showed that teachers could be effective models for pre-school children but only if they modelled 'enthusiastically', making favourable comments about the novel foods, and not if they modelled silently. Hobden and Pliner (1995) found that adult participants were influenced by exposure to a neophilic model, although the reduced neophobia did not generalize to non-modelled foods.

Type of food

Several studies have shown that individuals are more likely to reject novel foods of animal origin than those not of animal origin (Pliner and Pelchat, 1991; Pliner, 1994; Martins *et al.*, 1997). Further, participants' reactions to the novel animal foods resembled reactions to prototypical disgusting foods identified by Fallon and Rozin (1983) to a greater extent than did their reactions to the non-animal foods. Interestingly, the finding of a greater rejection of novel animal (versus non-animal) foods did not replicate in a group of children ranging in age from 5 to 11 years (Pliner, 1994). Since a study by Fallon *et al.* (1984) showed that disgust, as a category of rejection, had not fully achieved adult levels even in children aged 8 to 12 years, this finding is consistent with the notion that rejection of novel animal foods is mediated by disgust.

Studies on neophobia have traditionally focused on 'ethnic' foods, novel to one culture but familiar in others. In addition to ethnic cuisines, Tuorila (2001) identified four other kinds of novel foods: functional foods, genetically modified products, nutritionally modified foods and organic foods. The bases of rejection of these other 'kinds' of novel foods might be different from those related to unwillingness to eat ethnic foods. Although much more experimental research is needed, available data support this proposition. For instance, there is evidence suggesting that willingness to try ethnic novel foods is related to scores obtained on the Food Neophobia Scale (FNS), to be discussed later. However, Tuorila and her colleagues (Tuorila *et al.*, 2001) found little relationship between willingness to try functional foods and scores on the FNS, while Hursti and Magnusson (2002) found that attitudes towards organic and genetically modified foods were not related to FNS scores. Also, Backstrom *et al.* (2003) found that, although subjects in their study were reluctant to consume all kinds of novel foods, organic and ethnic foods were described in positive terms while biotechnological foods were associated with negative adjectives and metaphors (see also Magnusson and Koivisto-Hursti, 2002; Cardello, 2003; Koivisto Hursti and Magnusson, 2003 for data pertaining to negative attitudes towards food processing technologies). Furthermore, it is also the case that willingness to try novel ethnic foods seems to show a different relationship with age than does willingness to try the other kinds of novel foods. While many studies show that people become more willing to try novel ethnic foods as they get older (e.g. McFarlane and Pliner, 1997), people seem to become more reluctant to eat the other kinds of novel foods as they get older (de Jong *et al.*, 2002; Hursti and Magnusson, 2002). Given these differences, it might be expected that different kinds of novel foods might be differentially susceptible to the effects of different situational variables; however, there are no data available.

Amount of novelty in the situation

In a classic study, Archer and Sjoden (1979) found that rats were much more likely to accept a novel food when the surrounding environment was relatively familiar than when there were several novel cues present. Harper and Sanders

(1975) found that young children were more likely to accept a novel food from their mothers than from an unfamiliar experimenter. Rozin and Rozin's (1981) account of the functions of flavour principles, the characteristic seasonings used in various cuisines (Rozin, E., 1973), suggests that one such function is to facilitate the introduction of novel staple foods into a culture by adding sufficient familiarity to decrease the neophobia ordinarily produced by a new food. Stallberg-White and Pliner (1999; Pliner and Stallberg-White, 2000), examining flavour principles at the individual level, predicted and found that adding a familiar flavour to novel foods increased the willingness of both adults and children to taste them.

Arousal

Both the animal and the human literatures indicate that strong arousal produces a decrement in novelty preference. Making predictions from optimal level of arousal theories (e.g. Revelle et al., 1987), Pliner and colleagues (Pliner and Melo, 1997; Pliner and Loewen, 2002) found a negative relationship between willingness to taste novel foods and manipulated arousal. In addition, Pliner and Melo (1997) found that manipulated arousal interacted with individual differences in sensation seeking, often considered to be a measure of optimum level of arousal. Pliner et al. (1995) manipulated both fear and hunger and assessed willingness to try novel foods. In the condition in which arousal was presumably highest (high fear–high hunger), participants showed the greatest reluctance to try the novel foods. The findings in the previous section showing that willingness to try novel foods is greatest in situations that are otherwise relatively familiar are compatible with the arousal findings, if one simply assumes that arousal in a familiar situation is likely to be low (in comparison to a situation in which there is a large amount of novelty).

Individual Differences in Food Neophobia

Measures of individual differences

Although neophobia is a general characteristic of omnivores, there are clearly individual differences in the extent of it. To measure such individual differences, Pliner and Hobden (1992) developed the FNS (Food Neophobia Scale), a ten-item questionnaire consisting of such face valid items as 'I don't trust new foods'. Another approach was taken by Frank and his colleagues (Frank and van der Klaauw, 1994; Raudenbush et al., 1998), on whose revised Food Attitude Scale (FAS-R) participants' rated willingness to taste those foods on a presented list that they have never tried is the measure of food neophobia. To assess food neophobia in children, Loewen and Pliner (2000) developed the Food Situations Questionnaire (FSQ), on which children rate their feelings about trying particular novel foods in particular situations.

All three measures have been extensively validated. The FNS predicts choice of and rated willingness to eat novel foods both in and out of the laboratory (Pliner and Hobden, 1992; McFarlane and Pliner, 1997; Martins *et al.*, 1997; Raudenbush *et al.*, 1998; Raudenbush and Frank, 1999; Flight *et al.*, 2003), familiarity and experience with relatively exotic foods and 'foreign' cuisines (Pliner and Hobden, 1992; Flight *et al.*, 2003), willingness to explore food odours about which little information has been provided (Raudenbush *et al.*, 1998) and the serving of relatively uncommon foods at family mealtime (Koivisto and Sjoden, 1996; Hursti and Sjoden, 1997). Scores on the FAS/FAS-R are related to number of novel foods rejected on a questionnaire, the number of foods participants report having tried in the past, and a set of face valid questions querying reactions to novel foods (Frank and van der Klaauw, 1994; Raudenbush *et al.*, 1998). In addition, the FNS and the FAS-R are highly correlated with each other ($r = 0.73$; Raudenbush *et al.*, 1998). The FSQ predicts children's willingness to taste unfamiliar foods in the laboratory (Loewen and Pliner, 2000) and is significantly related to parents' ratings of their children's neophobia on the FNS.

Correlates of individual differences in food neophobia

Reactions to familiar and novel foods

Both Pliner's group and Frank's group have provided evidence suggesting that food neophobia and finickiness or pickiness (a tendency to reject familiar foods; Potts and Wardle, 1998) are distinct, although related, constructs. Pelchat and Pliner (1986) found that the two emerged as separate factors in mothers' reports of their children's eating behaviour. Kauer, Pelchat and Rozin (unpublished data) found that, although pickiness and neophobia items loaded on the same factor, when this factor was itself factor-analysed, the finickiness and neophobia items separated. In a study by Galloway *et al.* (2003) of 7-year-old girls, food neophobia was only modestly related to pickiness and had different predictors. Raudenbush *et al.* (1995) factor-analysed a set of questions pertaining to food and eating, obtaining three distinct factors, one consisting of items describing reactions to novel foods, labelled neophobia (e.g. 'I enjoy trying unusual foods') and another describing negative reactions to foods in general, labelled finickiness (e.g. 'I find many foods distasteful'). In a regression analysis, using scores on the neophobia and finickiness factors to predict the number of 'won't try' responses on the FAS (their original neophobia measure), they found the neophobia but not the finickiness factor to be a significant predictor. In a similar regression analysis, this time using the two factor scores to predict numbers of food likes and dislikes among familiar foods on the FAS, they found the finickiness but not the neophobia score to be a significant predictor. Taken together, these results strongly suggest that willingness to try novel foods (neophobia) and dislike for many familiar foods (finickiness) are distinct responses.

In support of this distinction, both groups have found that their measures of neophobia are related to willingness to taste novel foods but do not predict willingness to taste familiar foods or that the relationship between the neophobia measures and willingness is much stronger for novel than for familiar foods. Raudenbush and Frank (1999) carefully ensured that the novel and familiar foods they offered were equally familiar to high and to low scorers on the FNS, and found that the groups differed only in their willingness to taste the novel foods. In order to examine the relationships between food neophobia as measured by the FNS and various reactions to food, Pliner (unpublished data) computed correlations between FNS scores and these variables obtained in the studies from her laboratory and then averaged them, weighting each correlation by the number of subjects on which it was based. The average correlation between FNS scores and behaviouroid measures of willingness to try novel foods was –0.41, while the analogous correlation for familiar foods was only –0.09. These data can be seen in Table 5.1. Furthermore, neophobia is not only related to willingness to try novel foods, but also to expected liking for novel foods (Pliner and Hobden, 1992; Tuorila et al., 1994, 1998; Raudenbush and Frank, 1999). For studies from the Pliner laboratory, the average correlation between FNS scores and expected liking for novel foods was –0.34, while the analogous correlation for familiar foods was only –0.01. Further, several studies have found no relationship between scores on food neophobia measures and ratings of liking for familiar foods, actually tasted and/or rated from memory (Pliner and Hobden, 1992; Pliner and Loewen, 1997; Pliner et al., 1998; Potts and Wardle, 1998 [Study 2]; Raudenbush et al., 1998; but see Potts and Wardle, 1998, Study 1; Arvola et al., 1999). Again, examining correlations from several studies involving many participants, Pliner found an average correlation of –0.02 between FNS scores and liking for familiar foods actually tasted. However, the data relating food neophobia and liking for novel foods actually tasted are not straightforward. Several studies have demonstrated no relationship between the two (Pliner and Hobden, 1992), while others have demonstrated substantial relationships between them (Pliner and Loewen, 1997; Pliner et al., 1998). Once again averaging correlations from several studies, Pliner found that FNS scores were moderately correlated with liking for novel foods (mean $r = –0.22$). In summary, we believe that the pattern of relationships warrants treating neophobia and finickiness as separate constructs. Food neophobia, as measured by the FNS and other measures of neophobia, is strongly related to individuals' reactions to novel foods but has little to do with their reactions to familiar foods.

Table 5.1. Mean correlations between scores on the Food Neophobia Scale and reactions to novel and familiar foods. Note: The first number in parentheses in each cell refers to the number of correlations averaged to produce the mean; the second refers to the total number of participants involved in all the correlations averaged.

Type of food	Measure		
	Willingness to try	Expected liking	Actual liking
Novel	–0.41 (11, 1322)	–0.37 (5, 318)	–0.22 (7, 556)
Familiar	–0.09 (11, 1322)	–0.01 (3, 269)	–0.02 (10, 567)

Other food- and eating-related correlates of food neophobia

Raudenbush *et al.* (1995) examined several other potential food- and eating-related correlates of food neophobia, finding a modest positive correlation between FAS 'won't try' responses and scores on the Eating Attitudes Test, a measure of the symptoms of anorexia nervosa (Garner and Garfinkel, 1979), but no correlation between the FAS and scores on the Eating Disorder Inventory, a multidimensional eating disorder inventory (Garner *et al.*, 1983), or scores on the Restraint Scale, a measure of dieting (Herman *et al.*, 1978). In a series of interesting studies, Frank's group has also examined the relation between food neophobia (as measured by the FAS/FAS-R and the FNS) and hedonic evaluations of olfactory stimuli. They found that FAS scores are negatively correlated with rated pleasantness of the odours of familiar but concealed foods (Raudenbush *et al.*, 1995) and that FNS scores are negatively correlated with rated pleasantness of odorant solutions (Raudenbush *et al.*, 1998).

Sensation seeking

A number of studies have examined the relationship between food neophobia and the Sensation Seeking Scale, a measure of general willingness/unwillingness to approach novel, exciting and/or complex stimuli (Zuckerman, 1979). Several studies have shown that one or more of its subscales are negatively related to trait food neophobia measures (Pliner and Hobden, 1992; Walsh, 1993; Raudenbush *et al.*, 1995; Loewen and Pliner, 2000), to reported food attitudes (Terasaki and Imada, 1988) and to behavioural measures of neophobia (Otis, 1984). Food neophobia has also been shown to be related to a more general reluctance to approach novel stimuli, including unfamiliar people, places and activities (Pliner and Hobden, 1992; Raudenbush *et al.*, 1995).

Gender differences

Gender differences in food neophobia might be expected, given previous research that has demonstrated differences between males and females on such related variables as taste preferences (e.g. Desor *et al.*, 1975), food preferences (e.g. Logue and Smith, 1986) and food aversions (e.g. Babayan *et al.*, 1966). However, most research with the FNS, the FAS and the FSQ has produced no differences (Pliner and Hobden, 1992; Koivisto and Sjoden, 1996; Tuorila *et al.*, 1998; Meiselman *et al.*, 1999; Loewen and Pliner, 2000). When actual neophobic behaviour, as opposed to self-reported usual behaviour, is the measure, gender differences also fail to appear (Pliner, 1994; McFarlane and Pliner, 1997). There are some exceptions, however. Using the FAS, Frank and van der Klaauw (1994) found that women reported more 'won't try' responses than men, and Alley and Burroughs (1991) found that men were more likely than women to report seeking unusual and new foods (see also Magnusson and Koivisto-Hursti, 2002; Backstrom *et al.*, 2003; Cardello, 2003 for gender differences in attitudes towards other kinds of novel foods). In contrast, in two large Scandinavian samples, Hursti and Sjoden (1997) and Tuorila *et al.* (2001) found higher FNS scores in men than in women.

Age differences

The data on age differences in food neophobia are difficult to describe in any simple way. The various studies have used vastly different age ranges and age categories, different methods of testing for differences, and different measures of neophobia. When one examines actual neophobic behaviour, it appears that neophobia declines with age. Younger children accept fewer novel foods than older ones (Pliner and Loewen, 1997; Loewen and Pliner, 2000); junior high school students accept fewer novel foods than senior high school students (Pelchat and Pliner, 1995); and younger adults accept fewer novel foods than older adults (Otis, 1984; McFarlane and Pliner, 1997; Pelchat, 2000). There is, however, one clear exception; Harper and Sanders (1975) found that infants aged 1.5 years were more likely to accept a novel food than were children aged 3.5 years. This exception is interesting in light of Cashdan's (1994) hypothesis that there is a critical period for learning which foods are edible and that this period should occur during early childhood while the child is still protected by the parents. Accordingly, she predicted that food neophobia should be lowest in children younger than 24 months. Confirming this prediction, in a retrospective survey of parents of 1- to 10-year-old children she found that the children were most accepting of novel foods at age 2 years, with neophobia increasing sharply from 2 to 4 years of age. However, consistent with the data reported earlier, neophobia decreased from age 4 to 10 years.

When one examines the relationship between age and scores on various trait measures of food neophobia, there are many similar findings. In five student samples with age ranges of at least 10 years, FNS scores showed modest negative correlations with age (Pliner and Hobden, 1992); a group of children had higher FNS scores than their parents (Koivisto and Sjoden, 1996; Hursti and Sjoden, 1997); younger children had higher scores than older ones (Koivisto and Sjoden, 1996; Hursti and Sjoden, 1997; Pliner and Loewen, 2002); and in a longitudinal study mothers rated their children's willingness to eat novel foods as lower at 34 months than at 84 months (Carruth and Skinner, 2000). However, in several studies there were no differences between 7- to 9- and 10- to 12-year-olds (Pliner, 1994; Loewen and Pliner, 2000). In the most important exception to the general decline in food neophobia scores with age, Tuorila et al. (2001) tested a sample of Finns ranging in age from 16 to 80 years. Scores increased slightly but steadily until age 65 and then increased sharply in the 66–80 years age group. Although this finding is something of an outlier, it is difficult to dismiss, given that the sample upon which it is based is both large and representative.

Demographic variables

The relationships between food neophobia and several other demographic variables have been examined. In two studies, individuals living in rural areas were more neophobic than their more urban counterparts (Tuorila et al., 2001; Flight et al., 2003). In one of these studies (Tuorila et al., 2001) education was negatively related to FNS scores, while in the other a measure of socioeconomic status, based on education, was unrelated to food neophobia scores (Flight *et al.*, 2003).

Family Resemblance in Food Neophobia

Parents play an important role in the development of children's food habits. Several studies have examined family resemblance in terms of food preferences (e.g. Birch, 1980b; Pliner, 1983; Rozin *et al.*, 1984; Pliner and Pelchat, 1986; Logue *et al.*, 1988). Overall, these studies have shown only modest relationships between parents and their children with respect to food preferences, although similarities between parents and their children seem to increase as children get older (Birch, 1980b; Logue *et al.*, 1988). Resemblance appears to be stronger between siblings than between children and their parents (Pliner and Pelchat, 1986; Rozin and Millman, 1987). With regard to food neophobia, Pliner (1994) found a significant but modest relationship ($r = 0.31$) in neophobia scores between children and their mothers (see also Koivisto and Sjoden, 1996). Hursti and Sjoden (1997) found similar results using parental ratings of child food neophobia and an *ad hoc* food frequency questionnaire. Galloway *et al.* (2003) found that mothers' but not fathers' FNS scores were related to a trait measure of food neophobia in their daughters.

Mechanisms underlying food neophobia

Wong (1995) notes that, 'there have not been many systematic attempts to uncover the mechanisms of food neophobia'. One possibility is suggested by animal research on the effects of early pre-exposure to novelty in various modalities on subsequent reactions to novelty. Some of the research shows that pre-exposure to novel foods increases subsequent acceptance of different novel foods (Capretta *et al.*, 1975; Braveman, 1978). Another set of studies demonstrates that early pre-exposure to novel environmental stimuli (including handling) increases the willingness of adult rats to explore novel environments (e.g. Levine *et al.*, 1967; Weinberg *et al.*, 1978). Interestingly, there are also cross-modality effects. Weinberg *et al.* (1978) found that early handling increases consumption of a novel food by adults, and Braveman (1978) found that pre-exposure to novel flavours increases exploration of a novel environment by adults. Minor *et al.* (1994) found that individual differences in open field exploration predicted neophobic responses to a novel saccharine solution. Braveman (1978) postulated that these non-specific effects of pre-exposure on neophobia may be mediated by reduced emotional responsivity. In other words, pre-exposure to varied stimuli, including food stimuli, produces animals that are less emotionally responsive, and these animals are less neophobic in many domains, including the food domain.

Some of the data on individual differences in humans are consistent with these findings and theorizing. First of all, there is evidence for the same kind of cross-modal seeking or avoidance of novel stimuli as Minor *et al.* (1994) observed.

Raudenbush and Frank (1999) reported significant correlations between measures of willingness to try novel foods and willingness to engage in novel activities, while Pliner and Hobden (1992) reported correlations between scores on the FNS and scores on the General Neophobia Scale, a measure of willingness to approach novel people and situations. As noted earlier, several studies have shown that one or more of the subscales of the Sensation Seeking Scale (Zuckerman, 1979), a measure of willingness/unwillingness to approach novel, exciting and/or complex stimuli, are negatively related to food neophobia measures (Pliner and Hobden, 1992; Walsh, 1993; Raudenbush et al., 1995).

With respect to the role of anxiety, Pliner and Hobden (1992) reported several studies in which they obtained small but significant relationships between the FNS and trait anxiety (State–Trait Anxiety Inventory – Trait; Spielberger et al., 1970) in adults. Pliner and Loewen (1997), examining temperament in children, found that emotionality was significantly related to food neophobia. Galloway et al. (2003) found a highly significant correlation between a trait measure of food neophobia and anxiety. It should be noted, however, that such a relationship has failed to materialize in some studies (Raudenbush et al., 1995; Potts and Wardle, 1998).

Consistent with a general anxiety-mediation notion is the common finding that anxiolytic drugs, such as chlordiazepoxide, increase the intake of novel foods in rats (e.g. Cooper et al., 1981; Hodges et al., 1981; Britton et al., 1982). Indeed, degree of food neophobia is often used as a screen to assess the effects of benzodiazepine-like drugs (Poschel, 1971). The importance of anxiety as a mediator of food neophobia in humans can also be seen in the results of studies that involve acute manipulations of anxiety and assess state (as opposed to trait) neophobia. Pliner et al. (1995) found that increasing anxiety, by means conceptually unrelated to eating or food, increased food neophobic behaviour. In another study (Pliner et al., 1993) participants above the median in state anxiety were willing to taste fewer novel foods than their counterparts below the median. Thus, converging evidence points to a role for anxiety mediation in food neophobia.

Clinical Implications of Food Neophobia

Effects on health

Given that rejection of novel foods is likely to decrease diet breadth, it might be expected that there would be nutritional consequences of food neophobia. Galloway et al. (2003) found that food neophobia was negatively related to consumption of vegetables in 7-year-old girls. Similarly, Cooke et al. (2004) found that food neophobia was negatively related to the consumption of fruit and vegetables in pre-school children. Falciglia et al. (2000) compared three groups of children (neophobic, neophilic and average) and found that those in the first group were less likely to meet the recommended value for vitamin E than the others. In addition, an overall Healthy Eating Index score was significantly lower for the neophobic group, who also had a higher intake of saturated fat and less food variety than children in the other two groups.

Treatment of food neophobia

Because food neophobia, at least in extreme cases, might compromise health, devising means of reducing it would clearly be desirable. In a sense, the previous section on situational differences in food neophobia suggests possible means for interventions. That is, it would be expected that such situational manipulations as providing information, exposure to novel foods, presentation of novel foods in familiar contexts, and so on, might lead to a general reduction in neophobic behaviours. In more clinical settings, successful treatments of food neophobia in children (Singer *et al.*, 1992) and adults (Marcontell *et al.*, 2003) have taken the term 'neophobia' literally and adopted a phobic conceptualization of unwillingness to eat novel foods. Accordingly, treatments have involved a combination of techniques traditionally used with anxiety-related disorders, including relaxation training, development of a 'feared foods' hierarchy, systematic desensitization, cognitive restructuring and modelling, as well as nutritional counselling, education and *in vivo* exposure to feared foods. The idea is to gradually expose the individual to novel foods, while modelling appropriate eating behaviour, challenging negative cognitions (i.e. negative expectations regarding taste, texture or smell) and preventing avoidance. Generalization of reduction in neophobic behaviour is achieved by assigning homework and moving the sessions from the clinic to restaurants. Blissett and Harris (2002) added a paradoxical intervention to increase acceptance of novel foods with a child suffering from feeding problems. Parents were advised to introduce new foods as 'special', 'restricted' or 'only for grown-ups'.

Conclusion

Although food neophobia has clearly been adaptive for our species, it could be argued that culture has taken over much of the protective function of food neophobia. Except in rare circumstances, culture prevents encounters with dangerous ingestibles by removing them from the immediate environment and/or by labelling them as unsafe. In a sense, then, food neophobia may have outlived its usefulness. Indeed, as we have shown, it may be that the relatively neophobic among us might be at some nutritional risk. More research is clearly warranted to determine whether this is true. If so, then it will be advantageous to develop more efficacious techniques for reducing it.

References

Alley, T.R. and Burroughs, W.J. (1991) Do men have stronger preferences for hot, unusual, and unfamiliar foods? *Journal of General Psychology* 118, 201–214.
Archer, T. and Sjoden, P.-O. (1979) Neophobia in taste-aversion conditioning; individual differences and effects of contextual changes. *Physiological Psychology* 7, 364–369.

Arvola, A., Lahteenmaki, L. and Tuorila, H. (1999) Predicting the intent to purchase unfamiliar and familiar cheeses: the effects of attitudes, expected liking and food neophobia. *Appetite* 32, 113–126.

Babayan, S.Y., Budayr, B. and Lindgren, H.C. (1966) Age, sex, and culture as variables in food aversion. *Journal of Social Psychology* 68, 15–17.

Backstrom, A., Pirttila-Backman, A.-M. and Tuorila, H. (2003) Dimensions of novelty: a social representation approach to new foods. *Appetite* 40, 299–307.

Birch, L.L. (1980a) Effects of peer models' food choices and eating behaviors on preschoolers' food preferences. *Child Development* 51, 489–496.

Birch, L.L. (1980b) The relationship between children's food preferences and those of their parents. *Journal of Nutrition Education* 12, 14–18.

Birch, L.L. and Marlin, D.W. (1982) I don't like it; I never tried it: effects of exposure on two-year-old children's food preferences. *Appetite* 3, 353–360.

Birch, L.L., McPhee, L., Shoba, B.C., Pirok, E. and Steinberg, L. (1987) What kind of exposure reduces children's food neophobia? Looking vs. tasting. *Appetite* 9, 171–178.

Birch, L.L., Gunder, L., Grimm-Thomas, K. and Laing, D.G. (1998) Infants' consumption of a new food enhances acceptance of similar foods. *Appetite* 30, 283–295.

Blissett, J. and Harris, G. (2002) A behavioral intervention in a child with feeding problems. *Journal of Human Nutrition and Dietetics* 15, 255–260.

Braveman, N.S. (1978) Preexposure to feeding-related stimuli reduces neophobia. *Animal Learning & Behavior* 6, 417–422.

Britton, D.R., Koob, G.F., Rivier, J. and Vale, W. (1982) Intraventricular corticotropin-releasing factor enhances behavioral effects on novelty. *Life Sciences* 31, 363–367.

Capretta, P.J., Petersik, J.T. and Stewart, D.J. (1975) Acceptance of novel flavours is increased after early experience of diverse tastes. *Nature* 254, 689–691.

Cardello, A.V. (2003) Consumer concerns and expectations about novel food processing technologies: effects on product liking. *Appetite* 40, 217–233.

Carruth, B.R. and Skinner, J.D. (2000) Revisiting the picky eater phenomenon: neophobic behaviors of young children. *Journal of the American College of Nutrition* 19, 771–780.

Cashdan, E. (1994) A sensitive period for learning about food. *Human Nature* 5, 279–291.

Cooke, L.J., Wardle, J., Gibson, E.L., Sapochnik, M., Sheiham, A. and Lawson, M. (2004) Demographic, familial and trait predictors of fruit and vegetable consumption by pre-school children. *Public Health and Nutrition* 7, 295–302.

Cooper, S.J., Burnett, G. and Brown, K. (1981) Food preference following acute or chronic chlordiazepoxide administration: tolerance to an antineophobic action. *Psychopharmacology* 73, 70–74.

De Jong, N., Ocke, M., Branderhorst, H. and Friele, R. (2002) Functional food consumers in the Netherlands in the year 2000. Paper presented at the *10th Food Choice Conference*, Wageningen, The Netherlands, June–July.

Desor, J.A., Greene, L.S. and Maller, O. (1975) Preferences for sweet and salty in 9- and 15-year old and adult humans. *Science* 190, 686–687.

Duncker, K. (1938) Experimental modification of children's food preferences through social suggestion. *Journal of Abnormal and Social Psychology* 33, 489–507.

Falciglia, G.A., Couch, S.C., Gribble, L.S., Pabst, S.M. and Frank, R. (2000) Food neophobia in childhood affects dietary variety. *Journal of the American Dietetic Association* 100, 1474–1481.

Fallon, A. and Rozin, P. (1983) The psychological bases of food rejection by humans. *Ecology of Food and Nutrition* 13, 15–26.

Fallon, A.E., Rozin, P. and Pliner, P. (1984) The child's conception of food: the development of food rejections with special reference to disgust and contamination sensitivity. *Child Development* 55, 566–575.

Flight, I., Leppard, P. and Cox, D.N. (2003) Food neophobia and associations with cultural diversity and socio-economic status amongst rural and urban Australian adolescents. *Appetite* 41, 51–59.

Frank, R.A. and van der Klaauw, N.J. (1994) The contribution of chemosensory factors to individual differences in reported food preferences. *Appetite* 22, 101–123.

Galloway, A.T., Lee, Y. and Birch, L.L. (2003) Predictors and consequences of food neophobia and pickiness in young girls. *Journal of the American Dietetic Association* 103, 692–698.

Garner, D.M. and Garfinkel, P.E. (1979) The Eating Attitudes Test: an index of the symptoms of anorexia nervosa. *Psychological Medicine* 9, 273–279.

Garner, D.M., Olmstead, M.P. and Polivy, J. (1983) Development and validation of a multidimensional eating disorder inventory for anorexia nervosa and bulimia. *International Journal of Eating Disorders* 2, 15–34.

Haidt, J., McCauley, C. and Rozin, P. (1994) Individual differences in sensitivity to disgust. A scale sampling seven domains of disgust elicitors. *Personality and Individual Differences* 16, 701–713.

Harper, L. and Sanders, K. (1975) The effects of adults eating on young children's acceptance of unfamiliar foods. *Journal of Experimental Child Psychology* 20, 206–214.

Hendy, H.M. (2002) Effectiveness of trained peer models to encourage food acceptance in preschool children. *Appetite* 39, 217–225.

Hendy, H.M. and Raudenbush, B. (2000) Effectiveness of teacher modelling to encourage food acceptance in preschool children. *Appetite* 33, 1–16.

Herman, C.P., Polivy, J., Pliner, P. and Threlkeld, J. (1978) Distraction, emotionality, and the cognitive performance of dieters and nondieters. *Journal of Personality and Social Psychology* 36, 536–548.

Hobden, K. and Pliner, P. (1995) Effects of a model on food neophobia in humans. *Appetite* 25, 101–113.

Hodges, H.M., Green, S.E., Crewes, H. and Mathers, I. (1981) Effects of chronic chlordiazepoxide treatment on novel and familiar food preference in rats. *Psychopharmacology* 75, 311–314.

Hursti, U.-K.K. and Magnusson, M. (2002) Swedish consumers' opinions on genetically modified and organic foods. Paper presented at the *10th Food Choice Conference*, Wageningen, The Netherlands, June–July.

Hursti, U.-K.K. and Sjoden, P. (1997) Food and general neophobia and their relationship with self-reported food choice: familial resemblance in Swedish families with children of ages 7–17 years. *Appetite* 29, 89–103.

Kalat, J.W. and Rozin, P. (1973) 'Learned safety' as a mechanism in long-delay taste-aversion learning in rats. *Journal of Comparative and Physiological Psychology* 83, 198–207.

Koivisto, U.-K. and Sjoden, P.-O. (1996) Food and general neophobia in Swedish families: parent–child comparisons and relationships with serving specific foods. *Appetite* 26, 107–118.

Koivisto Hursti, U.-K. and Magnusson, M.K. (2003) Consumer perceptions of genetically modified and organic foods. What kind of knowledge matters? *Appetite* 41, 207–209.

Koster, E.P., Beckers, A.W.J.W. and Houben, J.H. (1987) The influence of health information on the acceptance of a snack in a canteen test. In: Martens, M., Dales, G.A.

and Russwurm, H. Jr (eds) *Flavour Science and Technology*. John Wiley, Chichester, UK, pp. 391–398.

Levine, S., Haltmeyer, G.C., Karas, G. and Denenberg, V. (1967) Physiological and behavioral effects of infantile stimulation. *Physiology & Behavior* 2, 55–59.

Loewen, R. and Pliner, P. (1999) Effects of prior exposure to palatable and unpalatable novel foods on children's willingness to taste other novel foods. *Appetite* 32, 351–366.

Loewen, R. and Pliner, P. (2000) The Food Situations Questionnaire: a measure of children's willingness to try novel foods in stimulating and non-stimulating situations. *Appetite* 35, 239–250.

Logue, A.W. and Smith, M.E. (1986) Predictors of food preferences in adult humans. *Appetite* 7, 109–125.

Logue, A.W., Logue, C.M., Uzzo, C.M., McCarty, M.J. and Smith, M.E. (1988) Food preferences in families. *Appetite* 10, 169–180.

McFarlane, T. and Pliner, P. (1997) Increasing willingness to taste novel foods: effects of nutrition and taste information. *Appetite* 28, 227–238.

Magnusson, M.K. and Koivisto-Hursti, U.-K. (2002) Consumer perceptions of foods produced by means of genetic engineering. *Appetite* 39, 9–24.

Marcontell, D.K., Laster, A.E. and Johnson, J. (2003) Cognitive–behavioral treatment of food neophobia in adults. *Journal of Anxiety Disorders* 17, 243–251.

Marinho, H. (1940) Social influence in the formation of enduring preferences. *Journal of Abnormal and Social Psychology* 37, 448–468.

Martins, Y., Pelchat, M.L. and Pliner, P. (1997) 'Try it; it's good and it's good for you': effects of taste and nutrition information on willingness to try novel foods. *Appetite* 28, 89–102.

Meiselman, H.L., Mastroianni, G., Buller, M. and Edwards, J. (1999) Longitudinal measurement of three eating behavior scales during a period of change. *Food Quality and Preference* 10, 1–8.

Minor, T.R., Dess, N.K., Ben-David, E. and Chang, W.-C. (1994) Individual differences in vulnerability to inescapable shock in rats. *Journal of Experimental Psychology: Animal Behavior Processes* 20, 402–412.

Otis, L. (1984) Factors influencing the willingness to taste unusual foods. *Psychological Reports* 54, 739–745.

Pelchat, M.L. (2000) You can teach an old dog new tricks: olfaction and responses to novel foods by the elderly. *Appetite* 35, 153–160.

Pelchat, M. and Pliner, P. (1986) Antecedents and correlates of feeding problems in young children. *Journal of Nutrition Education* 18, 23–29.

Pelchat, M.L. and Pliner, P. (1995) 'Try it. You'll like it'. Effects of information on willingness to try novel foods. *Appetite* 24, 153–165.

Pliner, P. (1982) The effects of mere exposure on liking for edible substances. *Appetite* 3, 283–290.

Pliner, P. (1983) Family resemblance in food likes and dislikes. *Journal of Nutrition Education* 15, 137–140.

Pliner, P. (1994) Development of measures of food neophobia in children. *Appetite* 23, 147–163.

Pliner, P. and Hobden, K. (1992) Development of a scale to measure the trait of food neophobia in humans. *Appetite* 19, 105–120.

Pliner, P. and Loewen, E.R. (1997) Temperament and food neophobia in children and their mothers. *Appetite* 28, 239–254.

Pliner, P. and Loewen, R. (2002) The effects of manipulated arousal on children's willingness to taste novel foods. *Physiology & Behaviour* 76, 551–558.

Pliner, P. and Melo, N. (1997) Food neophobia in humans: effects of manipulated arousal and individual differences in sensation seeking. *Physiology & Behavior* 61, 331–335.

Pliner, P. and Pelchat, M.L. (1986) Similarities in food preferences between children and their siblings and parents. *Appetite* 7, 333–342.

Pliner, P. and Pelchat, M. (1991) Neophobia in humans and the special status of foods of animal origin. *Appetite* 16, 205–218.

Pliner, P. and Stallberg-White, C. (2000) 'Pass the ketchup, please': familiar flavours increase children's willingness to taste novel foods. *Appetite* 34, 95–103.

Pliner, P., Pelchat, M. and Grabski, M. (1993) Reduction of neophobia in humans by exposure to novel foods. *Appetite* 20, 111–123.

Pliner, P., Eng, A. and Krishnan, K. (1995) The effects of fear and hunger on food neophobia in humans. *Appetite* 25, 77–87.

Pliner, P., Lahteenmaki, L. and Tuorila, H. (1998) Correlates of human food neophobia. *Appetite* 30, 93.

Poschel, B.P.H. (1971) A simple and specific screen for benzodiazepine-like drugs. *Psychoparamacologia* 19, 193–198.

Potts, H.W. and Wardle, J. (1998) The list heuristic for studying personality correlates of food choice behavior: a review and results from two samples. *Appetite* 30, 79–92.

Raudenbush, B. and Frank, R.A. (1999) Assessing food neophobia: the role of stimulus familiarity. *Appetite* 32, 261–271.

Raudenbush, B., van der Klaauw, N.J. and Frank, R.A. (1995) The contribution of psychological and sensory factors to food preference patterns as measured by the Food Attitudes Survey (FAS). *Appetite* 25, 1–15.

Raudenbush, B., Schroth, F., Reilley, S. and Frank, R.A. (1998) Food neophobia, odor evaluation and exploratory sniffing behavior. *Appetite* 31, 171–183.

Revelle, W., Anderson, K.J. and Humphreys, M.S. (1987) Empirical tests and theoretical extensions of arousal-based theories of personality. In: Strelau, J. and Eyesenck, H.J. (eds) *Personality Dimensions and Arousal*. Plenum Press, London, pp. 17–36.

Rozin, E. (1973) *The Flavour Principle Cookbook*. Hawthorne Books, New York.

Rozin, E. and Rozin, P. (1981) Culinary themes and variations. *Natural History* 90, 6–14.

Rozin, P. (1988) Cultural approaches to human food preferences. In: Morley, J.E., Sterman, M.B. and Walsh, J.T. (eds) *Nutritional Modulation of Neural Function*. Academic Press, New York, pp. 137–153.

Rozin, P. and Fallon, A. (1980) The psychological categorization of foods and non-foods: a preliminary taxonomy of food rejections. *Appetite* 1, 193–201.

Rozin, P. and Millman, L. (1987) Family environment, not heredity, accounts for family resemblances in food preferences and attitudes: a twin study. *Appetite* 8, 125–134.

Rozin, P., Fallon, A. and Mandell, R. (1984) Family resemblances in attitudes to foods. *Developmental Psychology* 20, 309–314.

Rozin, P., Haidt, J. and McCauley, C.R. (1993) Disgust. In: Lewis, M. and Haviland, J.M. (eds) *Handbook of Emotions*. Guilford Press, New York, pp. 575–594.

Schulze, G. and Watson, N.V. (1995) Comments on 'Flavor neophobia in selected rodent species'. In: Wong, R. (ed.) *Biological Perspectives on Motivated Activities*. Ablex Publishing Corporation, Norwood, New Jersey, pp. 229–230.

Singer, L.T., Ambuel, B., Wade, S. and Jaffe, A.C. (1992) Cognitive–behavioral treatment of health-impairing food phobias in children. *Journal of the American Academy of Child and Adolescent Psychiatry* 31, 847–852.

Spielberger, C.K., Gorsuch, R.L. and Lushene, R.E. (1970) *Manual for the State–Trait Anxiety Inventory (STAI)*. Consulting Psychologists Press, Palo Alto, California.

Stallberg-White, C. and Pliner, P. (1999) The effect of flavour principles on willingness to taste novel foods. *Appetite* 33, 209–221.

Sullivan, S. and Birch, L.L. (1990) Pass the sugar, pass the salt: experience dictates preferences. *Developmental Psychology* 26, 546–551.

Terasaki, M. and Imada, S. (1988) Sensation seeking and food preference. *Personality and Individual Differences* 9, 87–93.

Tuorila, H. (2001) Keeping up with the change: consumer responses to new and modified foods. Food Chain 2001 Programme Abstract, pp. 38–40.

Tuorila, H., Meiselman, H.L., Bell, R., Cardello, A.V. and Johnson, W. (1994) Role of sensory and cognitive information in the enhancement of certainty and liking for novel and familiar foods. *Appetite* 23, 231–246.

Tuorila, H., Andersson, A., Martikainen, A. and Salovaara, H. (1998) Effect of product formula, information and consumer characteristics on the acceptance of a new snack food. *Food Quality and Preference* 9, 313–320.

Tuorila, H., Lahteenmaki, L., Pohjalainen, L. and Lotti, L. (2001) Food neophobia among the Finns and related responses to familiar and unfamiliar foods. *Food Quality and Preference* 12, 29–37.

Walsh, L.L. (1993) 'I don't like it; I never tried it' in young adults. *Appetite* 20, 147.

Weinberg, J., Smotherman, W.S. and Levine, S. (1978) Early handling effects on neophobia and conditioned taste aversions. *Physiology & Behavior* 20, 589–596.

Wong, R. (1995) Flavor neophobia in selected rodent species. In: Wong, R. (ed.) *Biological Perspectives on Motivated Activities*. Ablex Publishing Corporation, Norwood, New Jersey, pp. 229–264.

Woodward, P. (1945) The relative effectiveness of various combinations of appeal in presenting a new food: soya. *American Journal of Psychology* 58, 301–323.

Zajonc, R.B. (1968) Attitudinal effects of mere exposure. *Journal of Personality and Social Psychology* 9, 1–27.

Zellner, D.A., Rozin, P., Aron, M. and Kulish, C. (1983) Conditioned enhancement of humans' liking for flavour by pairing with sweetness. *Learning and Motivation* 14, 338–350.

Zuckerman, M. (1979) *Sensation Seeking: Beyond the Optimal Level of Arousal*. Lawrence Erlbaum Associates, Hillsdale, New Jersey.

6 The Role of Learning in Development of Food Preferences

MARTIN R. YEOMANS

Department of Psychology, School of Life Sciences, University of Sussex, Falmer, Brighton BN1 9QG, UK

Introduction

Humans are born with few innate preferences for the diverse tastes and smells that are the principal elements of food and drink flavours. We are nevertheless able to acquire liking for a highly varied diet, incorporating an enormous range of gustatory and olfactory stimuli, often reversing innate influences, such as our natural dislike of bitter tastes. Although we are still some way from a full appreciation of the complex learning processes which underlie flavour preference development, the application of psychological principles and methodologies developed in the broader learning field has helped identify many of the key processes. This chapter clarifies the major learning concepts which underlie contemporary theories of flavour preference learning, and then evaluates the current status of the major relevant theories of preference development.

Why Learning Models are Needed

The problem of how to acquire specific preferences for nutritious foods while avoiding those that are harmful has been described as the omnivore's paradox (Rozin, 1977). To achieve this, while also learning what items are neither harmful nor beneficial and still make optimal use of available food resources, is seen as a major driving force for cognitive evolution. The huge variety of potential foodstuffs available to an omnivore precludes any genetic predisposition to like or dislike anything beyond those basic signals that act as reliable predictors of relevant and unambiguous post-ingestive effects. The only cues in nature for humans appear to be sweet and bitter tastes. Sweet tastes are generally liked, even by newborn infants (Desor *et al.*, 1973; Steiner, 1979; Berridge, 2000), and this has been explained in terms of the reliable relationship in nature between a sweet taste and safe, nutritious foods (Hladik *et al.*, 2002). Such explanations are attractive, but in humans any real test of these evolutionary hypotheses is extremely difficult, and this will always leave evolutionary explanations open to criticism. Evidence that sweet taste preferences are truly genetically determined are clearer in animal studies, where individual differences in preference for sweet tastes have allowed the breeding of sweet-preferring and sweet-disliking strains of rodents, with significant progress in identification of the specific receptors encoding for sweet taste (Bachmanov *et al.*, 2002). Taking the same evolutionary perspective, dislike for bitter tastes can be interpreted as the avoidance of items that are poisonous, since most poisons have a strong, bitter taste, and again significant progress has been made in identifying the relevant receptors and associated genes (Shi *et al.*, 2003). However, in the context of this chapter it is noteworthy that even these innate taste preferences can be modified by experience, so that people come to like bitter flavour components such as those produced by alcohol, caffeine, etc., where we are able to learn through experience that in these contexts bitterness not only predicts a safe (non-poisonous) item, but also one which has some form of desirable post-ingestive effect. This issue is explored in detail later. However, the limited scope for genetic explanations of flavour preference suggests that the majority of flavour preferences have to be acquired, and this chapter concentrates on the major psychological models of flavour preference development.

Major Learning Models Relating to Development of Food Preferences

Psychologists have put forward a number of theories to explain how learning principles may be applied to the problem of food preference development, and the four major theoretical positions are reviewed.

Mere exposure

The simplest learning concept to be applied to food preference development in humans was that of mere exposure (Zajonc, 1968). The essence of mere exposure is that repeated unreinforced exposure to any stimulus results in an increase in preference for that stimulus (the converse of the classic adage that familiarity breeds contempt). Mere exposure has been widely demonstrated outside the food preference literature (Bornstein, 1989), but specific studies examining this in human studies with food stimuli are more limited (Pliner, 1982; Crandall, 1984; Stevenson and Yeomans, 1995). Mere exposure remains a useful description of familiarity effects, but in itself offers no explanation for the nature of the underlying change. Thus explanations for mere exposure effects usually make reference to reduced neophobia (see Chapter 5), or other explanations such as opponent–process affective responses (Solomon and Corbit, 1974). Familiarity remains an important component of changes in preference, but in itself offers little explanation for the mechanism underlying preference change.

Neophobia and learned safety

The phrase 'learned safety' was one of the first learning concepts to be applied to food preference development and, in combination with the concept of neophobia (fear of new taste), was developed originally to explain the concept of bait shyness in rats and other rodents (Kalat and Rozin, 1973). Neophobia was seen as an innate tendency for rats to treat all new food items as potentially harmful. This resulted in a pattern of eating where potential new foods were consumed in small amounts when first encountered and then freely consumed only after a period of abstinence. The interpretation was that this behaviour allowed the animal to identify whether the food had harmful post-ingestive effects. If any illness was experienced following ingestion, the animal acquired a profound dislike for the food flavour, originally defined as a conditioned taste aversion (CTA; Garcia and Koelling, 1966) since the early studies combined basic tastes such as sweet or salty with illness, resulting in a long-lasting aversion to these tastes (Garcia *et al.*, 1966; Smith and Roll, 1967). How then do preferences develop? The learned safety model in essence suggested that a failure for a flavour to reliably predict illness effectively meant that the flavour predicted safety, and as neophobia came to be reduced by habituation so the flavour became preferred (Kalat and Rozin, 1973). This simplistic account holds many attractions, but explicit tests of the learned safety hypothesis are difficult. Essentially, the model simply predicts that any food which does not produce illness should become liked, and so it is hard to differentiate this explanation from mere exposure as an explanation of liking development. An obvious shortcoming of the learned safety model is that it cannot explain why humans do not develop a preference for items that are not deleterious but are not beneficial either (grass, sand, etc.). For this reason, this concept is generally seen as less useful as an explanation of food preference development than other models, but the concept should not be discarded entirely since it does provide a simple and elegant account of why we appear to learn more quickly to avoid foods that make us ill than to like foods that are beneficial. Moreover, the concept of neophobia is widely accepted, and detailed discussion of the importance of neophobia in human food preferences is provided elsewhere in this volume (see Chapter 5).

Flavour–consequence learning

The original discovery of CTA was crucial to the development of our understanding of flavour preferences, and indeed more broadly to our understanding of the very basis of learning in general. Essentially, flavour preferences can be thought of as associations between a neutral flavour stimulus and a hedonically significant post-ingestive event. Described in this way, flavour preference development can be seen as analogous to Pavlovian (classical) conditioning in learning models. Prior to the discovery of CTA, the most widely accepted models of Pavlovian conditioning were based on the simple notion that temporal contiguity between the neutral (conditioned stimulus; CS) and biologically relevant stimulus (unconditioned stimulus; UCS) was all that was needed for an association to develop.

The discovery of CTA was one of several key experimental findings which fundamentally challenged our understanding of the nature of associations underlying classical conditioning. The challenges from CTA were threefold. First, temporal contiguity predicted that learning should proceed when the two events occurred closely together in time, yet CTA could be seen even with 24 h elapsing between flavour exposure and induced nausea (Garcia et al., 1966; Smith and Roll, 1967). Secondly, CTA can occur after a single flavour–illness experience, whereas most examples of conditioned associations develop progressively over a number of learning trials. And finally, but importantly, there is a clear predisposition ('preparedness'; Seligman, 1970) to associate flavours with illness rather than other associated stimuli (Garcia and Koelling, 1966). After various claims that these characteristics set CTA as a unique form of learning (Bitterman, 1975), more recent models see CTA obeying the same fundamental laws of association, but adapted to meet the specific need to have a system of learning that allows rapid and robust learning of foods which are potentially harmful (Logue, 1979). This conclusion recognizes the functional value of CTA, but also sees the underlying associative mechanism as a modification of a more general associative learning system, rather than a separate and unique learning mechanism.

Flavour–consequence learning (FCL) broadens the original discovery of CTA into a generalized model for understanding changes in liking and preference based on the idea that we are pre-prepared to associate flavours with post-ingestive consequences. The ideas behind FCL are heavily influenced by broader concepts in associative learning, with the primary association being between the perceived sensory characteristics of the ingested food or drink (acting as CS) and the post-ingestive effects of the food or drink (UCS). One way of conceptualizing the associative substructure of FCL is shown in Fig. 6.1. Thus, as with other forms of learning, it is predicted that in most situations changes in preferences generated by FCL will proceed progressively, with repeated experiences of flavour and consequences strengthening the change in preference. Adopting an associative learning approach to FCL therefore leads to clear and testable hypotheses about how preferences should change with experience depending on the post-ingestive consequences. Therefore, most critical to the use of FCL as an explanation of flavour preference learning is identification of the nature of post-ingestive effects (the UCS) which lead to preference change, and accordingly this chapter focuses initially on the strength of evidence for FCL as a learning mechanism based on various different classes of UCS effects.

Flavour–consequence learning based on post-ingestive nutritive effects

There is a clear relationship between energy density and liking for foods (Drewnowski, 1998). When a wide range of participants rate their liking for foods from a wide variety of food classes, in every case there is a correlation between how much food is liked and the energy density of these foods (Fig. 6.2). Similar data are seen when considering children's preferences for fruit and vegetables, with a clear preference for those fruit that have higher energy density (Gibson and Wardle, 2003). These observations are entirely consistent with the idea that we are able, at some level, to associate food flavours with positive

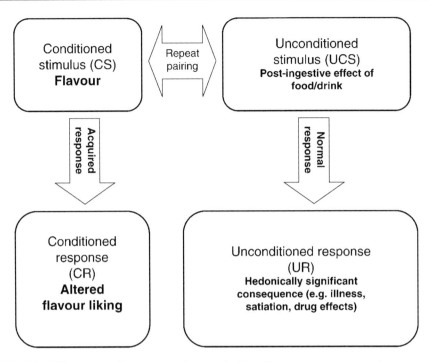

Fig. 6.1. The associative substructure underlying flavour–consequence learning.

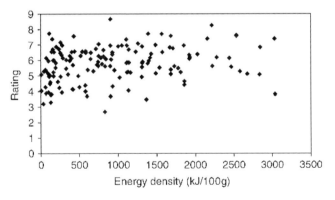

Fig. 6.2. The average rated pleasantness of 149 typical foods as a function of their energy density.

post-ingestive consequences: in this case, FCL would explain our generalized liking for foods as a consequence of our past experience of the extent to which these foods appease hunger. However, while such correlational data are consisent with the FCL concept, they do not offer any direct test of energy as the specific consequence which reinforces changes in flavour preference or liking.

The clearest evidence that energy can reinforce changes in flavour preferences comes from studies in animals, where neutral flavours are selectively paired with the post-ingestive delivery of energy (Capaldi, 1992; Sclafani, 1999). In the most sensitive designs, rats are given *ad libitum* access to two flavoured non-nutritive solutions. Consumption of one solution (the positive flavour cue, or CS$^+$ in Pavlovian conditioning terms) automatically leads to intragastric infusion of an energy-bearing liquid. In contrast, consumption of the alternative flavour leads to intragastric infusion of water. The outcome of these studies is a profound and durable preference for the CS$^+$ over the CS$^-$. This is true with a large number of energy-containing reinforcers: sucrose (Fedorchak and Bolles, 1987; Capaldi *et al.*, 1994; Harris *et al.*, 2000; Sclafani, 2002), glucose (Myers and Sclafani, 2001a, 2001b), starch (Elizalde and Sclafani, 1988; Sclafani and Nissenbaum, 1988; Ramirez, 1994), fats (Lucas and Sclafani, 1989) and alcohol (Ackroff and Sclafani, 2001, 2002a, 2003). These data lend very clear support to the FCL hypothesis, and clearly suggest that energy is a powerful reinforcer of food preferences in these highly controlled laboratory studies with animals.

While the data from animal research in support of FCL based on energy delivery is compelling, and FCL has been discussed as an important component of the development of liking for foods with high energy density (Stubbs and Whybrow, 2004), specific evidence of equivalent changes in flavour preference in controlled studies in humans is surprisingly weak. Relatively few studies have reported reliable increases in flavour preference in humans based on associations between flavours and nutrients in the 30 years since FCL was first discussed, contrasted with over 70 papers reporting successful studies in rodents. Perhaps the most convincing studies have been with children, with the reported increase in preference for high-energy (carbohydrate) drinks relative to low-energy drinks in children (Birch *et al.*, 1990) and two subsequent studies by the same group looking at FCL in relation to fat content in children (Johnson *et al.*, 1991; Kern *et al.*, 1993). However, in adults, the literature is surprisingly limited, with the clearest evidence for nutrient-related preferences coming in a study where two distinctly flavoured foods, one low and one high in protein, were consumed after a low-protein breakfast. Under these conditions a preference for the flavour associated with high protein emerged, with expression of this preference acutely sensitive to the current level of protein deprivation (Gibson *et al.*, 1995). This followed up on an earlier study, where preference for the flavour of a soup with added starch increased relative to a soup with no starch, provided participants were hungry when the soup was consumed (Booth *et al.*, 1982).

Why then is FCL so elusive in human studies? The problem in interpreting any situation where some studies report positive findings, and others (many of which will inevitably never be published) find no effect, is that it is always possible to posit *post hoc* reasons why a specific study may not have worked. In this way positive findings will always have greater impact than null results, and the existence of some published studies reporting evidence for FCL reinforced by nutrient delivery can be taken as adequate evidence for the existence of this learning mechanism in the development of human preferences. Closer inspection of the literature suggests that some of the reasons why evidence for FCL is not always found may itself be consistent with our understanding of the nature of associative learning in general. For example, it is well established that exposure to a potential CS prior to its actual pairing with a specific UCS slows down the rate at which an acquisition forms (Lubow and Moore, 1959; Reiss and Wagner, 1972). This phenomenon, which used to be referred to as latent learning but is often today simply called the CS pre-exposure effect, may be particularly relevant in studies of FCL in humans. The implication of CS pre-exposure is that the CS used as the target flavour in laboratory-based studies of FCL has to be novel to the consumer. In the studies which successfully reported FCL with energy as the consequence, the stimuli clearly met this criterion, but it is possible that prior familiarity with the CS prevented learning about the UCS in other studies. A counter-argument might be that some studies which used equally novel flavoured CS failed to find evidence of FCL (Stubenitsky *et al.*, 2000). However, in some cases studies defined novelty in terms of a flavour component presented in a food context that itself was a poor predictor of energy content. Thus prior learning that the context is a poor predictor of post-ingestive energy could interfere with (block) the specific association between the test flavour and the specific energy content of that product. This example illustrates the fundamental problem in researching FCL in adults, who bring to the laboratory studies a lifetime of prior associations which can always be used *post hoc* as potential explanations why specific studies failed to find evidence of FCL. In essence the problem is, as with most areas of science, that a failure to find an effect is never as powerful as a positive finding. That said, evidence for FCL in humans based on flavour–energy association remains far from compelling.

Flavour–consequence learning based on post-ingestive drug effects from foods and drinks

Some of the clearest flavour preferences are for drinks which contain substances with psychoactive consequences, such as alcohol and caffeine. Indeed, in these instances liking seems to be contrary to our natural instinct to dislike bitter tastes. FCL provides an obvious framework through which to explain this acquired liking: the specific flavour of the drink becomes a reliable and contingent predictor of the positive post-ingestive effect of the drink. In this respect, the research on flavour preferences in rats where alcohol was the reinforcer as an example of energy-based FCL (described in brief earlier) could be re-interpreted as rats showing a preference for the post-ingestive pharmacological effects of alcohol. This highlights the difficulty in dissociating these two aspects of the effects of alcohol: on one hand, alcohol is second only to fat in terms of the amount of energy delivered per unit mass, and on the other it is a psychoactive agent with well-defined and liked post-ingestive consequences. As discussed earlier, evidence for FCL with alcohol as UCS in rats is compelling (Ackroff and Sclafani, 2001, 2002a, 2002b, 2003), but despite its parsimony as an explanation of how humans acquire a liking for the flavour of alcoholic drinks, no studies have explicitly reported FCL with alcohol as UCS in humans.

In contrast to alcohol, FCL based on caffeine as post-ingestive consequence is now well established in laboratory models of FCL in humans (Rogers *et al.*, 1995; Richardson *et al.*, 1996; Yeomans *et al.*, 1998; Tinley *et al.*, 2003). Indeed, FCL with caffeine as the reinforcer is now being used as a convenient model through which to explore human associative learning in general (Yeomans *et al.*, 2000a).

The basic design of caffeine-based FCL studies is very straightforward: people consume a novel-flavoured drink which contains either caffeine (CS+) or an inert placebo (CS-) on several days, and either preference (Rogers et al., 1995; Tinley et al., 2004) or liking (Yeomans et al., 1998, 2000a, 2000b, 2001; Tinley et al., 2003) for the caffeine-paired flavour is measured. The consistent outcome is an increase in preference (Rogers et al., 1995) or liking (Yeomans et al., 1998, 2000a, 2000b, 2001; Tinley et al., 2003) for the CS+ relative to the CS-, consistent with the idea that the consumer has associated the flavour and consequence (caffeine), and adjusted liking accordingly. However, the degree to which this change in liking is seen in FCL studies with caffeine as the UCS depends crucially both on the extent of habitual caffeine consumption (Rogers et al., 1995; Tinley et al., 2004) and the degree to which consumers are caffeine-deprived at the time of testing (Yeomans et al., 1998). In terms of habitual caffeine use, only people who regularly consume caffeine showed an increased liking for a novel flavour paired with caffeine, whereas people who habitually consume little or no caffeine tended to develop an aversion for novel-flavoured caffeinated drinks (Rogers et al., 1995; Tinley et al., 2004). However, consumption of novel drinks containing caffeine did not lead to development of flavour liking in moderate consumers when they were not caffeine-deprived at the time of testing (Yeomans et al., 1998), even though the same consumers showed an acquired liking for the flavour of a caffeinated drink when caffeine-deprived. Thus the degree to which caffeine is an effective UCS depends crucially on the degree to which caffeine is habitually consumed.

Other examples of flavour–consequence learning

If FCL represents a general mechanism through which flavour preferences are acquired, FCL would be predicted to operate in any situation where a flavour predicts a post-ingestive effect that is interpretable as a positive or negative consequence. For example, FCL would predict that the distinctive flavour of a liquid which reliably appeases thirst should come to be liked. Recent data suggest this may be the case (Durlach et al., 2002), although the authors are cautious in interpreting these data as definitive evidence of FCL since an alternative explanation is possible whereby the flavour of the drink consumed when thirsty might itself have produced conditioned thirst. FCL could also be invoked as an explanation for the liking of the flavour of cigarettes by smokers, especially considering the distaste for the same sensory experience displayed by non-smokers. Recent research supports this interpretation: smokers developed a preference for a novel odour which was paired with nicotine delivery over a second odour predicting placebo (Rogers et al., 2002).

So far, the stimuli discussed as CS in FCL are complex flavours. However, even liking for the specific taste of salt can be interpreted in terms of FCL. Exercise has been reported to increase sodium palatability (Takamata et al., 1994; Leshem et al., 1999), and a recent study suggests conditioning of a sodium preference after exercise dependent on the amount of perspiration generated by the participant (Wald and Leshem, 2003). This notion of acquired liking for the taste of sodium as a consequence of salt need is further supported by increased sodium palatability in those congenital adrenal hyperplasia patients who are salt-wasting and not stabilized by medication (Kochli *et al.*, 2002).

The current status of flavour–consequence learning as a model of food preference development in humans

The early formulation of FCL as a model of flavour preferences was based almost exclusively on research with animals, and provided clear evidence that nutrients could reinforce changes in flavour preferences. The relative lack of success in equivalent studies in humans where the reinforcer was some form of energy source meant that many researchers started to question the importance of FCL in human food preferences. However, more recent studies using a variety of reinforcers (caffeine, thirst-reduction, etc.) now clearly demonstrate that FCL is evident in human flavour preferences, but also suggest that the specific conditions needed to bring this phenomenon under stimulus control in laboratory conditions are difficult to achieve in adults, who have already acquired a large repertoire of food preferences. So where does this leave FCL as a model of human flavour preference? Clearly, this form of learning can occur in humans, and this concept remains a parsimonious explanation for why preferences can be predicted by the energy they provide in the absence of any clear genetic predisposition. However, until further studies are published clearly showing FCL based on unambiguous flavour–nutrient associations, there will remain some doubt about the real importance of FCL in human food preference development.

Flavour–flavour models of evaluative conditioning

A second form of conditioned association which may contribute to changes in flavour preference and liking has been given the general name of evaluative conditioning (EC), which involves a change in evaluation of one stimulus by association with a second stimulus that is already liked or disliked (reviewed by Field and Davey, 1999; De Houwer *et al.*, 2001). Flavour-based EC involves pairing a neutral flavour CS with a liked or disliked flavour UCS. As with FCL, changes in liking are usually interpreted within an associative learning framework based on the principles of Pavlovian conditioning. The key features of this form of learning are highlighted in Fig. 6.3: the essential idea is that association of a previously hedonically neutral flavour or flavour component (interpreted as the CS) with a second flavour or flavour element which is already liked or disliked (interpreted as the UCS) results in an equivalent change in liking for the previously neutral flavour CS. EC is not restricted to learning about foods or drinks, but is generally seen as the explanation for changes in liking in any situation where a novel, neutral stimulus (CS) is contingently paired with a second, hedonically significant stimulus (UCS). Thus EC may represent a general form of affective learning, yet may be an important element of flavour preference development. For example, sweetness is innately liked (but see later) and the addition of sweetness to a wide variety of foods and drinks increases their immediate acceptability. EC therefore

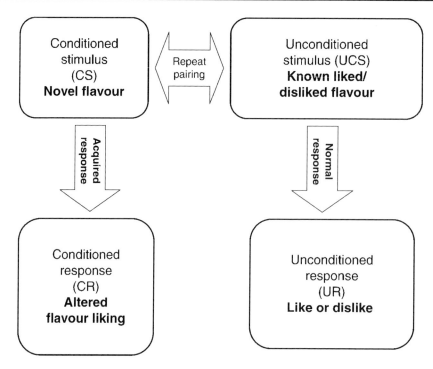

Fig. 6.3. The associative substructure underlying flavour–flavour learning.

predicts that this contingent association of flavour and sweetness results in increased liking for the sweet-associated flavour on its own. Despite the obvious attraction of this idea, for example as a possible explanation for the development of liking for flavours as diverse as coffee, tea, beer and wine, yoghurt, etc., all of which are initially consumed in a sweetened form, empirical evidence to support EC based on sweetness resulting in actual flavour preference acquisition in humans remains surprisingly scarce, with only one published study reporting EC based on sweetness (Zellner *et al.*, 1983) and others which failed to find this effect (Baeyens *et al.*, 1990; Rozin *et al.*, 1998). This issue is explored in more detail later.

In contrast to the paucity of evidence for flavour-based EC where the UCS is sweetness, studies have consistently reported reduced liking for a novel flavour that has been paired with an aversive UCS, such as the flavour produced by Tween (Baeyens *et al.*, 1990, 1995, 1996). Tween is a surfactant that generates a mildly unpleasant bitter and soapy flavour. The robustness of this acquired dislike, contrasted with the difficulty in finding equivalent changes based on sweetness in humans, perhaps implies that aversive flavours act more effectively as UCS in this type of learning. One explanation for this, discussed further later, is that the hedonic valance of a sweet UCS may depend on motivational state at the time of testing (i.e. sweet may be liked when hungry, but liking for sweetness is greatly reduced when sated; Cabanac and Duclaux, 1970; Cabanac, 1971), whereas the hedonic significance of an aversive UCS is independent of current motivational needs. If so, it would be expected that an aversive UCS will always be a more effective reinforcer of flavour-based EC than will UCS with potential positive post-ingestive consequences.

Although to date studies of EC in humans have concentrated on complex flavours, a more recent learning model explicitly paired specific olfactory CS with taste UCS (Stevenson *et al.*, 1995, 1998, 2000; Stevenson, 2003; Stevenson and Boakes, 2004) in an olfactory conditioning paradigm. The typical design of these studies was simple: odours were first presented orthonasally (i.e. were sniffed) on their own, and evaluations of various sensory characteristics, including those using gustatory descriptors (e.g. sweetness, sourness, saltiness, etc.), along with hedonic ratings, were made. The odour was then experienced repeatedly paired with a taste stimulus (e.g. 10% sucrose to give a sweet UCS). Finally, the odour was again presented orthonasally, and sensory and hedonic properties of the odour CS re-evaluated. The consistent finding in these studies was that ratings for the odour on the sensory dimension related to the trained UCS increased. For example, when an odour was paired with sucrose, the rated sweetness of the odour post-training was consistently higher than it was before training started (Stevenson *et al.*, 1995, 1998), even though the sucrose was not present when odours were rated orthonasally. More importantly in the present context, in none of these studies did the pairing of odour and taste UCS result in any change in hedonic evaluation or preference for the UCS. Thus, as with the examples of EC based on complex flavours discussed earlier, there was no evidence in these studies that sweetness acted as a reinforcer of hedonic change for a flavour element, even though the actual sensory properties of the odour CS were changed by repeated association with a sweet UCS.

The assumption in all tests of flavour preference change with a sweet UCS, both with flavour and odour CS, is that sweetness is liked. Although this is generally true, individuals vary in the degree to which they express liking for sweetness (Looy and Weingarten, 1991; Looy *et al.*, 1992), and since past studies failed to control for this, inclusion of both sweet likers and sweet dislikers could have resulted in very mixed responses. The corollary is that changes in liking for the sweet-paired CS should correlate with actual rated liking for the training sweet UCS: those participants who like the sweet taste should show increased liking for the sweet-paired odour, and those who dislike the sweet taste should show the converse. Recent data from our laboratory suggest this is the case. Briefly, participants rated liking for a novel odour CS presented orthonasally before and after four disguised training trials where the same odour was experienced retronasally in combination with a UCS of 10% sucrose. Although, in line with previous studies, overall liking was not increased by the odour–sweetness pairings, when overall changes were correlated with actual liking for the training odour–sweetness stimuli, a positive correlation was found (Fig. 6.4; Yeomans *et al.*, 2006). The implication is that overall liking for sweet-paired odours will be increased if the participants are preselected as sweet likers, and a subsequent study (Yeomans *et al.*, 2006) confirms this prediction (Fig. 6.5). Thus, the flavour–flavour model of EC can be shown to produce reliable changes in liking provided the actual hedonic tone of the UCS is factored into the study design.

Overall, development of a dislike for flavour components consistently paired with an aversive flavour UCS is robust, and may help explain how human flavour aversions develop. Flavour–flavour learning with sweet UCS may also be influential, particularly in consumers with strong sweet preferences. As with FCL,

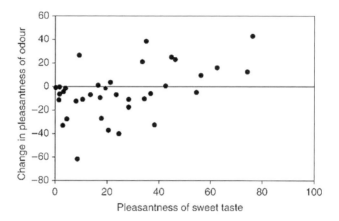

Fig. 6.4. Change in pleasantness of a novel odour paired with a sweet taste (10% sucrose) as a function of rated pleasantness of the sweet taste itself. (Adapted from Yeomans *et al.*, 2006 with permission.)

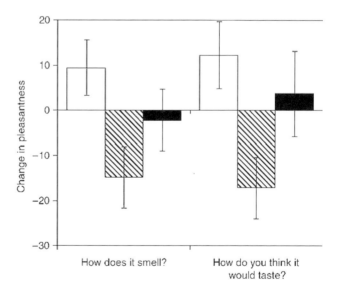

Fig. 6.5. Changes in the rated pleasantness of an odour paired with a sweet taste (10% sucrose: ☐), bitter (quinine: ▧) or water (■) for sweet likers who either rated how pleasant they found the odour or how pleasant they thought the solution would taste. (Adapted from Yeomans *et al.*, 2006 with permission.)

liking change with flavour–flavour learning requires relatively few pairings of CS and UCS flavours. Flavour–flavour learning may therefore be important in human flavour preference development, although as with FCL more research is needed to determine the full scope and importance of flavour–flavour associations.

The Role of Motivational State in Modulating Acquired Flavour Preferences

The preceding review identifies FCL and flavour–flavour conditioning as important mechanisms underpinning flavour preference development. However, equally important is the understanding of how the changes in preference produced by associations of this kind relate to the current nutritional needs of the consumer. First, consideration of this relationship might explain ambiguities in the existing literature on flavour preference development, such as the difficulty in finding evidence of FCL reinforced by nutrient delivery in human studies, and the disparity between acquired dislikes and likes seen in both FCL and flavour–flavour learning. Secondly, understanding the relationship between whether we like a particular flavour and our current nutritional needs (in terms of energy and/or macronutrients) is critical to our overall understanding of appetite control. For example, we know that liking is an important determinant of short-term intake (Yeomans, 1996; De Castro *et al.*, 2000), and in most cases studies of the impact of liking for the consumed food on appetite have used foods that are not innately preferred. This implies that once liking has been acquired, it has the potential to stimulate short-term over-consumption, and so contribute to a positive energy balance and ultimately obesity. In order to evaluate these issues, the final section of this chapter explores the relationship between acquired flavour preferences and nutritional needs at the time of testing.

The idea that the current motivational needs of a consumer influence their hedonic evaluation of a product makes intuitive sense. For instance, an acquired liking for a flavour predicting that a food has a high energy content would be appropriate when the consumer is hungry, but responding to that same acquired liking when sated could lead to overeating. Thus, it may be that the body has evolved a mechanism for not only acquiring food preferences, but determining whether expression of these acquired preferences is an appropriate response to a particular need state. This argument is easier to follow with some examples. In their classic study of conditioned preferences for a drink which predicted sugar-based energy, Birch *et al.* (1990) found that the acquired preference was much less when the children evaluated the drink when sated than when hungry. Thus although these children had acquired a preference for a flavour paired with energy when hungry, they expressed a lower preference for the energy-paired flavour when sated. Such a relationship makes nutritional sense: consuming a drink which predicts energy when not in need of energy goes against homeostasis. It also implies that increased liking acquired through FCL need not lead to over-consumption.

Another example of acquired preferences which were acutely sensitive to current need states was from the study of preferences for flavours paired with delivery of protein in adults (Gibson *et al.*, 1995). Again, the acquired preferences were much stronger when the consumer was acutely deprived of protein than when they had consumed a high-protein breakfast prior to evaluating the protein-paired flavour. This principle of expression of acquired preferences being sensitive to acute need state was also seen in the acquired like for novel drink flavours which predicted the presence or absence of caffeine (Yeomans *et al.*, 2000a, b). In this instance, state dependency was found in two ways. First, consumers had to be both caffeine-dependent (Rogers *et al.*, 1995; Tinley *et al.*, 2003, 2004) and acutely deprived of caffeine (Yeomans *et al.*, 1998) in order to develop liking for a novel flavour predictive of caffeine. Thus, the consumer had to be in an appropriate motivational state (both chronically dependent and acutely deprived of caffeine) in order for caffeine to be an effective reinforcer of FCL. Secondly, once caffeine consumers had acquired a liking for a novel caffeine-paired drink, they only continued to express that acquired liking when acutely in need of caffeine (Yeomans *et al.*, 2000a, b). Thus the body seems sensitive not only to the state needed to support the acquisition (learning) of conditioned preferences, but also is acutely sensitive to the relevance of these acquired preferences to the current need for caffeine. This leads to the question: can consumers develop an unexpressed (implicit) flavour liking? Put simply, if we consume something that has an effect on our body which is not relevant to our current needs but has the potential to be relevant to future needs, do we make the association between flavour and consequence and then express this as a sudden liking (or even craving) for that flavour when the anticipated consequence is of value to the consumer? For example, it has been suggested that the apocryphal craving for coal by pregnant women might reflect prior learning that the coal contains micronutrients which are then relevant to the particular nutritional demands of pregnancy. Attractive though this idea is, in practice there is no empirical evidence to support this type of implicit nutrient-based learning. The only published study to investigate this type of association in humans to date failed to find any implicit flavour liking (Yeomans *et al.*, 2001). In that study, undeprived moderate caffeine consumers were exposed to a novel caffeinated drink on four occasions. Since they were not caffeine-deprived, their liking for the drink flavour did not alter. Crucially, on a subsequent test day when they evaluated the drink when acutely deprived of caffeine, they again did not show any emergent liking for this drink.

Overall, human data suggest that current motivational state is crucial to the acquisition and expression of flavour preferences acquired through FCL. However, whether this is also true for flavour–flavour learning is largely untested in humans. The state dependence of flavour preferences acquired by association between a flavour and a post-ingestive consequence reported in humans has also been seen in animal-based studies of acquired flavour preferences for flavours paired with nutrient delivery. Thus rats that had developed a preference for a flavour paired with energy when hungry showed less preference for the energy-paired flavour when sated (Fedorchak and Bolles, 1987). However, in animal studies it has also been possible to explore state dependency in relation to FCL and flavour–flavour models of preference development (Capaldi, 1991; Fedorchak, 1997). The evidence here is that FCL is sensitive to motivational state but flavour–flavour learning is not. For example, when rats were conditioned to associate a flavour paired with sweet-tasting sucrose when hungry, this learning was unaffected by interspersed exposures to a non-caloric sweet taste (Harris *et al.*, 2000). However, attempts to train flavour–sucrose pairings in sated rats were disrupted by interspersed exposures to a non-caloric sweet taste. The implication is that when rats experience flavour–sucrose pairings, both FCL and flavour–flavour learning take place. When sated, the latter learning predominates, and is then disrupted by exposure to sweetness alone since this makes the flavour a poor predictor of sweetness delivery. When hungry, FCL predominates and this is not disrupted by exposure to sweetness without energy, making the flavour a reliable predictor of energy. Again, it would be interesting to see if the same distinction is found in human studies.

How then does the states-dependency of FCL explain why it is easier to condition flavour aversions than preferences in the laboratory? Most conditioned aversions are based on flavour–flavour learning, with an aversive UCS. This UCS will be aversive regardless of motivational state. In contrast, attempts to train FCL with energy as UCS in humans will be disrupted if the participants are not in the correct hungry or nutrient-deprived state when trained and tested. The issue remains, however, why flavour–flavour learning with sweetness as UCS is also complex in humans. As discussed earlier, the animal literature suggests that such learning should be independent of need state. However, in humans how pleasant we find sweet tastes depends on motivational state at the time of tasting: classically, sweet tastes are rated as more pleasant when hungry, and less so after ingestion of a high-energy preload (negative gustatory alliesthesia; Cabanac, 1971, 1989). If this is so, then it might be expected that a flavour which has become liked by association with a sweet taste also shows acute sensitivity to energetic needs at the time of rating. If so, past failures to find flavour–flavour conditioning with sweet tastes as UCS in humans (e.g. Baeyens *et al.*, 1990) may be in part a consequence a failure to control for need state during training. Thus, the possibility remains that both FCL and flavour–flavour conditioning are sensitive to need state, but further research is needed to confirm this.

Summary

The evolutionary pressures on animals, including humans, that have to identify appropriate foods by experience has led to the evolution of a highly complex but effective way of rapidly learning which flavours predict harmful consequences and which provide reliable signals of post-ingestive benefits. Once a flavour preference or aversion has been acquired, experience of that flavour with other flavours results in generalization of this acquired knowledge through flavour–flavour associations. We are still some way from fully understanding the associative structures which underlie flavour-based learning, and many questions remain about the degree to which the learning mechanisms seen in flavour preference development are equivalent to those seen in broader associative learning. This chapter has however shown that there is now a substantial body of research clearly demonstrating that flavour preferences can be acquired by association, and that multiple learning mechanisms are needed to fully explain flavour preference development.

References

Ackroff, K. and Sclafani, A. (2001) Flavor preferences conditioned by intragastric infusion of ethanol in rats. *Pharmacology, Biochemistry, and Behavior* 68, 327–338.

Ackroff, K. and Sclafani, A. (2002a) Flavor quality and ethanol concentration affect ethanol-conditioned flavor preferences. *Pharmacology, Biochemistry, and Behavior* 74, 229–240.

Ackroff, K. and Sclafani, A. (2002b) Ethanol flavor preference conditioned by intragastric carbohydrate in rats. *Pharmacology, Biochemistry, and Behavior* 74, 41–51.

Ackroff, K. and Sclafani, A. (2003) Flavor preferences conditioned by intragastric ethanol with limited access training. *Pharmacology, Biochemistry, and Behavior* 75, 223–233.

Bachmanov, A.A., Reed, D.R., Li, X. and Beauchamp, G.K. (2002) Genetics of sweet taste preference. *Pure and Applied Chemistry* 7, 1135–1140.

Baeyens, F., Eelen, P., Van Den Burgh, O. and Crombez, G. (1990) Flavor–flavor and color–flavor conditioning in humans. *Learning and Motivation* 21, 434–455.

Baeyens, F., Crombez, G., Hendrickx, H. and Eelen, P. (1995) Parameters of human evaluative flavor–flavor conditioning. *Learning and Motivation* 26, 141–160.

Baeyens, F., Crombez, G., De Houwer, J. and Eelen, P. (1996) No evidence for modulation of evaluative flavor–flavor associations in humans. *Learning and Motivation* 27, 200–241.

Berridge, K.C. (2000) Measuring hedonic impact in animals and infants: microstructure of affective taste reactivity patterns. *Neuroscience and Biobehavioral Reviews* 24, 173–198.

Birch, L.L., McPhee, L., Steinberg, L. and Sullivan, S. (1990) Conditioned flavor preferences in young children. *Physiology & Behavior* 47, 501–505.

Bitterman, M.E. (1975) The comparative analysis of learning. *Science* 188, 699–709.

Booth, D.A., Mather, P. and Fuller, J. (1982) Starch content of ordinary foods associatively conditions human appetite and satiation, indexed by intake and pleasantness of starch-paired flavours. *Appetite* 3, 163–184.

Bornstein, R.F. (1989) Exposure and affect: overview and meta-analysis of research, 1968–1987. *Psychological Bulletin* 106, 265–289.

Cabanac, M. (1971) Physiological role of pleasure. *Science* 173, 1103–1107.

Cabanac, M. (1989) Palatability of food and the ponderostat. *Annals of the New York Academy of Sciences* 575, 340–352.

Cabanac, M. and Duclaux, R. (1970) Specificity of internal signals in producing satiety for taste stimuli. *Nature* 229, 125–127.

Capaldi, E.D. (1991) Hunger and the learning of flavor preferences. In: Bolles, R.C. (ed.) *The Hedonics of Taste*. Lawrence Erlbaum Associates, Hillside, New Jersey, pp. 157–169.

Capaldi, E.D. (1992) Conditioned food preferences. *Psychology of Learning and Motivation* 28, 1–33.

Capaldi, E.D., Owens, J. and Palmer, K.A. (1994) Effects of food deprivation on learning and expression of flavor preferences conditioned by saccharin or sucrose. *Animal Learning & Behavior* 22, 173–180.

Crandall, C.S. (1984) The liking of foods as a result of exposure: eating doughnuts in Alaska. *Journal of Social Psychology* 125, 187–194.

De Castro, J.M., Bellisle, F., Dalix, A.-M. and Pearcey, S.M. (2000) Palatability and intake relationships in free-living humans: characterization and independence of influence in North Americans. *Physiology & Behavior* 70, 343–350.

De Houwer, J., Thomas, S. and Baeyens, F. (2001) Associative learning of likes and dislikes: a review of 25 years of research on human evaluative conditioning. *Psychological Bulletin* 127, 853–869.

Desor, J.A., Maller, O. and Turner, R.E. (1973) Taste in acceptance of sugars by human infants. *Journal of Comparative and Physiological Psychology* 84, 496–501.

Drewnowski, A. (1998) Energy density, palatability and satiety: implications for weight control. *Nutrition Reviews* 56, 347–353.

Durlach, P.J., Elliman, N.A. and Rogers, P.J. (2002) Drinking while thirsty can lead to conditioned increases in consumption. *Appetite* 39, 119–125.

Elizalde, G. and Sclafani, A. (1988) Starch-based conditioned flavor preferences in rats: influence of taste, calories and CS–US delay. *Appetite* 11, 179–200.

Fedorchak, P.M. (1997) The nature and strength of caloric conditioning. In: Bouton, M.E. and Fanselow, M.S. (eds) *Learning, Motivation and Cognition: The Functional Behaviourism of Robert C. Bolles*. American Psychological Association, Washington, DC, pp. 255–269.

Fedorchak, P.M. and Bolles, R.C. (1987) Hunger enhances the expression of calorie-but not taste-mediated conditioned flavour preferences. *Journal of Experimental Psychology. Animal Behavior Processes* 13, 73–79.

Field, A.P. and Davey, G.C.L. (1999) Re-evaluating evaluative conditioning: an exemplar comparison model of evaluative conditioning effects. *Journal of Experimental Psychology. Animal Behavior Processes* 25, 211–224.

Garcia, J. and Koelling, R.A. (1966) Relation of cue to consequence in avoidance learning. *Psychonomic Science* 4, 123–124.

Garcia, J., Ervin, F.R. and Koelling, R.A. (1966) Learning with prolonged delay of reinforcement. *Psychonomic Science* 5, 121–122.

Gibson, E.L. and Wardle, J. (2003) Energy density predicts preferences for fruit and vegetables in 4-year-old children. *Appetite* 41, 97–98.

Gibson, E.L., Wainwright, C.J. and Booth, D.A. (1995) Disguised protein in lunch after low-protein breakfast conditions food-flavor preferences dependent on recent lack of protein intake. *Physiology & Behavior* 58, 363–371.

Harris, J.A., Gorissen, M.C., Bailey, G.K. and Westbrook, R.F. (2000) Motivational state regulates the content of learned flavor preferences. *Journal of Experimental Psychology. Animal Behavior Processes* 26, 15–30.

Hladik, C.M., Pasquet, P. and Simmen, B. (2002) New perspectives on taste and primate evolution: the dichotomy in gustatory coding for perception of beneficent versus noxious substances as supported by correlations among human thresholds. *American Journal of Physical Anthropology* 117, 342–348.

Johnson, S.L., McPhee, L. and Birch, L.L. (1991) Conditioned preferences: young children prefer flavors associated with high dietary fat. *Physiology & Behavior* 50, 1245–1251.

Kalat, J.W. and Rozin, P. (1973) 'Learned safety' as a mechanism in long-delay taste-aversion learning in rats. *Journal of Comparative and Physiological Psychology* 83, 198–207.

Kern, D.L., McPhee, L., Fisher, J., Johnson, S. and Birch, L.L. (1993) The postingestive consequences of fat condition preferences for flavors associated with high dietary fat. *Physiology & Behavior* 54, 71–76.

Kochli, A., Rakover, Y. and Lesham, M. (2002) Perinatal dehydration correlates with adolescent salt preference. *Neural Plasticity* 9, 94.

Leshem, M., Abutbul, A. and Eilon, R. (1999) Exercise increases the preference for salt in humans. *Appetite* 32, 251–260.

Logue, A.W. (1979) Taste aversion and the generality of the laws of learning. *Psychological Bulletin* 86, 276–296.

Looy, H. and Weingarten, H.P. (1991) Effects of metabolic state on sweet taste reactivity in humans depend on underlying hedonic response profile. *Chemical Senses* 16, 123–130.

Looy, H., Callaghan, S. and Weingarten, H.P. (1992) Hedonic response of sucrose likers and dislikers to other gustatory stimuli. *Physiology & Behavior* 52, 219–225.

Lubow, R.E. and Moore, A.U. (1959) Latent inhibition: the effect of nonreinforced preexposure to the conditioned stimulus. *Journal of Comparative and Physiological Psychology* 52, 415–419.

Lucas, F. and Sclafani, A. (1989) Flavor preferences conditioned by intragastric fat infusions in rats. *Physiology & Behavior* 46, 403–412.

Myers, K.P. and Sclafani, A. (2001a) Conditioned enhancement of flavor evaluation reinforced by intragastric glucose. *Physiology & Behavior* 74, 495–505.

Myers, K.P. and Sclafani, A. (2001b) Conditioned enhancement of flavor evaluation reinforced by intragastric glucose. I. Intake acceptance and preference analysis. *Physiology & Behavior* 74, 481–493.

Pliner, P. (1982) The effect of mere exposure on liking for edible substances. *Appetite* 3, 283–290.

Ramirez, I. (1994) Flavor preferences conditioned with starch in rats. *Animal Learning & Behavior* 22, 181–187.

Reiss, S. and Wagner, A.R. (1972) CS habituation produces a 'latent inhibition' effect but no active conditioned inhibition. *Learning and Motivation* 3, 237–245.

Richardson, N.J., Rogers, P.J. and Elliman, N.A. (1996) Conditioned flavour preferences reinforced by caffeine consumed after lunch. *Physiology & Behavior* 60, 257–263.

Rogers, P.J., Richardson, N.J. and Elliman, N.A. (1995) Overnight caffeine abstinence and negative reinforcement of preference for caffeine-containing drinks. *Psychopharmacology* 120, 457–462.

Rogers, P.J., Prescott, A.P., Humphrey, C.L. and Hayward, R.C. (2002) Conditioned flavour preferences reinforced by nicotine. *Behavioral Pharmacology* 13, 502.

Rozin, P. (1977) The significance of learning in food selection: some biology, psychology and sociology of science. In: Barker, L.M., Best, M. and Domjan, M. (eds) *Learning Mechanisms in Food Selection*. Baylor University Press, Waco, Texas, pp. 557–589.

Rozin, P., Wrzesniewski, A. and Byrnes, D. (1998) The elusiveness of evaluative conditioning. *Learning and Motivation* 29, 397–415.

Sclafani, A. (1999) Macronutrient-conditioned flavor preferences. In: Berthoud, H.-R. and Seeley, R.J. (eds) *Neural Control of Macronutrient Selection*. CRC Press, Boca Raton, Florida, pp. 93–106.

Sclafani, A. (2002) Flavor preferences conditioned by sucrose depend upon training and testing methods: two-bottle tests revisited. *Physiology & Behavior* 76, 633–644.

Sclafani, A. and Nissenbaum, J.W. (1988) Robust conditioned flavor preference produced by intragastric starch infusions in rats. *American Journal of Physiology* 255, R672–R675.

Seligman, M.E.P. (1970) On the generality of the laws of learning. *Psychological Review* 77, 406–418.

Shi, P., Zhang, J., Yang, H. and Zhang, Y.P. (2003) Adaptive diversification of bitter taste receptor genes in mammalian evolution. *Molecular Biology and Evolution* 20, 805–814.

Smith, J.C. and Roll, D.L. (1967) Trace conditioning with X-rays as the aversive stimulus. *Psychonomic Science* 9, 11–12.

Solomon, R.S. and Corbit, J.D. (1974) An opponent–process theory of motivation: 1. Temporal dynamics of affect. *Psychological Review* 81, 119–145.

Steiner, J.E. (1979) Human facial expressions in response to taste and smell stimulation. In: Reese, H.W. and Lipsitt L.P. (eds) *Advances in Child Development and Behavior*, Vol. 13. Academic Press, New York, pp. 257–295.

Stevenson, R.J. (2003) Preexposure to the stimulus elements, but not training to detect them, retards odour–taste learning. *Behavioural Processes* 61, 13–25.

Stevenson, R.J. and Boakes, R.A. (2004) Sweet and sour smells: the acquisition of taste-like qualities by odors. In: Spence, C., Calvert, G. and Stein, B. (eds) *Handbook of Multisensory Processes*. MIT Press, Boston, Massachusetts, pp. 69–84.

Stevenson, R.J. and Yeomans, M.R. (1995) Does exposure enhance liking for the chilli burn? *Appetite* 24, 107–120.

Stevenson, R.J., Prescott, J. and Boakes, R.A. (1995) The acquisition of taste properties by odors. *Learning and Motivation* 26, 433–455.

Stevenson, R.J., Boakes, R.A. and Prescott, J. (1998) Changes in odor sweetness resulting from implicit learning of a simultaneous odor–sweetness association: an example of learned synesthesia. *Learning and Motivation* 29, 113–132.

Stevenson, R.J., Boakes, R.A. and Wilson, J.P. (2000) Resistance to extinction of conditioned odour perceptions: evaluative conditioning is not unique. *Journal of Experimental Psychology. Learning, Memory, and Cognition* 26, 423–440.

Stubbs, R.J. and Whybrow, S. (2004) Energy density, diet composition and palatability: influences on overall food energy intake in humans. *Physiology & Behavior* 81, 755–764.

Stubenitsky, K., Zandstra, L.H., Elliman, N.A., de Graaf, C., Smit, H.J., Rogers, P.J. and Mela, D.J. (2000) No development of energy-based conditioned flavour preferences in human adults under realistic eating conditions. *Appetite* 35, 311.

Takamata, A., Mack, G.W., Gillen, C.M. and Nadel, E.R. (1994) Sodium appetite, thirst, and body fluid regulation in humans during rehydration without sodium replacement. *American Journal of Physiology* 266, R1493–R1502.

Tinley, E.M., Yeomans, M.R. and Durlach, P.J. (2003) Caffeine does not reinforce conditioned flavour liking in fully abstinent caffeine consumers. *Psychopharmacology* 166, 416–423.

Tinley, E.M., Durlach, P.J. and Yeomans, M.R. (2004) How habitual caffeine consumption and dose influence flavour preference conditioning with caffeine. *Physiology & Behavior* 82, 317–324.

Wald, N. and Leshem, M. (2003) Salt conditions a flavor preference or aversion after exercise depending on NaCl dose and sweat loss. *Appetite* 40, 277–284.

Yeomans, M.R. (1996) Palatability and the microstructure of eating in humans: the appetiser effect. *Appetite* 27, 119–133.

Yeomans, M.R., Spetch, H. and Rogers, P.J. (1998) Conditioned flavour preference negatively reinforced by caffeine in human volunteers. *Psychopharmacology* 137, 401–409.

Yeomans, M.R., Jackson, A., Lee, M.D., Steer, B., Tinley, E.M., Durlach, P. and Rogers, P.J. (2000a) Acquisition and extinction of flavour preferences conditioned by caffeine in humans. *Appetite* 35, 131–141.

Yeomans, M.R., Jackson, A., Lee, M.D., Nesic, J.S. and Durlach, P.J. (2000b) Expression of flavour preferences conditioned by caffeine is dependent on caffeine deprivation state. *Psychopharmacology* 150, 208–215.

Yeomans, M.R., Ripley, T., Lee, M.D. and Durlach, P.J. (2001) No evidence for latent learning of liking for flavours conditioned by caffeine. *Psychopharmacology* 157, 172–179.

Yeomans, M.R., Mobini, S., Elliman, T.D., Walker, H.C. and Stevenson, R.J. (2006) Hedonic and sensory characteristics of odours conditioned by pairing with tastants. *Journal of Experimental Psychology: Animal Behavior Processes* (in press).

Zajonc, R.B. (1968) Attitudinal effects of mere exposure. *Journal of Personality and Social Psychology* 9, 1–27.

Zellner, D.A., Rozin, P., Aron, M. and Kulish, C. (1983) Conditioned enhancement of human's liking for flavor by pairing with sweetness. *Learning and Motivation* 14, 338–350.

7 Mood, Emotions and Food Choice

E.L. GIBSON

Clinical and Health Psychology Research Centre, School of Human and Life Sciences, Roehampton University, Whitelands College, Holybourne Avenue, London SW15 4JD, UK

Introduction

A link between food and mood has been espoused by every self-respecting sage for millennia; now, from recent research, some potential mechanisms are emerging. There is no doubt that mood and food choice interact with each other: the relationship can be anything from strong and overt to subtle and subconscious, and is more than just simple cause and effect. For example, mood could influence food choice via a change of appetite, or by changing other behaviour that constrains or alters food availability. On the other hand, alteration of mood may be an outcome – perhaps even consciously sought – of food choice. That is more akin to a psychological conceptualization of food choice, and appetite in general, as being motivated by anticipation of shifting internal state (nutritional, cognitive or emotional) from current (need) to required (ideal/sated) state (Booth, 1994). Thus, mood could provide an internal stimulus or state that elicits a beneficial, e.g. corrective, food choice. Furthermore, eating a particular food, or combination, can alter mood via sensory (including hedonic) effects, associated social context, cognitive expectations, changes in appetite or nutritional modulation of brain function, for example. These possibilities are considered in more detail below. First, we need to consider what is meant by mood and emotion.

What are Mood and Emotion?

Mood is typically characterized as a psychological arousal state lasting at least several minutes and usually longer, with dimensions related to energy, tension and pleasure (hedonic tone; Thayer, 1989; Matthews and Deary, 1998; Reid and Hammersley, 1999). Moods have been distinguished from emotions, in that

emotions can be defined as short-term affective responses to appraisals of particular stimuli, situations or events having reinforcing potential, whereas moods
may appear and persist in the absence of obvious stimuli, and may be more
covert to observers (Matthews and Deary, 1998; Rolls, 1999). However, this
distinction has been more theoretical than empirical (Fredrickson, 2004).

In this chapter, both moods and emotions are considered in relation to food,
since there is evidence for involvement of both types of affect, and instances
where the distinction is unclear – research on food and mood lags behind
neuropsychological research on mood and emotion (Small *et al.*, 2001). The
term 'affect' is meant here to refer to either mood or emotion. Food may alter or
induce emotions by rapid sensory stimulation or relief of hunger, or as a result of
cognitive appraisal of the change in internal state or its expectation, but can also
alter mood by slower changes in brain chemistry.

Thayer (1989) proposed the existence of two main mood dimensions, energetic and tense arousal. The sleep–wakefulness circadian rhythm is considered a
prime example of the energetic arousal dimension, with the peak in this arousal
cycle usually observed in the late morning (Smith, 1992). The tense arousal
dimension is conceived of as representing mood changes in response to perceived threats, in concert with 'fight or flight' responses or behavioural inhibition
as appropriate. The dimensions do not occur in isolation, but rather can interact;
so for example, moderate tension can be energizing, whereas high tension can
reduce energy. Other mood concepts can be characterized in terms of these
dimensions: for instance, positive affect and pleasant mood are related to low
tension and higher energy, whereas negative affect, unpleasant mood, depression and anxiety are related to high tension and lower energy. Research in this
area relating nutrition and mood has employed a variety of measures of mood,
but largely based on either analogue rating scales or adjective check lists.

However, Reid and Hammersley (1999), in reviewing the effects of carbohydrates on arousal, argued that recent theories of mood and emotion suggest
that mood changes do not necessarily follow from changes in neurophysiological
arousal. Instead, the affective significance of a given level of arousal will depend
on the person's current subjective and motivational state. The interaction of
physiology, arousal and emotion may also be moderated by personality factors,
which have even been shown to influence effects of stress on taste perception (Dess and Edelheit, 1998). In particular, the major personality traits of
extraversion and neuroticism are known to moderate mood changes (Matthews
and Deary, 1998), and to interact with mood and responses to emotional stimuli
(Canli *et al.*, 2004). Thus, personality and cognitive factors could substantially
modulate any impact of physiological change induced by food. It will be seen
that these concerns might explain some of the variability in findings, and need to
be borne in mind when interpreting results in this area.

General Effects of Hunger and Eating on Mood

The most common way in which food can affect behaviour is the change in
mood and arousal that occurs from before to after eating a meal. This might

sound trite, but it is not trivial: this general meal effect is probably the most reli- able example of an effect of diet on behaviour. Many animals, including human beings, tend to be aroused, alert and even irritable when hungry. This encour- ages their search for food. However, their mental efforts can become distracted by this task, to the detriment of other behaviours. After eating a satiating meal, we and other animals typically become calm, lethargic and may even sleep. Nutrient absorption is rapidly detected by the brain, as afferent information is conveyed by the vagus nerve from the gut and liver. The potential influence of this internal information route on emotional behaviour is beginning to be acknowledged (Zagon, 2001): indeed, artificial vagal stimulation is being devel- oped as a treatment for depression (George *et al.*, 2002). When mood and eat- ing context were randomly sampled ten times a day for a week, eating a meal was more likely to result in a positive mood than either a neutral or negative mood (Macht *et al.*, 2004), at least in the short term. Indeed, it would be an awkward, not to say unsustainable life if eating mainly resulted in bad moods.

Nevertheless, even this seemingly straightforward phenomenon can be dis- torted, and can vary across individuals and situations. The impact of a food or drink will depend on the person's initial state, expectations and attitudes. For example, thirsty people improved their vigilance when allowed to drink water, whereas when people were asked to drink when not thirsty, their performance deteriorated (Rogers *et al.*, 2001). One might predict a similar result for eating when hungry versus full, although this comparison does not appear to have been studied.

Meal size, timing and habit

Numerous experiments have shown that manipulation of the structure of meals results in variation in postprandial changes in mood and mental function. One obvious facet of meals that has been investigated is what is eaten, i.e. nutrient composition and/or sensory aspects, which is discussed below.

Besides any nutritional effects, two other influences are known to interact with attempts to measure dietary effects on behaviour. First, most people are very habitual in their choice of food and size and timing of meals. As a result, they have learned a set of beliefs and expectations about the impact of their habitual dietary regime. Therefore, particularly in short-term tests, these expectations may override or mitigate physiological changes. Dietary experiences that differ from a person's habitual eating could lead their behaviour to change through cognitive rather than (or as well as) physiological influences. For example, whilst there is some evidence that larger meals may reduce arousal and impair vigilance, this effect can depend on the meal size being different from that habitually consumed (Craig, 1986). In fact, meal size per se seems to have little impact on mood unless too little is eaten (Gibson and Green, 2002), whereas Macht (1996) found that a larger meal prevented deterioration in mood in people being stressed by noise.

Secondly, there are circadian rhythms and sleep–wake cycles in arousal and performance, which complicate interpretation of meal effects. As mentioned, there is a tendency for levels of arousal and alertness to rise during the morning, reaching a peak near midday. Some evidence suggests that breakfast may help to control this arousal, so that attention can be successfully focused on the task in hand. Conversely, omitting breakfast may increase autonomic reactivity (Conners and Blouin, 1983), leading to less focused attention, especially when associated with increasing hunger. This effect could explain one finding that children without breakfast showed better recall of objects to which they had not been asked to attend (Pollitt et al., 1983): such attention to irrelevant stimuli is also known to occur with increased anxiety (Dusek et al., 1976).

The drop in arousal and ability to sustain attention after the midday meal has been termed the 'post-lunch dip' (Folkard and Monk, 1985). However, this may not simply be an effect of eating, because vigilance has also been found to decline from late morning to early afternoon in subjects not eating lunch (Smith and Miles, 1986). That is, there is an underlying circadian rhythm that is confounded with the effect of a midday meal. In fact, using noise stress to arouse subjects during a midday meal prevented any decline in performance due to the meal (Smith and Miles, 1986). It has also been shown that the more anxious one is feeling prior to lunch, the less one will experience any post-lunch dip. In support of this, studies have found that subjects scoring highly on a personality measure of extraversion and low on neuroticism were more likely to be affected by post-lunch dip (Craig et al., 1981; Smith and Miles, 1986). Thus, stable extraverts may be more easily calmed by lunch but their post-lunch performance can suffer. This is in line with recent evidence that brain activity related to working memory interacts with emotional state and these personality traits (Gray and Braver, 2002). These are examples of the importance of individual differences and context in predicting meal effects.

Sensation, Expectation and Mood

The sensation of sweetness is innately pleasant, whereas some other sensations derived from tasting food are innately aversive, such as bitterness and sourness. It is relevant that, together with evidence of ingestion or rejection, these conclusions depend on observing facial expressions in newborn babies that we adults interpret as reflecting positive or negative emotions. Pleasure and displeasure are of course fundamental concepts underlying motivation to choose to eat particular foods. However, it is important to recognize that sensory qualities of foods do not have invariant hedonic attributes; rather, these are dependent on context and experience. Within a given context, of course, one can make predictions about the hedonic reactions to different foods or tastes, but even then there will be variation due to differential experience and attitudes among the eaters (Booth, 1994).

Expectations about food are obviously personal predictions of the consequences of eating a food, which depend on experience with that food in a variety of contexts. Such expectations are not just impotently 'all in the mind', but can have real influence on both behaviour and physiology. For instance, at the group level, labelling a drink of glucose solution as placebo prevented any beneficial effects of the glucose load on performance (Green et al., 2001); at the individual level, Melanson *et al.* (1999) found that changes in plasma glucose after a zero-energy aspartame-sweetened drink (i.e. no glucose was ingested) were correlated with perceived sweetness of the drink – falls in blood glucose being associated with greater perceived sweetness.

Emotional responses to food may be at least as sensitive to expectations. In a laboratory study, Macht *et al.* (2003) asked women to rate various emotions immediately after eating small amounts (5 g) of nine different foods, three being low in energy, three medium and three high in energy (in counterbalanced order). Intensity of negative moods (sad, ashamed, anxious, sleepy) increased with increasing energy density of the foods, and more so for overweight than normal-weight women. Moreover, medium- and high-energy foods were rated less healthy and more dangerous than low-energy foods. These effects were independent of rated pleasantness of the foods. It is most likely that these effects were psychological rather than physiological in nature, given the small amounts of food eaten and the immediacy of the ratings. The negative effects of the high-energy foods presumably reflect concerns about their impact on health and weight gain. Interestingly, though, stronger increases in negative mood were seen for women reporting greater tendencies to eat in response to emotional state. This would imply that any reinforcing effect of eating such foods on prior emotional state must occur during rather than after eating – a beneficial effect of a real meal would not have been detected by this design.

These results are similar to the finding that self-identified chocolate 'addicts' felt more guilty after eating chocolate than did a control group (Macdiarmid and Hetherington, 1995). The chocolate 'addicts' also reported lower positive and higher negative affect prior to eating. By contrast, in healthy men, experimental induction of sadness decreased appetite, whereas when cheerful, chocolate tasted more pleasant and stimulating, and more of it was eaten (Macht *et al.*, 2002). This gender difference is likely to be confounded by dispositional differences (see section after next).

Nevertheless, there is evidence that sweet, and perhaps fatty, tastes or sensations in particular may have an ability to influence mood, at least in some individuals some of the time, and might be a key determinant of affective influences on food choice. This evidence is considered in the next sections.

Sweet Taste, Reward, Distress, Analgesia and Neural Substrates

Eating food when hungry is satisfying a fundamental drive, like breathing or breeding. Inevitably, this will involve activation of brain pathways of 'reward', which might be experienced as positive affect, so reinforcing approach to, and contact with, a goal such as a food source. Research has shown that eating activates neural substrates in a similar manner to drugs of abuse, although with important differences of degree. The most evidenced neural substrates of reward are the dopamine, opioid and benzodiazepine/γ-aminobutyric acid neurotransmitter systems. Recent evidence supports a possible dissociation of these systems, such that dopamine may principally underlie motivational aspects of eating ('wanting'), whereas opioid and benzodiazepine systems may mediate hedonic evaluation of food sensory stimuli ('liking'; Berridge and Robinson, 1998).

Endogenous opioid neuropeptides are released during stress, and are known to be important for adaptive effects such as resistance to pain. They are also involved in motivational and reward processes in eating behaviour, such as stimulation of appetite by palatable foods (Doyle et al., 1993; Mercer and Holder, 1997a). One might therefore expect a link between opioid action, mood and food choice. Perhaps the best evidence for opioid involvement in an interaction between mood, stress and eating is the finding that, in animals and human infants, the ingestion of sweet and fatty foods, including milk, alleviates crying and other behavioural signs of distress (Blass et al., 1989). Recently, this effect was shown to depend on sweet taste rather than calories, as non-nutritive sweeteners also reduce crying (Barr et al., 1999). This stress-reducing effect of sweet tastants can be blocked by opioid antagonists, and opioid analgesia can be enhanced by chronic intake of sucrose solutions or fat (Blass et al., 1989; Kanarek et al., 1991; D'Anci et al., 1997). However, there is also evidence, in rats and humans, that analgesic effects of sweet-tasting solutions may be mediated by cholinergic mechanisms (Kanarek and Carrington, 2004).

In human neonates, sucking on a pacifier (dummy) is also very effective in reducing signs of pain or 'spontaneous' crying (hence the name; Carbajal et al., 1999). Happily, so is brief exposure to breast milk (Upadhyay et al., 2004). Interestingly, as babies grow older, sweet taste becomes less effective at calming than does pacifier-sucking, which might reflect a maturational separation of taste and emotion (Blass and Camp, 2003), or a difference in opportunities to learn the instrumental emotional value of the two experiences. Furthermore, the extent to which adults (whether rat or human) retain an analgesic effect of sweet taste remains controversial, but this might again reflect variation in retention of this phenomenon through a combination of predisposition and experience, as well as methodological differences. Perceived palatability (liking) may be important, as well as gender and duration and timing of exposure (Mercer and Holder, 1997b; Kanarek and Carrington, 2004). Using the cold pressor test (holding the hand in very cold water), pain threshold latency (but not tolerance) was extended by concurrent sweet taste in 8- to 11-year-old children (Miller et al., 1994). However, in adults, pain tolerance, not threshold, was increased by prior tasting of a sucrose solution, although only in participants with lower blood pressure: those with higher blood pressure were already more tolerant (whether for peripheral vascular or more complex neural reasons is unclear) when tasting only water, so a ceiling effect may have prevented further tolerance induced by sweetness (Lewkowski et al., 2003). Predictors of maturational differences in these effects remain a fertile area for research.

It remains speculative to conclude that adults select sweet, fatty, palatable foods for opioid-mediated relief of stress. Also, such behaviour would need to be explained in the context of stress itself enhancing endogenous opioid release. Nevertheless, it is intriguing to note that stress reinstates opiate drug abuse in humans and rats in which the habit had been extinguished (Shaham et al., 2000). Moreover, repeated intake of a sweet, fatty, energy-dense food was found to down-regulate an opioid pathway (ventral striatum) involved in food reward in rats, suggesting an adaptation to chronic activation of this appetitive pathway (Kelley *et al.*, 2003).

Similarly, over-consumption of palatable energy-dense (e.g. high-fat, high-sugar) food may down-regulate dopamine (D2) receptors, since their availability in the striatum has been shown to be inversely correlated to body mass index (Wang *et al.*, 2001), and a questionnaire measure of 'sensitivity to reward' was found to be less in obese than in overweight people (Davis *et al.*, 2004). This latter finding was interpreted as suggesting that chronic overeating may eventually induce a more anhedonic state (i.e. less sensitivity to reward), although this measure was also correlated to emotional eating. However, it seems possible that obese respondents may report less pleasure from various activities as a result of social stigma and physical disability. Rather, Wang *et al.* (2001) argued that their findings were in line with a neurochemical predisposition that may cause over-eating of palatable foods so as to enhance dopamine release. In support of this, energy-dense snack food appears to reinforce greater effort to obtain it in obese than non-obese women (Saelens and Epstein, 1996), and young children of obese parents showed greater 'enjoyment of food', as well as higher preference for high-fat energy-dense foods, than did the offspring of non-obese parents (Wardle *et al.*, 2001). It may also be relevant that binge eating, and other eating disorders, are associated with greater risk of substance abuse, as well as susceptibility to negative affect (Yanovski *et al.*, 1993): dopamine also mediates stress sensitivity and depression (Pani *et al.*, 2000).

Negative Affect, Comfort Eating and Food Choice

There has been a longstanding interest in the relationship between emotions and eating behaviour in human beings. Much of this derived from early psychosomatic and psychoanalytic clinical models of overeating and obesity, at a time when obese patients were relatively scarce and often treated in therapy (Rand and Stunkard, 1978): this contrasts markedly with the current situation in the USA and UK, where obesity afflicts almost a quarter of the adult population (York *et al.*, 2004). These models were based on the notion that obese people may overeat by confusing emotional arousal with hunger and/or seeking comfort or distraction from emotional distress by eating (Schachter *et al.*, 1968; Bruch, 1974; see Chapter 20). These ideas became less popular when, in the 1980s and 1990s, studies designed to induce negative affect, e.g. using frightening films or ego-threatening challenges, found different effects on eating depending on the level of dietary restraint (the conscious attempt to restrict food intake; Heatherton *et al.*, 1991). However, more recent evidence suggests that restrained and emotional eating may have been conflated by some rather muddled psychometrics (Oliver *et al.*, 2000; Williams *et al.*, 2002; see discussion under 'Dietary restraint, emotional eating and stress'). This, together with the neurochemical evidence discussed in the previous section, has contributed to a resurgence of interest in the role of negative affect and emotional eating as predictors of problematic eating and poor control of weight (Waters *et al.*, 2001; Chua *et al.*, 2004; Fulkerson *et al.*, 2004).

A related area of study, that of the impact of stress on eating, has emerged in part from animal studies of psychopathology, especially depression (Robbins and Fray, 1980; Willner *et al.*, 1998), as well as the aforementioned studies testing effects of negative affect on eating. Most of this work addresses whether stress alters overall food intake, rather than food choice, although some evidence supports a predilection for sweet taste in depression or during chronic stress (Wardle and Gibson, 2002). Therefore, this chapter concentrates on studies that shed light on any relationship between stress, emotion and food choice, or at least specific nutrient or dietary effects, rather than simply overall changes in intake.

Naturalistic studies of stress and food choice

Naturally occurring stressful circumstances can provide a predictable context in which to study stress-related variations in diet. Examples include examinations or periods of high workload. It should be borne in mind that the nature of the stressor may determine the findings. The animal literature suggests that physical, more prolonged and uncontrollable stressors might be more likely to suppress eating, whereas brief arousing and/or psychosocial stressors might elicit overeating (Robbins and Fray, 1980). However, it is obviously difficult to study effects of severe stressors for ethical reasons, and grief or family life stress cannot be accurately modelled, only surveyed.

Also, in real-world stressful situations, there will often be other consequences of stress beyond the emotional and physiological domain which may not be under the control of the stressed individual. For instance, stress at work may include increased time pressure and demands on attention. These changes could reduce the available range of food to a person no matter what they actually felt like eating. Such factors may also affect choice in favour of foods that could be rapidly procured and eaten, i.e. from a pragmatic rather than sensory perspective.

McCann *et al.* (1990) examined the effects of variation in workload on food intake and serum lipids with a small group of female office workers. The workers reported a higher energy intake and a higher percentage of energy as fat in two high workload periods compared with the normal work period. Michaud *et al.* (1990) also found higher energy intake from 24 h food records for a day of examination, compared with a month later, among 15- to 19-year-old high school students. Increased academic workload and negative affect were associated with a less healthy diet in a study of health behaviours among university students (Weidner *et al.*, 1996). Conversely, in another study, positive affect during exam periods was associated with improved diet (Griffin *et al.*, 1993).

Two epidemiological surveys of adolescents support a relationship between stress, depression and unhealthy changes in eating habits. In US teenagers, depressive symptoms were associated with perceived barriers to healthy eating, meal skipping and more disordered eating, although the only significant change in diet appeared to be increased consumption of soft drinks in more depressed school children (Fulkerson *et al.*, 2004). In a study of health behaviours in 11- to 13-year-old school children in London, greater perceived stress was associated with more fatty food intake, less fruit and vegetable intake, more snacking, and a reduced likelihood of daily breakfast consumption (Cartwright *et al.*, 2003).

Lowe and Fisher (1983) analysed mood ratings prior to eating, over 13 days, and found that overweight women ate more snacks during negative than positive moods. Similarly, when nurses and teachers completed diaries of their diet and stress levels, intake of high-fat 'fast foods' was found to be greater during high stress than during low stress periods (Steptoe *et al.*, 1998). In a Finnish population-based study, 'stress-driven eaters' ate more energy-dense high-fat foods and had higher body mass indices (Laitinen *et al.*, 2002).

Bellisle *et al.* (1990) compared the midday-meal intake on the day before a surgical operation with intake at a comparable time of day a few weeks later in 12 middle-aged men, and found no difference either in energy intake or dietary composition. However, the men showed considerable variation, ranging from one man eating 125% more on the pre-surgery day to another who ate 53% less.

A few studies have included non-stressed control groups, so as to disconfound high and low stress periods from sequential changes in the environment unrelated to stress. This helps to exclude the possibility that the dietary changes associated with the high stress periods were the result of different foods being available at the school or workplace, rather than the individual's choices in the low and high stress periods. In a study of examination stress which included a control group, Pollard *et al.* (1995) found no overall nutritional difference between students taking examinations and others for whom there were no examinations scheduled at that time. O'Donnell *et al.* (1987) also failed to find significant differences in the diets of 13 medical students between 3 months and 1 week prior to exams, or compared with a non-student control group. Even so, their plasma cholesterol and catecholamines were raised during the stressful pre-exam week: stress is well known to produce unfavourable changes in blood lipids independently of diet (Brindley *et al.*, 1993). Macht *et al.* (2005) compared changes in emotional state and eating behaviour of 22 students, 3–4 weeks and 3–4 days before an exam, with a control group, using pagers to cue random sampling of mood and eating. The students awaiting an exam had increased negative affect and decreased positive affect, together with an increase in reported eating for distraction. However, no differences were found for food intake or choice. In a recent study in which time sequence was not a confounding factor, high work load in department store workers was associated with higher fat, sugar and total energy intakes, but only in people who habitually restrained their food intake (Wardle *et al.*, 2000); emotional eating was not assessed but might be an important mediator (see next section).

On balance, these naturalistic studies provide some evidence that stress or negative affect can result in an increase in unhealthy food choices, if not an increase in overall intake. The inconsistency of these findings is reflected in results of surveys of the influence of stress or negative affect on eating behaviour in non-clinical populations. So far as overall food intake is concerned, surveys of self-reported changes in eating behaviour reveal a bidirectional effect across the samples, but consistency within individuals. Thus, 38–72% of sampled populations reported eating less when stressed, whereas slightly fewer, 28–50%, reported eating more, with a minority in each survey believing stress did not alter their food intake (Willenbring et al., 1986; Stone and Brownell, 1994; Weinstein et al., 1997; Oliver and Wardle, 1999).

There is also evidence to suggest that a pattern of change in food choice under stress might be expected. Oliver and Wardle (1999) asked about perceived changes in intake of a number of specific foods or food categories during stress. This revealed an interesting pattern of effects of stress, which was partly independent of whether participants were grouped as reporting eating more, the same or less overall when stressed. That is, sweets and chocolate were reported to be eaten more under stress by all groups, even those eating less overall; conversely, intakes of fruit and vegetables, and meat and fish, were reported as less or unchanged under stress in all groups (Fig. 7.1). The changes for the staple

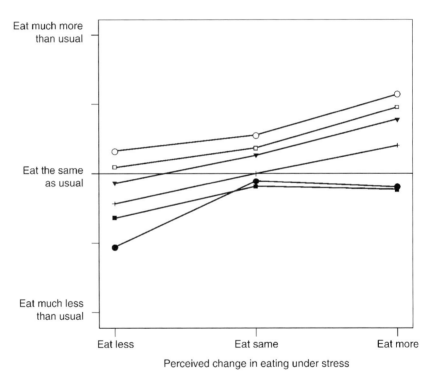

Fig. 7.1. Reported changes in intake of various food categories (○, sweets and chocolate; □, cake and biscuits; ▼, savoury snacks; +, bread; ■, fruit and vegetables; ●, meat and fish) during stress (y-axis) for three groups of people (x-axis): those who perceive eating less overall, those who perceive eating the same overall and those who perceive eating more overall under stress. The non-overlapping lines illustrate a consistent relative pattern in the change in intake under stress for different foods. Note that intake of sweets and chocolate is raised significantly by stress even in the group who perceived their overall intake to be less under stress. Data are from a survey of 212 students. (Adapted from Oliver and Wardle, 1999.)

food, bread, matched the overall group self-perceptions of changes in eating due to stress. These data imply that mechanisms governing effects of stress on food choice may be somewhat separate from those influencing overall appetite under stress, and that foods such as sweets and chocolate may be particularly useful in ameliorating stress.

The next section considers possible psychometric explanations for differences in susceptibility to stress-induced eating.

Dietary restraint, emotional eating and stress

An important question is whether certain psychological or physiological characteristics predispose a person to change their food choice in an unhealthy direction. For example, there was also evidence that those reporting eating more when stressed were more likely to be dieters or restrained eaters (Weinstein *et al.*, 1997; Oliver and Wardle, 1999). This is consistent with a number of experimental studies which were based on the premise that the adaptive response to stress should be reduced appetite and eating, but that the obese, overweight or restrained eaters may be unresponsive to their internal physiological influences on appetite (Rodin, 1981; Craighead and Allen, 1995), or normally dominant cognitive strategies for restraint may be disinhibited or overridden during negative affect or stress (Schachter *et al.*, 1968; Herman and Polivy, 1975). In support of this, Rutledge and Linden (1998) found that incidental snacking during recovery from a stressful task was greatest in subjects showing the least signs of physiological arousal during the task, but this relationship was attenuated among highly cognitively restrained subjects.

Two aspects of this area of research may limit the validity of the findings. First, most studies only report overall food intake, and the food is usually palatable snack food presented as a 'taste test' or as an incidental snack, rather than a meal where substantial food choice is possible. Secondly, dietary restraint was measured in most studies by the Restraint Scale (Herman and Polivy, 1980), which includes the tendency for eating to be disinhibited by emotional states. When separate scales were used to measure restraint and emotional eating (Dutch Eating Behaviour Questionnaire; van Strien *et al.*, 1986), the latter was the better predictor of stress-induced eating (Oliver *et al.*, 2000). That is, Oliver *et al.* (2000) tested the effects of public-speaking stress on intake of a variety of foods from sweet, salty and bland taste categories, and in addition, high- and low-fat examples within those sensory groups. Analysing effects by taste category may be important because stress and mood have been shown to affect taste perception (Amsterdam *et al.*, 1987; Dess and Edelheit, 1998). The food was presented as a buffet-style meal during preparation of the speech task. Stress did not alter overall intake: however, stressed emotional eaters ate more sweet high-fat foods (chocolate and cake) and a more energy-dense meal, than either unstressed emotional eaters or non-emotional eaters in either condition. This supports the survey findings of Oliver and Wardle (1999) that sweet fatty foods such as chocolate may be preferentially sought during stress or negative affect, at least in a subgroup of susceptible individuals.

Emotional eating may underlie previous reports that dietary restraint or female gender predicts stress-induced eating (Grunberg and Straub, 1992; Waters et al., 2001; Chua et al., 2004). Moreover, emotional eaters may be more susceptible to effects of stress: women who ate more from a selection of snack foods after a stressful task also showed the greatest release of the stress-sensitive hormone, cortisol (Epel et al., 2001), and more stress-induced negative affect. These high reactors also showed a preference for sweet foods. So it seems that emotional eaters may be more likely to experience mood disturbance when challenged. Indeed, it has been argued recently that dietary restraint contributes to emotional eating by increasing the likelihood that goals will be violated (Williams et al., 2002). Dietary restraint also seems to contribute to stress-induced eating of sweet fatty foods by women classified as disinhibited eaters (Haynes et al., 2003).

Williams et al. (2002) also found that, unlike emotional eating, dietary restraint per se impairs attention through cognitive resource competition independently of mood. Similarly, other findings suggest that cognitively challenging tasks may elicit eating in restrained eaters by focusing attention on the salient food cues, whilst disrupting 'diet monitoring', with little emotional involvement (Ward and Mann, 2000; Lattimore and Caswell, 2004). By comparison, Wallis and Hetherington (2004) found that highly restrained/low emotional eaters ate more chocolate after both ego-threatening and cognitively demanding tasks, whereas low restraint/high emotional eaters ate more chocolate only after the ego threat.

Thus, restrained and emotional eating are clearly distinguishable: in the former group, stress alters eating via cognitive routes, but stress acts on eating via emotional needs in the latter group.

Meal Composition and Effects of Specific Nutrients

What is it about the properties of less healthy foods that encourages their selection by some people when stressed? The importance of sensory qualities has already been discussed above (section on 'Sweet Taste, Reward, Distress, Analgesia and Neural Substrates'). The present section now considers other possible mechanisms, such as nutritional properties and their influence on brain function related to mood and emotion. By contrast, direct pharmacological manipulation of mood by substances in food, as is often proposed for chocolate for instance, would normally be unlikely for reasons of quantity and availability to the brain (Rogers and Smit, 2000).

Carbohydrate versus protein

The effects on mood of varying the macronutrient composition of meals have been studied extensively. This is largely because of evidence that plasma and brain levels of precursor amino acids for synthesis of monoamine neurotransmitters, strongly implicated in mood disorders, can depend on carbohydrate : protein ratios in the diet (Fernstrom, 1983). Synthesis of the neurotransmitter serotonin (or 5-hydroxy-tryptamine; 5-HT) depends on dietary availability of the precursor essential amino acid, tryptophan (TRP), due to a lack of saturation of the rate-limiting enzyme, tryptophan hydroxylase, which converts TRP to 5-hydroxytryptophan.

An important complication is that TRP competes with several other amino acids, the large neutral, primarily branched-chain, amino acids (LNAA), for the same transport system from blood to brain. If the protein content of a meal is sufficiently low, such as 5% or less total energy as protein, then relatively few amino acids will be absorbed from the food in the gut. At the same time, insulin will stimulate tissue uptake of competing amino acids from the circulation, and the plasma ratio of TRP to those amino acids (TRP : LNAA) will rise, favouring more TRP entry to the brain (Yokogoshi and Wurtman, 1986). Conversely, a high-protein meal, which would be less insulinogenic, results in absorption of large amounts of competing amino acids into the blood, especially the branched-chain amino acids, leucine, isoleucine and valine. On the other hand, TRP is scarce in most protein sources, and is readily metabolized on passage through the liver: thus, the plasma ratio of TRP to competing amino acids falls after a protein-rich meal. Indeed, the protein-induced reduction in plasma TRP ratio often seems to be more marked than any carbohydrate-induced rise (Lieberman *et al.*, 1986; Lyons and Truswell, 1988; Wolever *et al.*, 1988; Christensen and Redig, 1993). Such effects also depend on the interval since, and nutrient content of, the last meal (Fernstrom and Fernstrom, 1995).

This evidence is particularly relevant to dietary effects on mood and arousal, because 5-HT has long been implicated in sleep, as well as affective disorders such as depression and anxiety (Cowen, 1996). There is experimental evidence that people feel more calm and sleepy after snacks or meals rich in carbohydrate but virtually free of protein (an unusual situation) than after protein-rich meals with little carbohydrate (reviewed by Benton, 2002). This is compatible with changes in 5-HT function, but typically these studies did not determine whether this was due to an increase in 5-HT after the carbohydrate-rich meal or a decrease after the protein meal, which could prevent the postprandial sleepiness. Furthermore, adding more than 5 or 6% protein (of total energy) to the carbohydrate meal has been shown to prevent the increased synthesis of central 5-HT, relative to fasted levels, in both rats and people (Fernstrom and Fernstrom, 1995; Benton and Donohoe, 1999). Also, even pure carbohydrate does not appear to induce sleepiness in everyone.

It is notable that chocolate, often chosen during stress, is high in sugar and stimulates insulin release (Brand Miller *et al.*, 2003), but has only 3–6% of energy as protein. Thus, if eaten in sufficient amounts on an empty stomach, chocolate might increase TRP availability to the brain and so enhance 5-HT-mediated mood. However, the mood-enhancing actions recently demonstrated for caffeine and theobromine in chocolate (Smit *et al.*, 2004), together with sensory and social reinforcement, are more probable mechanisms.

Another difficulty in comparing effects of carbohydrate and protein intake is that relative changes in mood and performance might be due to protein-induced raised plasma tyrosine (TYR; Fernstrom and Fernstrom, 1994; Markus *et al.*, 1998), the precursor amino acid for synthesis of the catecholamine neurotransmitters, which also competes with LNAA for entry into the brain. In catecholamine systems where the neurones are firing rapidly, acute physiological increases in brain TYR, e.g. by feeding a high-protein diet, can raise TYR hydroxylation rate and catecholamine turnover (Fernstrom and Fernstrom, 1994). These neurotransmitters – adrenaline, noradrenaline, dopamine – are involved in mood, arousal, attention and motivation. Nevertheless, high-protein meals in human beings do not always raise the plasma TYR : LNAA ratio, depending on nutritional status or time of day, for example (Schweiger et al., 1986a).

Differential effects on performance have been seen with less extreme variations in protein and carbohydrate intake. A lunch of 55% energy as protein and 15% as carbohydrate produced faster responses to peripheral stimuli, but greater susceptibility to distraction, compared with eating the reverse proportions of protein and carbohydrate (Smith et al., 1988). With these protein : carbohydrate ratios, the plasma TRP : LNAA ratio could still be lowered by the protein-rich meal relative to the carbohydrate-rich one (Wurtman et al., 2003). However, mood and sleepiness were not affected by macronutrient composition in that study.

A delay of at least 1 h after eating may be necessary to allow neurotransmitter precursor changes to influence mood and behaviour (Gibson et al., 1999; Wurtman et al., 2003). Earlier effects might be related to changes in glucose availability, vagal afferent signals of nutrient absorption, and secretion of insulin or other hormones.

An interesting question is whether chronic intake of high or low ratios of carbohydrate to protein has any effects on mood: there is some evidence that it might. De Castro (1987) found that, when mood was averaged over 9 days, a high proportion of protein predicted greater depression, whereas a high proportion of carbohydrate predicted less depression. This might reflect changes in 5-HT function: Schweiger et al. (1986b) found that, after 6 weeks on either a high- or low-carbohydrate diet, mood in women had deteriorated on the latter diet and better mood was associated with higher average 24 h plasma TRP : LNAA ratio. In obese women eating their regular diet freely, lower levels of anxiety and depression at baseline predicted greater intake of carbohydrate and less protein over 4 days (Pellegrin et al., 1998).

Effects of dietary fat

Most studies of effects of fat have varied its level with that of carbohydrate while keeping protein constant, so allowing isoenergetic meals. Comparisons have been made for low-fat (e.g. 11–29% of energy as fat), medium-fat (e.g. 45%) and high-fat (e.g. 56–74%) breakfasts, mid-morning snacks and midday meals, as well as intraduodenal infusions of lipid or saline. On balance, high-fat meals appear likely to increase subsequent fatigue and reduce alertness and attention, relative to high-carbohydrate/low-fat meals (Dye et al., 2000; Gibson and Green, 2002). However, there are inconsistencies relating to changes in specific moods and effects of meal timing: for instance, feelings of drowsiness, confusion and uncertainty were found to increase after both low- and high-fat lunches but not after a medium-fat lunch (Lloyd *et al.*, 1994). One possibility is that mood may be adversely affected by meals that differ substantially in macronutrient composition from habitual ones. An alternative is that similar mood effects could be induced (albeit by different mechanisms) by high carbohydrate in one meal and high fat in the other. For example, 1.67 MJ (400 kcal) drinks of pure fat or carbohydrate taken in the morning both increased an objective measure of fatigue relative to a mixed-macronutrient drink, even though the two single-nutrient drinks had opposite effects on plasma TRP : LNAA ratios (Cunliffe *et al.*, 1997).

In many of these studies, the meals were designed to disguise variation in fat level from participants. So, effects on mood may have resulted from discrepancies between subjects' expectations of certain post-ingestive effects and the actual effects that resulted from neurohormonal responses to detection of specific nutrients in the duodenum and liver. This could explain the increase in tension, 90 min post-lunch, with increasing fat intake reported predominantly by female subjects (Lloyd *et al.*, 1994), which might reflect an aversive reaction to (unexpected) fat-related post-ingestive sensations.

Other specific nutrient effects

In principle, food choice could be driven by the need to replenish a particular essential nutrient, such as a vitamin, mineral, fatty acid or amino acid (or at least protein). There is certainly a long history of evidence that animals can learn to select diets for just these reasons (Thibault and Booth, 1999; Gibson, 2001; see Chapter 6). The assumption is that eating a diet that replenishes a nutritional need reinforces liking for the flavours of that diet. Therefore, one might expect that such an experience would be rewarding, and may involve some sense of positive affect or well-being. As most of this research has been conducted in rats, we cannot be sure of their mood state (not that anyone asked). However, there are a few relevant studies in humans, which are now considered.

Essential micronutrients

There is growing interest in a possible effect on mood of a number of essential micronutrients, especially the omega-3 and omega-6 essential fatty acids, B vitamins including thiamine, B_6 and B_{12}, and the essential mineral cofactor selenium (Benton and Donohoe, 1999). However, despite the likelihood that these nutrients can influence brain function, the evidence for their effects on mood via dietary intake remains equivocal (Gibson and Green, 2002; Ness *et al.*, 2003). Furthermore, it is not known whether such micronutrients have any influence on human food choice, although there is an intriguing finding that some dietary preferences of rats are influenced by their ability to sense essential fatty acids on the tongue (Gilbertson *et al.*, 1998).

Protein

Numerous species have been shown capable of learning to choose a good source of protein or an essential amino acid when lacking that nutrient, including

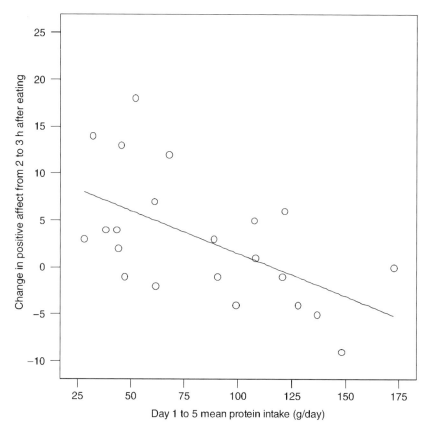

Fig. 7.2. Scattergraph of individual subjects' data for the change in positive affect
from 2 to 3 h after eating a protein-rich meal versus average daily protein intake over
the preceding 5 days when subjects were asked to eat either a high- or low-protein
diet (E.L. Gibson, unpublished data). Lower prior protein intake significantly predicts
a greater rise in positive affect ($r = -0.57$, $P < 0.01$), which might underlie the ability
of a protein meal eaten during protein shortage to reinforce liking for the flavours of
that meal (c.f. Gibson *et al.*, 1995).

human beings (Gibson *et al.*, 1995). However, we have recently reported the
first study of the effects on mood of eating a protein-rich meal when lacking protein (Gibson, 2003). Participants ate a protein-rich lunch after 5 days of either a
low- or high-protein diet. Changes in positive and negative affect, and cortisol,
were measured from before the meal to 3 h afterwards. Not surprisingly, there
was little effect of the meal in those participants already adapted to a high-protein
diet. Negative affect was low before the meal and continued to fall slightly after
the meal. By contrast, in the low-protein diet group there was a sharp rise in positive affect 2 h after starting to eat. Furthermore, this improvement in mood was
positively correlated ($r = 0.77$, $P < 0.01$) with the amount of cortisol secreted in
response to the meal in this group. Because the change in mood occurred more
than an hour after eating, it is not likely to be due to immediate appraisal of the

meal, but rather to some post-ingestive consequence. We believe this increase in well-being is related to the reinforcing effect of eating a good source of protein when it is a needed nutrient (Gibson *et al.*, 1995). This is supported by the finding that the rise in positive affect from 2 to 3 h after the meal was predicted by the average daily protein intake in the preceding 5 days for all participants – lower prior protein intake being associated with a greater rise in mood after the protein-rich meal (Fig. 7.2).

Susceptibility to Mood Enhancement by Diet

How do these findings on effects of nutrients relate to food choice? Presumably, one would need to learn to recognize that certain foods or meals – and hence proportions of macronutrients – would produce particular mood changes in particular situations. These may be beneficial or harmful, but the eater might in principle learn to eat a protein-rich meal when needing to be aroused, or a low-protein carbohydrate-rich meal when needing to be calmed (Gibson and Green, 2002). In healthy people, there seems to be little direct evidence for such corrective food choice, although data are scarce (Møller, 1986; Fernstrom and Fernstrom, 1994). By contrast, in the next section, evidence is presented which suggests that certain people, especially those with emotional disorders, may be susceptible to beneficial effects of specific proportions of macronutrients.

Anxiety, depression and neuroticism

The possibility that a carbohydrate-rich low-protein meal could raise 5-HT function gave rise to the proposal that some depressed people may self-medicate by eating high proportions of carbohydrate (Wurtman and Wurtman, 1989). It was suggested that this would lead to increased 5-HT release in a manner reminiscent of antidepressant drugs, which enhance aspects of 5-HT function by inhibiting removal of 5-HT from the synaptic cleft between nerve cells. For the most part, early behavioural and pharmacological evidence for such a phenomenon was not very convincing (Booth, 1987; Benton and Donohoe, 1999).

Importantly, however, there is evidence that availability of TRP can influence brain function in humans. For instance, feeding a TRP-free diet acutely, which considerably reduced plasma TRP (and so could be expected to impair 5-HT function), induced depressed mood in previously recovered depressives or in people with a genetic predisposition to depression (Heninger *et al.*, 1996), as well as in relatives of patients suffering from bipolar disorder (Quintin *et al.*, 2001). This dietary TRP-depletion method also disrupted performance of healthy volunteers on emotionally meaningful cognitive tasks, similarly to depressed patients (Murphy *et al.*, 2002). Even so, the reduction of TRP achieved by this method is far greater than that seen after eating a high-carbohydrate/ low-protein meal (Gibson and Green, 2002).

Other recent research provides some further support for beneficial effects of carbohydrate-rich/protein-poor meals on mood and emotion in some people.

When participants were divided into high or low stress-prone groups, as defined by a questionnaire measure of neuroticism, carbohydrate-rich/protein-poor meals (which raised plasma TRP : LNAA ratios) prior to a stressful task were found to block task-induced depressive feelings and release of the glucocorticoid stress hormone, cortisol, but only in the high stress-prone group (Markus *et al.*, 1998). This finding was replicated using high- versus low-TRP-containing proteins (α-lactalbumin and casein, respectively; Markus *et al.*, 2000). It was argued that, because stress increases 5-HT activity, the poor stress-coping of this sensitive group might indicate a deficit in 5-HT synthesis that is improved by this dietary intervention. However, despite recent links between genetic differences in 5-HT function and stress-related personality variables, findings on genetic vulnerability of the 5-HT system to stress are currently too variable to draw definite conclusions (Munafo *et al.*, 2003). One possible source of confusion may arise from genetic and phenotypic differences between peripheral and central 5-HT systems (Russo *et al.*, 2003; Walther and Bader, 2003).

Another group which may be sensitive to dietary manipulation of 5-HT function is women suffering from the luteal phase-dependent mood disorder, premenstrual syndrome (PMS). Pharmacological activation of the central 5-HT system appears to reduce PMS dysphoria (Parry, 2001), and women may be more physiologically reactive to stress during the luteal phase (Collins *et al.*, 1985), which could implicate 5-HT. There is some experimental evidence that carbohydrate-rich, protein-poor meals or beverages can improve mood in women with PMS (Wurtman *et al.*, 1989; Sayegh *et al.*, 1995). Thus, food choice during the late luteal phase of the menstrual cycle could, in some women, be motivated by a need to improve their mood, and this might occur through dietary manipulation of 5-HT function. However, evidence for such menstrual cycle-dependent self-medicating food choice is equivocal (Rogers and Smit, 2000).

Hypothalamic–pituitary–adrenal axis, serotonin and depression

There is another link between macronutrient intake, stress and mood. Chronic dysfunction of the stress-sensitive hormone, cortisol, and its controlling hypothalamic–pituitary–adrenal (HPA) axis, is associated with depression and anxiety, as well as abdominal obesity (Björntorp, 2001). Moreover, protein-rich meals that prevent a meal-induced fall in arousal also stimulate release of cortisol in unstressed people, and the size of this effect is correlated positively with poor psychological well-being (Gibson *et al.*, 1999). Over 10 days, a carbohydrate-rich diet was associated with lower average plasma cortisol than a high-protein diet (Anderson *et al.*, 1987). Acutely, a carbohydrate preload, but not protein or fat load, enhances cortisol release during stress (Gonzalez-Bono *et al.*, 2002). So, the contrasting acute and chronic effects of carbohydrate may reflect an adaptive change in HPA axis function.

Raised levels of cortisol in stressed people contribute to abdominal obesity, which in turn promotes insulin resistance (Björntorp, 2001). However, insulin resistance may increase the likelihood that high-carbohydrate/low-protein foods would raise brain TRP and 5-HT levels, because of increased levels of plasma free fatty acids which, by competing for binding to albumin, could result in more unbound TRP in plasma. This might underlie recent findings that insulin-resistant people are less prone to suicide and depression, both of which are believed to be increased by low 5-HT function (Golomb *et al.*, 2002; Lawlor *et al.*, 2003). However, this could also depend on normalization of HPA axis function and cortisolaemia by increased intake of high-carbohydrate energy-dense foods (Dallman *et al.*, 2003), and possibly an improvement in mood. Conversely, high baseline cortisol predicts depression induced by dietary depletion of TRP (Åberg-Wistedt *et al.*, 1998), and stress causes both worsening of mood and reduced TRP : LNAA ratio (Tuiten *et al.*, 1995), which might in part be due to greater diversion of TRP to peripheral metabolism by cortisol (Russo *et al.*, 2003). It may be relevant that patients with seasonal affective disorder show increased insulin resistance in the winter, together with a greater predilection for sugar-rich foods (Kräuchi *et al.*, 1999). Unfortunately, despite this protective effect, insulin resistance is a substantial risk to health by promotion of cardiovascular disease.

Conclusion

Mood can alter food choice, and food choice can alter mood, for a variety of reasons. The view is taken that these phenomena are often two sides of the same behavioural coin. In other words, where the relationship is consistent, predictable, perhaps habitual, this would usually indicate that the effect of one on the other involves some reinforcing outcome. This might be a reduction in negative mood, e.g. by assuaging hunger, or an increase in positive mood through sensory pleasure; or it might be mediated by enhanced resilience under stress, or the removal of aversive physiological symptoms. In stressful 'fight or flight' situations, eating any more than a small amount might have aversive consequences for an unwilling gut. Figure 7.3, with its bidirectional pathways, is an attempt to illustrate how some of this circularity might lead to the sorts of predictable effects that have been discussed here. The direction of an association between mood and food choice, or whether it exists at all, will depend upon an individual's psychological and neurohormonal dispositions.

The point is that the eater will often have learnt, consciously or subconsciously, their best food choice strategy depending on their current mood and the outcome sought. An obvious example is the lifting of mood, or calming of stressed 'nerves', by eating foods having hedonic sensory qualities that elicit pleasure and activation of palliative neural substrates: chocolate may spring to mind for most people, although it has been pointed out that some people suffer later for indulging this particular 'sin' (but they would not be 'addicts' without reinforcement).

Another reinforcing outcome might follow from eating those foods which, via effects on precursor amino acid availability, raise 5-HT synthesis in susceptible people having deficits in serotoninergic influence on stress coping. Intake of other nutrients might also alter mood, although the only case where there is some

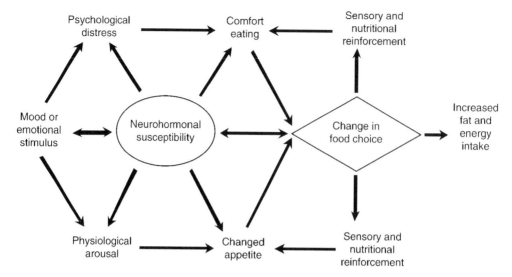

Fig. 7.3. Pathways for susceptibility to mood-dependent unhealthy changes in food choice. The bidirectionality of many arrows indicates the likely circularity in the relationships between food choice and mood. A key point is the role of individual psychological and neurophysiological dispositions in determining these relationships and their outcomes. Negative affect is likely to be associated with unhealthy food choice.

support for a nutrient actually reinforcing subsequent food choice in human beings is when adequate protein is eaten during acute protein insufficiency.

Exceptions to this reinforcement-based model include situations where mood is altered by circumstances that also restrict food choice (having to work late in the office, for example), so the link is not directly mediatory. However, such a mechanism is probably of less interest to readers of this book.

Throughout this chapter, the role of individual differences has been emphasized, particularly in stress-coping, eating attitudes and personality traits. Indeed, much of the evidence on relationships between food choice, stress and negative affect suggests that there may be little point in seeking general phenomena, since relevant behavioural responses are clearly very divergent. Thus, it seems that the interesting questions for the future should try to characterize more reliably the predictive traits, and psychophysiological mechanisms, underlying the link between food choice and mood, so that adverse consequences can be avoided. The era of foods tailored to our personal emotional needs may soon be upon us.

References

Åberg-Wistedt, A., Hasselmark, L., Stain-Malmgren, R., Apéria, B., Kjellman, B.F. and Mathé, A.A. (1998) Serotonergic 'vulnerability' in affective disorder: a study of the tryptophan depletion test and relationships between peripheral and central serotonin indexes in citalopram-responders. *Acta Psychiatrica Scandinavica* 97, 374–380.

Amsterdam, J.D., Settle, R.G., Doty, R.L., Abelman, E. and Winokur, A. (1987) Taste and smell perception in depression. *Biological Psychiatry* 22, 1481–1485.

Anderson, K.E., Rosner, W., Khan, M.S., New, M.I., Pang, S., Wissel, P.S. and Kappas, A. (1987) Diet–hormone interactions: protein–carbohydrate ratio alters reciprocally the plasma levels of testosterone and cortisol and their respective binding globulins in man. *Life Sciences* 40, 1761–1768.

Barr, R.G., Pantel, M.S., Young, S.N., Wright, J.H., Hendricks, L.A. and Gravel, R. (1999) The response of crying newborns to sucrose: is it a 'sweetness' effect? *Physiology & Behavior* 66, 409–417.

Bellisle, F., Louis-Sylvestre, J., Linet, N., Rocaboy, B., Dalle, B., Cheneau, F., L'Hinoret, D. and Guyot, L. (1990) Anxiety and food intake in men. *Psychosomatic Medicine* 52, 452–457.

Benton, D. (2002) Carbohydrate ingestion, blood glucose and mood. *Neuroscience and Biobehavioral Reviews* 26, 293–308.

Benton, D. and Donohoe, R.T. (1999) The effects of nutrients on mood. *Public Health Nutrition* 2, 403–409.

Berridge, K.C. and Robinson, T.E. (1998) What is the role of dopamine in reward: hedonic impact, reward learning, or incentive salience? *Brain Research. Brain Research Reviews* 28, 309–369.

Björntorp, P. (2001) Do stress reactions cause abdominal obesity and comorbidities? *Obesity Reviews* 2, 73–86.

Blass, E.M. and Camp, C.A. (2003) Changing determinants of crying termination in 6- to 12-week-old human infants. *Developmental Psychobiology* 42, 312–316.

Blass, E.M., Shide, D.J. and Weller, A. (1989) Stress-reducing effects of ingesting milk, sugars, and fats. A developmental perspective. *Annals of the New York Academy of Sciences* 575, 292–305.

Booth, D.A. (1987) Central dietary feedback onto nutrient selection – not even a scientific hypothesis. *Appetite* 8, 195–201.

Booth, D.A. (1994) *Psychology of Nutrition*. Taylor and Francis, London.

Brand Miller, J.C., Holt, S.H., de Jong, V. and Petocz, P. (2003) Cocoa powder increases postprandial insulinemia in lean young adults. *Journal of Nutrition* 133, 3149–3152.

Brindley, D.N., McCann, B.S., Niaura, R., Stoney, C.M. and Suarez, E.C. (1993) Stress and lipoprotein metabolism: modulators and mechanisms. *Metabolism* 42(Suppl. 1), 3–15.

Bruch, H. (1974) *Eating Disorders: Anorexia, Obesity and The Person Within*. Routledge and Kegan Paul, London.

Canli, T., Amin, Z., Haas, B., Omura, K. and Constable, R.T. (2004) A double dissociation between mood states and personality traits in the anterior cingulate. *Behavioral Neuroscience* 118, 897–904.

Carbajal, R., Chauvet, X., Couderc, S. and Olivier-Martin, M. (1999) Randomised trial of analgesic effects of sucrose, glucose, and pacifiers in term neonates. *British Medical Journal* 319, 1393–1397.

Cartwright, M., Wardle, J., Steggles, N., Simon, A.E., Croker, H. and Jarvis, M.J. (2003) Stress and dietary practices in adolescents. *Health Psychology* 22, 362–369.

Christensen, L. and Redig, C. (1993) Effect of meal composition on mood. *Behavioral Neuroscience* 107, 346–353.

Chua, J.L., Touyz, S. and Hill, A.J. (2004) Negative mood-induced overeating in obese binge eaters: an experimental study. *International Journal of Obesity and Related Metabolic Disorders* 28, 606–610.

Collins, A., Eneroth, P. and Landgren, B.M. (1985) Psychoneuroendocrine stress responses and mood as related to the menstrual cycle. *Psychosomatic Medicine* 47, 512–527.

Conners, C.K. and Blouin, A.G. (1983) Nutritional effects on behavior of children. *Journal of Psychiatric Research* 17, 193–201.

Cowen, P.J. (1996) The serotonin hypothesis: necessary but not sufficient. In: Feighner, J.P. and Boyer, W.F. (eds) *Selective Serotonin Re-uptake Inhibitors: Advances in Basic Research and Clinical Practice*, 2nd edn. John Wiley, London, pp. 63–86.

Craig, A. (1986) Acute effects of meals on perceptual and cognitive efficiency. *Nutrition Reviews* 44, 163–171.

Craig, A., Baer, K. and Diekmann, A. (1981) The effects of lunch on sensory-perceptual functioning in man. *International Archives of Occupational and Environmental Health* 49, 105–114.

Craighead, L.W. and Allen, H.N. (1995) Appetite awareness training: a cognitive behavioral intervention for binge eating. *Cognitive and Behavioral Practice* 2, 249–270.

Cunliffe, A., Obeid, O.A. and Powell-Tuck, J. (1997) Post-prandial changes in measures of fatigue: effect of a mixed or a pure carbohydrate or pure fat meal. *European Journal of Clinical Nutrition* 51, 831–838.

Dallman, M.F., Pecoraro, N., Akana, S.F., la Fleur, S.E., Gomez, F., Houshyar, H., Bell, M.E., Bhatnagar, S., Laugero, K D. and Manalo, S. (2003) Chronic stress and obesity: a new view of 'comfort food'. *Proceedings of the National Academy of Sciences USA* 100, 11696–11701.

D'Anci, K.E., Kanarek, R.B. and Marks-Kaufman, R. (1997) Beyond sweet taste: saccharin, sucrose, and polycose differ in their effects upon morphine-induced analgesia. *Pharmacology, Biochemistry, and Behavior* 56, 341–345.

Davis, C., Strachan, S. and Berkson, M. (2004) Sensitivity to reward: implications for overeating and overweight. *Appetite* 42, 131–138.

De Castro, J.M. (1987) Macronutrient relationships with meal patterns and mood in the spontaneous feeding behavior of humans. *Physiology & Behavior* 39, 561–569.

Dess, N.K. and Edelheit, D. (1998) The bitter with the sweet: the taste/stress/temperament nexus. *Biological Psychology* 48, 103–119.

Doyle, T.G., Berridge, K.C. and Gosnell, B.A. (1993) Morphine enhances hedonic taste palatability in rats. *Pharmacology, Biochemistry, and Behavior* 46, 745–749.

Dusek, J.B., Mergler, M.L. and Kermis, M.D. (1976) Attention, encoding, and information processing in low- and high-test-anxious children. *Child Development* 47, 201–207.

Dye, L., Lluch, A. and Blundell, J.E. (2000) Macronutrients and mental performance. *Nutrition* 16, 1021–1034.

Epel, E., Lapidus, R., McEwen, B. and Brownell, K. (2001) Stress may add bite to appetite in women: a laboratory study of stress-induced cortisol and eating behavior. *Psychoneuroendocrinology* 26, 37–49.

Fernstrom, J.D. (1983) Role of precursor availability in control of monoamine biosynthesis in brain. *Physiological Reviews* 63, 484–546.

Fernstrom, J.D. and Fernstrom, M.H. (1994) Dietary effects on tyrosine availability and catecholamine synthesis in the central nervous system: possible relevance to the control of protein intake. *Proceedings of the Nutrition Society* 53, 419–429.

Fernstrom, M.H. and Fernstrom, J.D. (1995) Brain tryptophan concentrations and serotonin synthesis remain responsive to food consumption after the ingestion of sequential meals. *American Journal of Clinical Nutrition* 61, 312–319.

Folkard, S. and Monk, T.H. (1985) *Hours of Work: Temporal Factors in Work Scheduling*. Wiley, Chichester, UK.

Fredrickson, B.L. (2004) The broaden-and-build theory of positive emotions. *Philosophical Transactions of the Royal Society of London, Series B, Biological Sciences* 359, 1367–1378.

Fulkerson, J.A., Sherwood, N.E., Perry, C.L., Neumark-Sztainer, D. and Story, M. (2004) Depressive symptoms and adolescent eating and health behaviors: a multifaceted view in a population-based sample. *Preventive Medicine* 38, 865–875.

George, M.S., Nahas, Z., Li, X.B., Kozel, F.A., Anderson, B. and Yamanaka, K. (2002) Potential new brain stimulation therapies in bipolar illness: transcranial magnetic stimulation and vagus nerve stimulation. *Clinical Neuroscience Research* 2, 256–265.

Gibson, E.L. (2001) Learning in the development of food cravings. In: Hetherington, M.M. (ed.) *Food Cravings and Addiction*. Leatherhead Publishing, Leatherhead, UK, pp. 193–234.

Gibson, E.L. (2003) Learnt protein appetite in human beings: involvement of cortisol in postingestive reinforcement by protein intake. *Appetite* 40, 334.

Gibson, E.L. and Green, M.W. (2002) Nutritional influences on cognitive function: mechanisms of susceptibility. *Nutrition Research Reviews* 15, 169–206.

Gibson, E.L., Wainwright, C.J. and Booth, D.A. (1995) Disguised protein in lunch after low-protein breakfast conditions food-flavor preferences dependent on recent lack of protein intake. *Physiology & Behavior* 58, 363–371.

Gibson, E.L., Checkley, S., Papadopoulos, A., Poon, L., Daley, S. and Wardle, J. (1999) Increased salivary cortisol reliably induced by a protein-rich midday meal. *Psychosomatic Medicine* 61, 214–224.

Gilbertson, T.A., Liu, L., York, D.A. and Bray, G.A. (1998) Dietary fat preferences are inversely correlated with peripheral gustatory fatty acid sensitivity. *Annals of the New York Academy of Sciences* 855, 165–168.

Golomb, B.A., Tenkanen, L., Alikoski, T., Niskanen, T., Manninen, V., Huttunen, M. and Mednick, S.A. (2002) Insulin sensitivity markers – predictors of accidents and suicides in Helsinki Heart Study screenees. *Journal of Clinical Epidemiology* 55, 767–773.

Gonzalez-Bono, E., Rohleder, N., Hellhammer, D.H., Salvador, A. and Kirschbaum, C. (2002) Glucose but not protein or fat load amplifies the cortisol response to psychosocial stress. *Hormones and Behavior* 41, 328–333.

Gray, J.R. and Braver, T.S. (2002) Personality predicts working-memory-related activation in the caudal anterior cingulate cortex. *Cognitive, Affective, and Behavioral Neuroscience* 2, 64–75.

Green, M.W., Taylor, M.A., Elliman, N.A. and Rhodes, O. (2001) Placebo expectancy effects in the relationship between glucose and cognition. *British Journal of Nutrition* 86, 173–179.

Griffin, K.W., Friend, R., Eitel, P. and Lobel, M. (1993) Effects of environmental demands, stress, and mood on health practices. *Journal of Behavioral Medicine* 16, 643–661.

Grunberg, N.E. and Straub, R.O. (1992) The role of gender and taste class in the effects of stress on eating. *Health Psychology* 11, 97–100.

Haynes, C., Lee, M.D. and Yeomans, M.R. (2003) Interactive effects of stress, dietary restraint, and disinhibition on appetite. *Eating Behaviour* 4, 369–383.

Heatherton, T.F., Herman, C.P. and Polivy, J. (1991) Effects of physical threat and ego threat on eating behaviour. *Journal of Personality and Social Psychology* 60, 138–143.

Heninger, G.R., Delgado, P.L. and Charney, D.S. (1996) The revised monoamine theory of depression: a modulatory role for monoamines, based on new findings from monoamine depletion experiments in humans. *Pharmacopsychiatry* 29, 2–11.

Herman, C.P. and Polivy, J. (1975) Anxiety, restraint and eating behavior. *Journal of Abnormal Psychology* 84, 666–672.

Herman, C.P. and Polivy, J. (1980) Restrained eating. In: Stunkard, A.J. (ed.) *Obesity.* Saunders, Philadelphia, Pennsylvania, pp. 208–225.

Kanarek, R.B. and Carrington, C. (2004) Sucrose consumption enhances the analgesic effects of cigarette smoking in male and female smokers. *Psychopharmacology* 173, 57–63.

Kanarek, R.B., White, E.S., Biegen, M.T. and Marks-Kaufman, R. (1991) Dietary influences on morphine-induced analgesia in rats. *Pharmacology, Biochemistry, and Behavior* 38, 681–684.

Kelley, A.E., Will, M.J., Steininger, T.L., Zhang, M. and Haber, S.N. (2003) Restricted daily consumption of a highly palatable food (chocolate Ensure®) alters striatal enkephalin gene expression. *European Journal of Neuroscience* 18, 2592–2598.

Kräuchi, K., Keller, U., Leonhardt, G., Brunner, D.P., van der Veld, P., Haug, H.J. and Wirz-Justice, A. (1999) Accelerated post-glucose glycaemia and altered alliesthesia-test in seasonal affective disorder. *Journal of Affective Disorders* 53, 23–26.

Laitinen, J., Ek, E. and Sovio, U. (2002) Stress-related eating and drinking behavior and body mass index and predictors of this behavior. *Preventive Medicine* 34, 29–39.

Lattimore, P. and Caswell, N. (2004) Differential effects of active and passive stress on food intake in restrained and unrestrained eaters. *Appetite* 42, 167–173.

Lawlor, D.A., Davey Smith, G. and Ebrahim, S. (2003) Association of insulin resistance with depression: cross-sectional findings from the British women's heart and health study. *British Medical Journal* 327, 1383–1384.

Lewkowski, M.D., Ditto, B., Roussos, M. and Young, S.N. (2003) Sweet taste and blood pressure-related analgesia. *Pain* 106, 181–186.

Lieberman, H.R., Spring, B.J. and Garfield, G.S. (1986) The behavioral effects of food constituents: strategies used in studies of amino acids, protein, carbohydrate and caffeine. *Nutrition Reviews* 44, 61–70.

Lloyd, H.M., Green, M.W. and Rogers, P.J. (1994) Mood and cognitive performance effects of isocaloric lunches differing in fat and carbohydrate content. *Physiology & Behavior* 56, 51–57.

Lowe, M.R. and Fisher, E.B. (1983) Emotional reactivity, emotional eating and obesity: a naturalistic study. *Journal of Behavioral Medicine* 6, 135–148.

Lyons, P.M. and Truswell, A.S. (1988) Serotonin precursor influenced by type of carbohydrate meal in healthy adults. *American Journal of Clinical Nutrition* 47, 433–439.

McCann, B.S., Warnick, G.R. and Knopp, R.H. (1990) Changes in plasma lipids and dietary intake accompanying shifts in perceived workload and stress. *Psychosomatic Medicine* 52, 97–108.

Macdiarmid, J.I. and Hetherington, M.M. (1995) Mood modulation by food: an exploration of affect and cravings in 'chocolate addicts'. *British Journal of Clinical Psychology* 34, 129–138.

Macht, M. (1996) Effects of high- and low-energy meals on hunger, physiological processes and reactions to emotional stress. *Appetite* 26, 71–88.

Macht, M., Roth, S. and Ellgring, H. (2002) Chocolate eating in healthy men during experimentally induced sadness and joy. *Appetite* 39, 147–158.

Macht, M., Gerer, J. and Ellgring, H. (2003) Emotions in overweight and normal-weight women immediately after eating foods differing in energy. *Physiology & Behavior* 80, 367–374.

Macht, M., Haupt, C. and Salewsky, A. (2004) Emotions and eating in everyday life: application of the experience-sampling method. *Ecology of Food and Nutrition* 43, 327–337.

Macht, M., Haupt, C. and Ellgring, H. (2005) The perceived function of eating is changed during examination stress: a field study. *Eating Behaviors* 6, 109–112.

Markus, C.R., Panhuysen, G., Tuiten, A., Koppeschaar, H., Fekkes, D. and Peters, M.L. (1998) Does carbohydrate-rich, protein-poor food prevent a deterioration of mood and cognitive performance of stress-prone subjects when subjected to a stressful task? *Appetite* 31, 49–65.

Markus, C.R., Olivier, B., Panhuysen, G.E.M., Van der Gugten, J., Alles, M.S., Tuiten, A., Westenberg, H.G.M., Fekkes, D., Kopeschaar, H.F. and de Haan, E.E.H.F. (2000) The bovine protein α-lactalbumin increases the plasma ratio of tryptophan to the other large neutral amino acids, and in vulnerable subjects raises brain serotonin activity, reduces cortisol concentration, and improves mood under stress. *American Journal of Clinical Nutrition* 71, 1536–1544.

Matthews, G. and Deary, I.J. (1998) *Personality Traits*. Cambridge University Press, Cambridge, UK.

Melanson, K.J., Westerterp-Plantenga, M.S., Campfield, L.A. and Saris, W.H. (1999) Blood glucose and meal patterns in time-blinded males, after aspartame, carbohydrate, and fat consumption, in relation to sweetness perception. *British Journal of Nutrition* 82, 437–446.

Mercer, M.E. and Holder, M.D. (1997a) Food cravings, endogenous opioid peptides, and food intake: a review. *Appetite* 29, 325–352.

Mercer, M.E. and Holder, M.D. (1997b) Antinociceptive effects of palatable sweet ingesta on human responsivity to pressure pain. *Physiology & Behavior* 61, 311–318.

Michaud, C., Kahn, J.P., Musse, N., Burlet, C., Nicolas, J.P. and MeJean, L. (1990) Relationships between a critical life event and eating behaviour in high-school students. *Stress Medicine* 6, 57–64.

Miller, A., Barr, R.G. and Young, S.N. (1994) The cold pressor test in children: methodological aspects and the analgesic effect of intraoral sucrose. *Pain* 56, 175–183.

Møller, S.E. (1986) Carbohydrate/protein selection in a single meal correlated with plasma tryptophan and tyrosine ratios to neutral amino acids in fasting individuals. *Physiology & Behavior* 38, 175–183.

Munafo, M.R., Clark, T.G., Moore, L.R., Payne, E., Walton, R. and Flint, J. (2003) Genetic polymorphisms and personality in healthy adults: a systematic review and meta-analysis. *Molecular Psychiatry* 8, 471–484.

Murphy, F.C., Smith, K.A., Cowen, P.J., Robbins, T.W. and Sahakian, B.J. (2002) The effects of tryptophan depletion on cognitive and affective processing in healthy volunteers. *Psychopharmacology* 163, 42–53.

Ness, A.R., Gallacher, J.E., Bennett, P.D., Gunnell, D.J., Rogers, P.J., Kessler, D. and Burr, M.L. (2003) Advice to eat fish and mood: a randomised controlled trial in men with angina. *Nutritional Neuroscience* 6, 63–65.

O'Donnell, L., O'Meara, N., Owens, D., Johnson, A. and Collins, P. (1987) Plasma catecholamines and lipoproteins in chronic psychological stress. *Journal of the Royal Society of Medicine* 80, 339–342.

Oliver, G. and Wardle, J. (1999) Perceived effects of stress on food choice. *Physiology & Behavior* 66, 511–515.

Oliver, G., Wardle, J. and Gibson, E.L. (2000) Stress and food choice: a laboratory study. *Psychosomatic Medicine* 62, 853–865.

Pani, L., Porcella, A. and Gessa, G.L. (2000) The role of stress in the pathophysiology of the dopaminergic system. *Molecular Psychiatry* 5, 14–21.

Parry, B.L. (2001) The role of central serotonergic dysfunction in the aetiology of premenstrual dysphoric disorder – therapeutic implications. *CNS Drugs* 15, 277–285.

Pellegrin, K.L., O'Neil, P.M., Stellefson, E.J., Fossey, M.D., Ballenger, J.C., Cochrane, C.E. and Currey, H.S. (1998) Average daily nutrient intake and mood among obese women. *Nutrition Research* 18, 1103–1112.

Pollard, T.M., Steptoe, A., Canaan, L., Davies, G.J. and Wardle, J. (1995) The effects of academic examination stress on eating behaviour and blood lipid levels. *International Journal of Behavioral Medicine* 2, 299–320.

Pollitt, E., Lewis, N.L., Garza, C. and Shulman, R.J. (1983) Fasting and cognitive function. *Journal of Psychiatric Research* 17, 169–174.

Quintin, P., Benkelfat, C., Launay, J.M., Arnulf, I., Pointereau-Bellenger, A., Barbault, S., Alvarez, J.C., Varoquaux, O., Perez-Diaz, F., Jouvent, R. and Leboyer, M. (2001) Clinical and neurochemical effect of acute tryptophan depletion in unaffected relatives of patients with bipolar affective disorder. *Biological Psychiatry* 50, 184–190.

Rand, C. and Stunkard, A.J. (1978) Obesity and psychoanalysis. *American Journal of Psychiatry* 135, 547–551.

Reid, M. and Hammersley, R. (1999) The effects of carbohydrates on arousal. *Nutrition Research Reviews* 12, 3–23.

Robbins, T.W. and Fray, P.J. (1980) Stress-induced eating: fact, fiction or misunderstanding? *Appetite* 1, 103–133.

Rodin, J. (1981) Current status of the internal/external hypothesis for obesity: what went wrong? *American Psychologist* 36, 361–372.

Rogers, P.J. and Smit, H.J. (2000) Food craving and food 'addiction': a critical review of the evidence from a biopsychosocial perspective. *Pharmacology, Biochemistry, and Behavior* 66, 3–14.

Rogers, P.J., Kainth, A. and Smit, H.J. (2001) A drink of water can improve or impair mental performance depending on small differences in thirst. *Appetite* 36, 57–58.

Rolls, E.T. (1999) *The Brain and Emotion*. Oxford University Press, Oxford, UK.

Russo, S., Kema, I.P., Fokkema, M.R., Boon, J.C., Willemse, P.H.B., de Vries, E.G.E., den Boer, J.A. and Korf, J. (2003) Tryptophan as a link between psychopathology and somatic states. *Psychosomatic Medicine* 65, 665–671.

Rutledge, T. and Linden, W. (1998) To eat or not to eat: affective and physiological mechanisms in the stress–eating relationship. *Journal of Behavioral Medicine* 21, 221–240.

Saelens, B.E. and Epstein, L.H. (1996) Reinforcing value of food in obese and non-obese women. *Appetite* 27, 41–50.

Sayegh, R., Schiff, I., Wurtman, J., Spiers, P., McDermott, J. and Wurtman, R. (1995) The effect of a carbohydrate-rich beverage on mood, appetite, and cognitive function in women with premenstrual syndrome. *Obstetrics and Gynecology* 86, 520–528.

Schachter, S., Goldman, R. and Gordon, A. (1968) Effects of fear, food deprivation, and obesity on eating. *Journal of Personality and Social Psychology* 10, 91–97.

Schweiger, U., Warnhoff, M., Pahl, J. and Pirke, K.M. (1986a) Effects of carbohydrate and protein meals on plasma large neutral amino acids, glucose, and insulin plasma levels of anorectic patients. *Metabolism* 35, 938–943.

Schweiger, U., Laessle, R., Kittl, S., Dickhaut, B., Schweiger, M. and Pirke, K.M. (1986b) Macronutrient intake, plasma large neutral amino acids and mood during weight-reducing diets. *Journal of Neural Transmission* 67, 77–86.

Shaham, Y., Erb, S. and Stewart, J. (2000) Stress-induced relapse to heroin and cocaine seeking in rats: a review. *Brain Research. Brain Research Reviews* 33, 13–33.

Small, D.M., Zatorre, R.J., Dagher, A., Evans, A.C. and Jones-Gotman, M. (2001) Changes in brain activity related to eating chocolate: from pleasure to aversion. *Brain* 124, 1720–1733.

Smit, H.J., Gaffan, E.A. and Rogers, P.J. (2004) Methylxanthines are the psychopharmacologically active constituents of chocolate. *Psychopharmacology* 176, 412–419.

Smith, A.P. (1992) Time of day and performance. In: Smith, A.P. and Jones, D.M. (eds) *Handbook of Human Performance*. Vol. 2. *Health and Performance*. Academic Press, London, pp. 217–235.

Smith, A.P. and Miles, C. (1986) Acute effects of meals, noise and nightwork. *British Journal of Psychology* 77, 377–387.

Smith, A.P., Leekham, S., Ralph, A. and McNeill, G. (1988) The influence of meal composition on post-lunch performance efficiency and mood. *Appetite* 10, 195–203.

Steptoe, A., Lipsey, Z. and Wardle, J. (1998) Stress, hassles and variations in alcohol consumption, food choice and physical exercise: a diary study. *British Journal of Health Psychology* 3, 51–63.

Stone, A. and Brownell, K.D. (1994) The stress-eating paradox: multiple daily measurements in adult males and females. *Psychology and Health* 9, 425–436.

Thayer, R.E. (1989) *The Biopsychology of Mood and Arousal*. Oxford University Press, Oxford, UK.

Thibault, L. and Booth, D.A. (1999) Macronutrient-specific dietary selection in rodents and its neural bases. *Neuroscience and Biobehavioral Reviews* 23, 457–528.

Tuiten, A., Panhuysen, G., Koppeschaar, H., Fekkes, D., Pijl, H., Frolich, M., Krabbe, P. and Everaerd, W. (1995) Stress, serotonergic function, and mood in users of oral contraceptives. *Psychoneuroendocrinology* 20, 323–334.

Upadhyay, A., Aggarwal, R., Narayan, S., Joshi, M., Paul, V.K. and Deorari, A.K. (2004) Analgesic effect of expressed breast milk in procedural pain in term neonates: a randomized, placebo-controlled, double-blind trial. *Acta Paediatrica* 93, 518–522.

Van Strien, T., Frijters, J.E.R., Bergers, G.P.A. and Defares, P.B. (1986) Dutch Eating Behaviour Questionnaire for assessment of restrained, emotional and external eating behaviour. *International Journal of Eating Disorders* 5, 295–315.

Wallis, D.J. and Hetherington, M.M. (2004) Stress and eating: the effects of ego-threat and cognitive demand on food intake in restrained and emotional eaters. *Appetite* 43, 39–46.

Walther, D.J. and Bader, M. (2003) A unique central tryptophan hydroxylase isoform. *Biochemical Pharmacology* 66, 1673–1680.

Wang, G.J., Volkow, N.D., Logan, J., Pappas, N.R., Wong, C.T., Zhu, W., Netusil, N. and Fowler, J.S. (2001) Brain dopamine and obesity. *The Lancet* 357, 354–357.

Ward, A. and Mann, T. (2000) Don't mind if I do: disinhibited eating under cognitive load. *Journal of Personality and Social Psychology* 78, 753–763.

Wardle, J. and Gibson, E.L. (2002) Impact of stress on diet: processes and implications. In: Stansfeld, S. and Marmot, M.G. (eds) *Stress and the Heart: Psychosocial Pathways to Coronary Heart Disease*. BMJ Books, London, pp. 124–149.

Wardle, J., Steptoe, A., Oliver, G. and Lipsey, Z. (2000) Stress, dietary restraint and food intake. *Journal of Psychosomatic Research* 48, 195–202.

Wardle, J., Guthrie, C., Sanderson, S., Birch, L. and Plomin, R. (2001) Food and activity preferences in children of lean and obese parents. *International Journal of Obesity and Related Metabolic Disorders* 25, 971–977.

Waters, A., Hill, A. and Waller, G. (2001) Bulimics' responses to food cravings: is binge-eating a product of hunger or emotional state? *Behaviour Research and Therapy* 39, 877–886.

Weidner, G., Kohlmann, C.W., Dotzauer, E. and Burns, L.R. (1996) The effects of academic stress on health behaviors in young adults. *Anxiety, Stress and Coping: An International Journal* 9, 123–133.

Weinstein, S.E., Shide, D.J. and Rolls, B.J. (1997) Changes in food intake in response to stress in men and women: psychological factors. *Appetite* 28, 7–18.

Willenbring, M.L., Levine, A.S. and Morley, J.E. (1986) Stress-induced eating and food preference in humans: a pilot study. *International Journal of Eating Disorders* 5, 855–864.

Williams, J.M.G., Healy, H., Eade, J., Windle, G., Cowen, P.J., Green, M.W. and Durlach, P. (2002) Mood, eating behaviour and attention. *Psychological Medicine* 32, 469–481.

Willner, P., Benton, D., Brown, E., Cheeta, S., Davies, G., Morgan, J. and Morgan, M. (1998) 'Depression' increases 'craving' for sweet rewards in animal and human models of depression and craving. *Psychopharmacology* 136, 272–283.

Wolever, T.M.S., Jenkins, D.J.A. and Anderson, G.H. (1988) Metabolic response to test meals containing different carbohydrate foods: 2. Plasma amino acid responses and amino acid ratios. *Nutrition Research* 8, 583–592.

Wurtman, J.J., Brzezinski, A., Wurtman, R.J. and Laferrere, B. (1989) Effect of nutrient intake on premenstrual depression. *American Journal of Obstetrics and Gynecology* 161, 1228–1234.

Wurtman, R.J. and Wurtman, J.J. (1989) Carbohydrates and depression. *Scientific American* 260, 68–75.

Wurtman, R.J., Wurtman, J.J., Regan, M.M., McDermott, J.M., Tsay, R.H. and Breu, J.J. (2003) Effects of normal meals rich in carbohydrates or proteins on plasma tryptophan and tyrosine ratios. *American Journal of Clinical Nutrition* 77, 128–132.

Yanovski, S.Z., Nelson, J.E., Dubbert, B.K. and Spitzer, R.L. (1993) Association of binge eating disorder and psychiatric comorbidity in obese subjects. *American Journal of Psychiatry* 150, 1472–1479.

Yokogoshi, H. and Wurtman, R.J. (1986) Meal composition and plasma amino acid ratios: effect of various proteins or carbohydrates, and of various protein concentrations. *Metabolism* 35, 837–842.

York, D.A., Rossner, S., Caterson, I., Chen, C.M., James, W.P., Kumanyika, S., Martorell, R. and Vorster, H.H. (2004) Prevention Conference VII: Obesity, a worldwide epidemic related to heart disease and stroke: Group I: worldwide demographics of obesity. *Circulation* 110, e463–e470.

Zagon, A. (2001) Does the vagus nerve mediate the sixth sense? *Trends in Neurosciences* 24, 671–673.

8 Food Cravings and Addictions

SUZANNE HIGGS

School of Psychology, University of Birmingham, Edgbaston, Birmingham B15 2TT, UK

Prevalence of Food Cravings

Food cravings are common experiences. Questionnaire-based studies have reported that 60–97% of participants experience regular cravings for a specific food (Rodin *et al.*, 1991; Rozin *et al.*, 1991; Weingarten and Elston, 1991). Although only a few studies have been published on the cross-cultural incidence of food cravings, there is no evidence to suggest that cravings are restricted to particular cultures or ethnic groups (Zellner *et al.*, 1999; Cepeda-Benito *et al.*, 2000; Parker *et al.*, 2003). However, there are data suggesting that women report more cravings than men (Weingarten and Elston, 1991; Pelchat, 1997) and that the frequency of cravings declines with age (Pelchat, 1997).

Cravings and Food Choice

Cravings can influence food choice by increasing the likelihood that the craved food is consumed. This has been confirmed in experimental studies showing that cravings are associated with increased intake of the desired food (Fedoroff *et al.*, 1997, 2003). In reality though, the relationship between cravings and food intake is likely to be complex because cravings can be successfully resisted, and there may be other barriers to desired intake such as availability. In support of this, self-report diary studies of food cravings reveal a less reliable relationship between food cravings and consumption (Harvey *et al.*, 1993; Tuomisto *et al.*, 1999). Nevertheless, given the widespread and ubiquitous nature of food cravings, even a modest correlation between cravings and intake would still be expected to translate into a sizeable influence on everyday food choice.

Explanations of Food Cravings

Despite the suggestion that cravings have a significant impact on food choice, little is known about what causes food cravings, and what purpose they serve. Contrary to popular belief, most food cravings are unlikely to serve a simple homeostatic function to maintain nutritional balance, or avoid a biological need state. Although there are a few rare cases in the literature that document cravings associated with a pathological need for salt (e.g. Wilkins and Richter, 1940), the induction of a similar need state in healthy volunteers by salt depletion has not been shown to induce cravings (Beauchamp et al., 1990). Additionally, many food cravings are experienced in the absence of a deprivation state (Pelchat and Schaefer, 2000), and even when it has been assumed that a state of depletion underlies certain food cravings, it has been difficult to demonstrate that consumption of the craved food reliably reverses this need state (Teff et al., 1989) or satisfies the cravings (Michener and Rozin, 1994). While there is some consensus that homeostasis-based theories of craving fail to provide a comprehensive explanation of the phenomenon, it has been difficult to distinguish between alternatives due to a lack of direct and unambiguous supporting evidence.

It is frequently observed that there are striking similarities in the phenomenology of food cravings and cravings for drugs of abuse. Both are characterized by strong urges to consume a specific substance, and addicts frequently report that cravings can persist long after drug use has been discontinued (Mucha et al., 1999); in other words, in the absence of any disruption to body homeostasis such as a drug-induced need state. These strong parallels indicate that drug and food cravings may arise from similar underlying processes, and suggest that explanations of food cravings might fruitfully focus on the mechanisms common to the control of both eating and drug-taking.

Mechanisms of Motivation and Reward and their Relevance to Cravings

Eating and drug-taking are motivated behaviours that are controlled by learning processes (for a review see Cardinal and Everitt, 2004). Repeated consumption of a food or drug in the presence of a salient cue can lead to an association being formed in memory between the cue (known as the conditioned stimulus) and the rewarding consequences of consuming the food or drug, such as feelings of pleasure (known as the unconditioned stimulus). By this process, the occurrence of the unconditioned stimulus can be predicted by the conditioned stimulus, and behaviour may be modified based on this learned expectancy (known as the conditioned response; Bolles, 1972). The conditioned response is likely to serve an adaptive function: preparing the body for the delivery of the reward and facilitating consumption via an increase in arousal and food-seeking behaviour (Cardinal et al., 2002). Via association, conditioned stimuli may also take on some of the properties of the reward itself and thus acquire hedonic properties (Bindra, 1974). For example, a food flavour (conditioned stimulus) can come to be preferred if it predicts the delivery of energy (unconditioned stimulus; Sclafani, 1995). The important point is that cues that have been reliably paired with eating and drug-taking in the past can come to exert control over behaviour in the future by triggering responses that both anticipate and mimic the effects of the reward. Moreover, these responses are likely to be accompanied by an emotional state, which could manifest as a desire to consume the food or drug; in other words, a craving. Thus, one way of conceptualizing food and drug cravings is as the emotional expression of a cue-elicited learned appetite.

One advantage of this idea is that it can account for the fact that cravings occur in the absence of a need state. Deprivation has been shown to enhance the learned response to food presentation but it is not necessary for conditioned stimuli to elicit eating (Weingarten, 1983, 1984; Holland *et al.*, 2002). Specific support for the theory is lacking though, because most studies of appetitive learning have been conducted using rodents. While it is possible to model craving processes in non-human animals, the relationship between the unconditioned and conditioned responses of laboratory rats and the human experience of craving is difficult to determine. Human studies have shown that cravings can be elicited by exposing participants to food-related cues (Fedoroff *et al.*, 1997; Tuomisto *et al.*, 1999). These data are consistent with an interpretation of cravings as a learned appetite, but do not provide conclusive evidence, because cue reactivity responses may be subject to demand characteristics, or may reflect unconditioned effects of food-related stimuli on arousal. Nevertheless, the theory predicts that manipulations that alter the impact of conditioned rewards on behaviour should elicit or inhibit accompanying food cravings. There is a large body of data suggesting that certain psychopharmacological agents specifically alter the rewarding properties of food, and so one way of testing this hypothesis is to examine the effect of these drugs on the expression of food cravings in humans.

The Psychopharmacology of Food Reward and Cravings

The study of food reward has traditionally involved examination of the behavioural response of laboratory animals to palatable foods while trying to minimize post-ingestive physiological changes such as the accumulation of food in the stomach. Much attention in this area has focused on the role of benzodiazepine/γ-aminobutyric acid (GABA) and endogenous opioid systems in mediating food reward. More recently, with the discovery that there are compounds in the brain that mimic the effects of the main pharmacologically active ingredient in the recreational drug cannabis (Gaoni and Mechoulam 1964; Devane *et al.*, 1992), attention has been drawn to the role of cannabinoids in mediating food reward. Finally, there is a large body of evidence to suggest that activation of dopamine systems in the brain serves as common substrate for many different types of rewards. Rather than provide a general overview of the neuropharmacology of appetite, this chapter outlines the mechanisms likely to underlie the rewarding properties of food, and reviews the evidence that activity in these systems is related to changes in food cravings. The focus is on drugs acting at benzodiazepine, opioid, cannabinoid and dopamine receptors.

Benzodiazepines/γ-aminobutyric acid

Benzodiazepine receptor (BZR) agonists are synthetic drugs like the tranquilizer diazepam that act to enhance GABAergic inhibitory neurotransmission in the brain (Ticku, 1991). They are commonly used to treat anxiety and sleep disorders, but in addition to these well-known effects, BZR agonists stimulate robust increases in food intake in many species including cats (Fratta et al., 1976), rabbits (Mansbach et al., 1984), non-human primates (Foltin et al., 1985) and people (Kelly et al., 1992; Haney et al., 1997).

It has been suggested that specific modulation of the hedonic impact or palatability of food explains benzodiazepine-induced hyperphagia. This view is based on a considerable amount of data, and benzodiazpines are considered an exemplary case of drug-induced enhancement of palatability. First, benzodiazepines are effective in the taste reactivity test. This test involves the analysis of the distinctive facial reactions elicited by taste solutions (e.g. sucrose, salt, quinine or citric acid solutions). Because small volumes of the tastants are infused directly into the mouth, post-ingestive effects are minimized and the pattern of reactions elicited is thought to indicate whether it is evaluated as either positively hedonic or aversive (Berridge, 2003). It is significant therefore that the BZR agonist chlordiazepoxide has been shown on several occasions to enhance positive hedonic reactions in the rat, while leaving aversive reactions unaffected (Berridge and Treit, 1986; Treit et al., 1987; Berridge, 1988; Treit and Berridge, 1990; Pecina and Berridge, 1996). Benzodiazepines also enhance sucrose sham-feeding in the rat (Cooper et al., 1988). Post-ingestional influences on feeding are reduced in sham feeding because a tube is implanted in the rat's stomach, which prevents the normal accumulation of fluids. Thus, the effectiveness of drugs to alter sham feeding is unlikely to be due to modulation of satiety signals.

Another method that has been used to study palatability is microstructural analysis of ingestive behaviour. The timing of licks emitted by rats consuming a liquid diet can be logged by a computer, enabling detailed analysis of the temporal and structural pattern of the behaviour. The effects of experimental manipulations on these licking profiles can then be characterized. It has been shown that the number of licks emitted early in the test session, and the duration of bouts (runs of licks that cluster together into naturally occurring 'units'), increases linearly as the concentration of saccharin added to a glucose solution is increased (Breslin et al., 1996). This manipulation increases the palatability of a solution without affecting its nutritive or osmotic properties. On the other hand, decreasing palatability by adding quinine (a bitter-tasting substance) has the opposite effect on licking profiles (Davis and Levine, 1977). Consistent with an effect of benzodiazepines to increase palatability, the BZR agonist midazolam increases licking in a brief exposure test via an increase in mean bout duration (Higgs and Cooper, 1996, 1997, 1998a, 2000), an effect that is reversed by the specific benzodiazepine antagonist flumazenil (Higgs and Cooper, 1997).

Interestingly, benzodiazepine drugs that have opposite pharmacological effects to agonists (inverse agonists) decrease early licking responses and mean bout duration (Higgs and Cooper, 1996, 1998a). This suggests that bidirectional modulation of palatability can be achieved via action at BZRs.

There is also evidence that the BZR agonists diazepam and chlordiazepoxide increase appetitive behaviour directed towards procuring food reinforcers. Both drugs have been shown to increase operant responding (lever pressing) under a progressive ratio schedule of reinforcement in rats: an effect that is thought to reflect increased food-seeking behaviour (Higgs *et al.*, 2004). This effect of benzodiazepines is consistent with the view that changes in the hedonic assessment of rewards are usually associated with alterations in appetitive behaviours.

There are no published studies that have directly examined the mechanisms underlying the effects of BZR agonists on ingestion in humans, but an increase in the number of eating episodes in male volunteers living in a residential laboratory has been demonstrated following treatment with alprazolam (Kelly *et al.*, 1992). This effect was not associated with any decrease in anxiety (which is entirely consistent with the suggestion that the hyperphagic effects of these drugs can be dissociated from their tranquilizing actions). Most interestingly, a study of food cravings in women with premenstrual dysphoric disorder showed that alprazolam increased food intake in the premenstrual period. This effect was not accompanied by any changes in mood, and was specific for craved foods (Evans *et al.*, 1999).

Opioids

It is well known that administration of opiate-like drugs alters food intake in humans and other animals (for a recent review see Yeomans and Gray, 2002). Furthermore, there is clear evidence for opioid modulation of palatability responding in rodents (Cooper and Kirkham, 1993). Both central and peripheral administration of opioid agonists increases palatable food intake in the rat (Morley *et al.*, 1982; Gosnell *et al.*, 1983; Levine and Billington, 1989; Zhang *et al.*, 1998; Kelley *et al.*, 2002; Zhang and Kelley, 2000), whereas antagonist administration decreases intake (Holtzman, 1974; Cooper, 1980; Apfelbaum and Mandenoff, 1981; Bodnar *et al.*, 1995; Kelley *et al.*, 1996). Although it has been suggested that opioid agonists may preferentially enhance intake of high-fat foods (Marks-Kaufman and Kanarek, 1980), more recent data point to an explanation in terms of increased intake of a preferred diet as opposed to macronutrient-specific effects (Giraudo *et al.*, 1993). Consistent with this argument is the finding that the anorectic action of naloxone is enhanced in rats ingesting a more palatable food (Glass *et al.*, 2001). Further support for opioid modulation of taste hedonics is provided by the observation that opioid antagonists are effective in reducing sham feeding (Rockwood and Reid, 1982; Kirkham and Cooper, 1988a, 1988b; Kirkham, 1990). Lastly, the effects of opioid agonists and antagonists to respectively enhance and reduce hedonic taste reactivity responding are also consistent with the idea that opioids are involved in mediating the hedonic evaluation of foodstuffs (Parker et al., 1992; Doyle et al., 1993; Pecina and Berridge, 1995, 2000; Rideout and Parker, 1996), as is the observation of early modulation of licking response for palatable solutions (Higgs and Cooper, 1998b).

The effectiveness of opioid antagonists to decrease hedonic reactivity suggests that the release of endogenous opioids may be part of the neural response that determines palatability. A prediction that therefore arises is that intake of palatable food should be associated with opioid release in relevant brain areas. One way of addressing this issue is to assess brain opioid levels indirectly by measuring behavioural responses to opioid drugs in animals that have been exposed to palatable foods. If palatable food intake causes opioid release then it is expected that the well-known analgesic or pain-relieving effects of exogenously administered opioid agonists should be enhanced. In other words, less morphine should be required to achieve the same analgesic effect due to the presence of already circulating endogenous opioids. This has been established in a number of studies (D'Anci et al., 1996; Kanarek et al., 1997; Kanarek and Homoleski, 2000), along with the related finding that consumption of sucrose and milk has analgesic effects in both humans and rats (Blass and Fitzgerald, 1988; Blass and Hoffmeyer, 1991).

Another approach is to take biochemical measures of opioid activity. For example, levels of endogenous opioids can be measured following consumption of palatable foods. In addition, changes in opioid receptor numbers can be taken as an index of endogenous neurotransmitter activity. An early study reported changes in receptor binding consistent with increased levels of the endogenous opioid β-endorphin in the hypothalamus of the rat (Dum et al., 1983). More recently it has been shown that endogenous dynorphin is increased in the brains of rats fed a palatable diet (Welch et al., 1996). But this effect is probably linked to dietary-induced obesity, because it was not observed in rats that ate the same amount of palatable diet but did not gain weight (due to the fact that their intake was yoked to the control group). This suggests that the effects of overfeeding on endogenous opioid activity may be different from those due to palatable food consumption per se. Hence, the biochemical evidence is consistent with the notion that palatable food intake increases endogenous opioid activity, but also indicates that other adaptive changes occur in response to diet-induced obesity. That these effects can be dissociated has been confirmed by a study showing that activation of opioid systems in sucrose-fed rats occurs independently of changes in body weight (Shabir and Kirkham, 1999).

The possibility that opioid manipulations affect food-seeking behaviour has been confirmed in both pharmacological (Zhang et al., 2003) and genetic models (Hayward et al., 2002). In this latter study, non-deprived mice lacking certain endogenous opioids made fewer responses in order to obtain food pellets under a progressive ratio schedule of reinforcement.

Human data relating to the effects of opioid antagonists also support the notion that these drugs alter hedonic aspects of eating. The majority of human studies report that opioid antagonist administration lowers the rated pleasantness of eaten foods without altering taste perception (Yeomans et al., 1990; Yeomans and Wright, 1991; Drewnowski et al., 1992; Yeomans and Gray,

1996; Arbisi *et al.*, 1999). The application of microstructural analysis to human eating behaviour indicates that opioid antagonists reduce rated palatability (Yeomans and Gray, 1997). There is only one report to suggest that the opioid antagonist naloxone decreased food cravings in depressed patients (Zimmermann *et al.*, 1997), but naltrexone has been shown to be effective in reducing craving for alcohol (Volpicelli *et al.*, 1995; Weinrieb and O'Brien, 1997).

Cannabinoids

The active ingredient in cannabis, Δ^9-tetrahydrocannabinol (Δ^9-THC), is known to bind to a specific receptor in the brain known as the CB1 receptor (Pertwee, 1997). This receptor is also the binding site for several cannabinoid compounds that occur naturally in the brain, including anandamide and 2-arachidonoyl-glycerol (2-AG; Devane *et al.*, 1992). The suggestion that cannabinoids have a powerful effect on food intake is supported by historical accounts of the use of the drug to enhance appetite and anecdotal reports that marijuana intoxication is associated with increased consumption (colloquially known as the 'munchies'). Perhaps surprisingly, rigorous empirical investigation of cannabinoid effects on feeding has only been undertaken relatively recently. This may be in part due to the fact that specific antagonists, which are necessary to probe the pharmacological specificity of any effects, were not available before the 1990s. The first demonstration of a robust and dose-related hyperphagia in response to administration of Δ^9-THC in rats was published by Kirkham and colleagues in 1998 (Williams *et al.*, 1998). This effect has been shown to be mediated by action at CB1 receptors (Williams and Kirkham, 2002), and there have been similar reports of increases in food intake induced by the endocannabinoids anandamide (Williams and Kirkham, 1999; Hao *et al.*, 2000; Jamshidi and Taylor, 2001) and 2-AG (Kirkham *et al.*, 2002).

More recent behavioural studies indicate that changes in the hedonic properties of food may underlie cannabinoid-induced hyperphagia. The cannabinoid agonists Δ^9-THC and anandamide increase licking for sucrose in rats, primarily via an increase in mean bout duration, which as discussed previously may provide an index of palatability. Conversely, the CB1 antagonist SR141716 decreases mean bout duration (Higgs *et al.*, 2003a). These results are consistent with reports that cannabinoid agonists enhance the effectiveness of other rewarding stimuli such as electrical brain stimulation (Gardner and Vorel, 1998). Although there are no data available concerning the effects of cannabinoids in the taste reactivity test, it will be interesting to examine whether they elicit changes in hedonic responding.

There is also evidence that cannabinoids affect food-seeking behaviour. McGregor and colleagues have shown that SR141716 decreases the motivation of rats to respond for palatable fluids in a lick-based progressive ratio study (Gallate and McGregor, 1999). A subsequent study demonstrated increased operant responding for sucrose following administration of the synthetic cannabinoid agonist CP 55,940 (Gallate *et al.*, 1999). Consistent with these findings is the effect of Δ^9-THC to increase progressive ratio responding for food pellets (Higgs *et al.*, 2003b).

Ethical issues relating to examination of the effects of recreationally abused drugs have probably contributed to that fact that there have been few well-controlled studies examining the effects of cannabinoid agonists on appetite in humans. Nevertheless, the consensus is that Δ^9-THC increases intake of sweet snack foods rather than staple meals, which could be consistent with an enhancement of palatability (Foltin *et al.*, 1988; Mattes *et al.*, 1994). Given the obvious interest in developing drugs to treat obesity, greater attention has been paid to the effects of cannabinoid antagonists. The preliminary results of phase III clinical trials suggest that the cannabinoid antagonist SR141716 (rimonabant) is effective in inducing significant weight loss in obese participants. There are no data relating to the effect of rimonabant on food cravings, but the drug is being tested as an aid to smoking cessation. Early reports indicate that it may enhance quitting by reducing tobacco cravings, although these have yet to be published in full.

Dopamine

There is an extensive literature suggesting that manipulations of brain dopamine systems affect food reward (for reviews see Berridge and Robinson, 1998; Wise, 2004). For example, blockade of dopamine systems using antagonists has been consistently shown to reduce reward-related consumption, preference and operant responding for food reinforcers (Rolls *et al.*, 1974; Wise *et al.*, 1978; Wise and Colle, 1984; Bailey *et al.*, 1986; Wise and Raptis, 1986; Towell *et al.*, 1987; Ettenberg, 1989; Wilner *et al.*, 1990; Hsiao and Smith, 1995; Smith, 1995; Berridge and Robinson, 1998; Zhang *et al.*, 2003). What is more, consumption of palatable foods and exposure to cues associated with palatable food delivery increases brain dopamine levels (Hernandez and Hoebel, 1988; Blackburn *et al.*, 1989; Schultz *et al.*, 1993; Bassareo and Di Chiara, 1999; Hajnal and Norgren, 2001, 2002; Roitman *et al.*, 2004). It was initially suggested that dopamine mediates the hedonic impact of food (Wise, 1982). In support of this, there is ample evidence that dopamine antagonists reduce, whereas agonists enhance, sham feeding (Geary and Smith, 1985; Schneider *et al.*, 1986; Smith and Schneider, 1988). In particular, it has been shown that sucrose sham-feeding results in a concentration-dependent increase in brain dopamine (Hajnal *et al.*, 2004). Recent microstructural data also implicate dopamine in palatability responding (Higgs and Cooper, 2000; Genn *et al.*, 2003). However, the hedonia hypothesis has been challenged by data suggesting that dopamine manipulations do not reliably alter taste reactivity responding. Berridge and colleagues found that rats whose dopamine systems had been severely depleted, by administration of a specific neurotoxin, responded similarly to controls in terms of their facial reactions to an infusion of sucrose, even though they did not voluntarily approach food (Berridge *et al.*, 1989). In non-depleted rats, administration of the dopamine agonist apmorphine, and the antagonist pimozide, similarly failed to modify hedonic palatability responses (Treit and Berridge, 1990).

Furthermore, mice with genetic mutations resulting in elevated dopamine levels did not show enhanced taste reactivity responses to sucrose (Pecina *et al.*, 2003). Reductions in hedonic reactions to pimozide have been observed by some authors (Parker and Lopez, 1990; Leeb *et al.*, 1991), but it has been suggested that these effects may be explained by sensorimotor deficits (Pecina *et al.*, 1997).

These data have been taken to suggest that dopamine is not involved in the process by which hedonic value is assigned to rewards (Berridge, 1996; Berridge and Robinson, 1998). Whether the taste reactivity test provides a definitive measure of hedonic evaluation has been questioned though. It has been argued that because these responses occur in decerebrate rats and anencephalic human babies they may constitute sensory reflexes rather than hedonic responses (Di Chiara, 2002; Wise, 2004; although see Berridge and Robinson, 1998 for counter-arguments).

While the role of dopamine in hedonic evaluation may be debatable, there is strong evidence that it is important for normal appetitive responses to rewarding stimuli. For example, the ability of conditioned stimuli to elicit approach behaviour and promote operant responding for food rewards is dependent upon dopamine (Dickinson *et al.*, 2000; Wyvell and Berridge, 2000, 2001; Parkinson *et al.*, 2002). On the basis of this and other evidence it has been hypothesized that dopamine systems are important for the energizing properties of rewards (Salamone *et al.*, 1997), and are critically involved in learning about rewards (Everitt *et al.*, 2001; Di Chiara, 2002; Schultz, 2002). Another suggestion is that dopamine mediates the incentive salience of rewarding stimuli or enables them to attract attention and become 'wanted' (Berridge and Robinson, 1998; Robinson and Berridge, 2003).

Despite the widespread use of drugs with antagonistic action at dopamine receptors in the treatment of schizophrenia, the effects of dopamine modulation on food intake and cravings have been difficult to determine because most of these drugs possess significant activity at receptors other than dopamine. There is a lot of evidence to suggest that antipsychotic treatment is associated with substantial weight gain in patients, but recent data point towards the involvement of serotonergic rather than dopaminergic mechanisms in these effects (Casey and Zorn, 2001). However, evidence that dopamine manipulations affect food craving in people comes from a recent brain imaging study. Volkow *et al.* (2002) showed that exposure to food cues in combination with administration of the dopamine agonist methylphenidate induced a significant increase in dopamine levels that was positively correlated with ratings of desire to eat. Interestingly, amphetamine, which acts to increase brain dopamine concentrations, also increases craving for drugs (Leyton *et al.*, 2002).

Implications for Food Addictions

The data reviewed so far suggest that modulation of brain GABA, opioid, cannabinoid and dopamine systems affects food reward. There is also some evidence (albeit limited) that pharmacological manipulations of brain reward systems produce concomitant changes in food cravings, thus providing support for the suggestion that food cravings may be an emotional response associated with reward-related behaviour. In accordance with the suggestion that feeding and drug-taking are controlled by similar motivational processes, there is a great deal of overlap between the pathways underlying drug and food reward. In fact, it has been argued that drugs of abuse hijack the brain's natural reward systems by either mimicking the effects of reinforcers such as food or sex, or producing exaggerated responses in specific reward systems (Koob, 1992; Kelley and Berridge, 2002). Because the rewarding effects of drugs of abuse are thought to contribute to their dependence-inducing properties, food addiction has been proposed as a new and prevalent disorder. The popular media has actively reinforced this view, and it has even been suggested that food addiction may underlie recent rises in obesity in the USA and the UK. It is certainly the case that the effects of food on brain neurochemistry are similar to those of drugs of abuse. Both food and stimulant drugs like cocaine and nicotine increase dopamine release in the brain (Di Chiara, 1995), while opioid agonists like heroin act indirectly to increase brain dopamine, and alcohol enhances the effects of GABA (Koob, 1992). But it should be noted that there are differences in food- and drug-induced neurochemical effects too. Drugs of abuse generally evoke much greater release of dopamine when measured using microdialysis techniques and the dopamine response to drugs of abuse does not habituate to the same extent as for food (Di Chiara, 2002). These differences suggest that drugs of abuse may induce dependence via mechanisms that differentiate them from food reinforcers. Another key difference between drugs of abuse and food relates to sensitization. The incentive salience theory of addiction suggests that sensitization of dopamine-dependent drug 'wanting' underlies addiction. It is argued that repeated administration of drugs of abuse increases cue-elicited craving, leading to compulsive use (Robinson and Berridge 1993, 2003). While acute, *ad libitum* exposure to palatable foods does not appear to induce sensitization, there is evidence that chronic and restricted access to highly palatable foods results in escalating levels of intake and adaptive changes in dopamine and opioid systems that are similar to those observed following sensitization to drugs of abuse (Uhl *et al.*, 1988; Georges *et al.*, 1999; Colantuoni *et al.*, 2001; Kelley *et al.*, 2003; Viganò *et al.*, 2003; Spangler *et al.*, 2004). Furthermore, cross-sensitization between chronic sugar intake and drugs of abuse has been shown recently (Avena and Hoebel 2003a, 2003b). Thus, binge-like patterns of palatable food intake can induce neurochemical changes similar to those thought to underlie addiction to drugs of abuse. In addition, abrupt withdrawal from chronic intermittent consumption of sugar has been shown to induce effects that mimic those observed following withdrawal from opiate drugs of abuse (Colantuoni *et al.*, 2002). A case could be made to suggest that repeated restriction of food intake followed by excessive consumption (a pattern that is sometimes observed in bulimia) results in behavioural and neurochemical changes that resemble an addicted state. In support of this, food cravings have been identified as an antecedent to bingeing in some bulimic patients (Mitchell *et al.*, 1985) and there are often high rates of co-morbid drug abuse in bulimia (Bulik *et al.*, 1992).

Concluding Comments

The evidence presented in this chapter suggests that food cravings may arise from activation of brain systems associated with food reward. Manipulations of GABAergic, opioid, cannabinoid and dopamine systems, which are important in mediating reward-related behaviours, can induce or inhibit cravings. These systems have also been implicated in drug craving and addiction, raising the possibility that people can become addicted to food in the same way they can become dependent upon drugs. There are many similarities between the effects of palatable food consumption and drugs of abuse on brain neurochemistry, but the effects of drugs that are relevant to their dependence-inducing liability may only be replicated by very specific feeding regimens. This suggests a possible distinction between pathological and everyday cravings. The latter may be related to normal appetite mechanisms that encourage the consumption of foods that have been experienced as rewarding in the past. Given that these are likely to be energy-rich foods, cravings may serve an important function in the selection of foods that are important for survival. Neural adaptations in brain opioid and dopamine systems consequent upon binge-like or excessive patterns of palatable food consumption may underlie more intense cravings that could contribute to compulsive behaviour, but this is likely to be limited to individuals with highly disordered eating patterns, rather than being a widespread phenomenon. Clearly, further investigation into the relationship between food cravings and brain reward mechanisms is warranted. In this regard, assessment of the neural correlates of food craving and reward in humans using imaging techniques such as positron emission tomography and functional magnetic resonance imaging could prove informative. Finally, the development of pharmacological interventions aimed at blocking, for example, cannabinoid- and dopamine-mediated effects on food reward could be useful in the treatment and management of pathological food cravings.

References

Apfelbaum, M. and Mandenoff, A. (1981) Naltrexone suppresses hyperphagia induced in the rat by a highly palatable diet. *Pharmacology, Biochemistry, and Behavior* 15, 89–91.

Arbisi, P.A., Billington, C.J. and Levine, A.S. (1999) The effect of naltrexone on taste detection and recognition threshold. *Appetite* 32, 241–249.

Avena, N.M. and Hoebel, B.G. (2003a) A diet promoting sugar dependency causes behavioral cross-sensitization to a low dose of amphetamine. *Neuroscience* 122, 17–20.

Avena, N.M. and Hoebel, B.G. (2003b) Amphetamine-sensitized rats show sugar-induced hyperactivity (cross-sensitization) and sugar hyperphagia. *Pharmacology, Biochemistry, and Behavior* 74, 635–639.

Bailey, C.S., Hsiao, S. and King, J.E. (1986) Hedonic reactivity to sucrose in rats: modification by pimozide. *Physiology & Behavior* 38, 447–452.

Bassareo, V. and Di Chiara, G. (1999) Differential responsiveness of dopamine transmission to food-stimuli in nucleus accumbens shell/core compartments. *Neuroscience* 89, 637–641.

Beauchamp, G.K., Bertino, M., Burke, D. and Engelman, K. (1990) Experimental sodium depletion and salt taste in normal human volunteers. *American Journal of Clinical Nutrition* 51, 881–889.

Berridge, K.C. (1988) Brain-stem systems mediate the enhancement of palatability by chlordiazepoxide. *Brain Research* 447, 262–268.

Berridge, K.C. (1996) Food reward: brain substrates of wanting and liking. *Neuroscience and Biobehavioral Reviews* 20, 1–25.

Berridge, K.C. (2003) Pleasures of the brain. *Brain and Cognition* 52, 106–128.

Berridge, K.C. and Robinson, T.E. (1998) What is the role of dopamine in reward: hedonic impact, reward learning, or incentive salience? *Brain Research Reviews* 28, 309–369.

Berridge, K.C. and Treit, D. (1986) Chlordiazepoxide directly enhances positive ingestive reactions in rats. *Pharmacology, Biochemistry, and Behavior* 24, 217–221.

Berridge, K.C., Venier, I.L. and Robinson, T.E. (1989) Taste reactivity analysis of 6-hydroxydopamine-induced hyperphagia: implications for arousal and anhedonia hypotheses of dopamine function. *Behavioural Neuroscience* 103, 36–45.

Bindra, D. (1974) A motivational view of learning, performance, and behavior modification. *Psychological Review* 81, 199–213.

Blackburn, J.R., Phillips, A.G., Jakubovic, A. and Fibiger, H.C. (1989) Dopamine and preparatory behavior. 2. A neurochemical analysis. *Behavioral Neuroscience* 103, 15–23.

Blass, E.M. and Fitzgerald, E. (1988) Milk-induced analgesia and comforting in 10-day-old rats: opioid mediation. *Pharmacology, Biochemistry, and Behavior* 29, 9–13.

Blass, E.M. and Hoffmeyer, L.B. (1991) Sucrose as an analgesic for newborn infants. *Pediatrics* 87, 215–218.

Bodnar, R.J., Glass, M.J., Ragnauth, A. and Cooper, M.L. (1995) General μ and κ opioid antagonists in the nucleus accumbens alter food intake under deprivation, glucoprivic and palatable conditions. *Brain Research* 700, 205–212.

Bolles, R.C. (1972) Reinforcement and expectancy learning. *Psychological Review* 79, 394–409.

Breslin, P.A.S., Davis, J.D. and Rosenak, R. (1996) Saccharin increases the effectiveness of glucose in stimulating ingestion in rats but has little effect on negative feedback. *Physiology & Behavior* 60, 411–416.

Bulik, C.M., Sullivan, P.F., Epstein, L.H., Mckee, M., Kaye, W.H., Dahl, R.E. and Weltzin, T.E. (1992) Drug-use in women with anorexia and bulimia-nervosa. *International Journal of Eating Disorders* 11, 213–225.

Cardinal, R.N. and Everitt, B.J. (2004) Neural and psychological mechanisms underlying appetitive learning: links to drug addiction. *Current Opinion in Neurobiology* 14, 156–162.

Cardinal, R.N., Parkinson, J.A., Hall, J.A. and Everitt, B.J. (2002) Emotion and motivation: the role of the amygdala, ventral striatum and prefrontal cortex. *Neuroscience and Biobehavioral Reviews* 26, 321–352.

Casey, D.E. and Zorn, S.H. (2001) The pharmacology of weight gain with antipsychotics. *Journal of Clinical Psychiatry* 62, 4–10.

Cepeda-Benito, A., Gleaves, D.H., Fernandez, M.C., Vila, J. and Reynoso, J. (2000) The development and validation of Spanish versions of the state and trait food cravings questionnaires. *Behaviour Research and Therapy* 38, 1125–1138.

Colantuoni, C., Schwenker, J., McCarthy, J., Rada, P., Ladenheim, B., Cadet, J.L., Schwartz, G.J., Moran, T.H. and Hoebel, B.G. (2001) Excessive sugar intake alters binding to dopamine and μ-opioid receptors in the brain. *NeuroReport* 12, 3549–3552.

Colantuoni, C., Rada, P., McCarthy, J., Patten, C., Avena, N.M., Chadeayne, A. and Hoebel, B.G. (2002) Evidence that intermittent, excessive sugar intake causes endogenous opioid dependence. *Obesity Research* 10, 478–488.

Cooper, S.J. (1980) Naloxone: effects on food and water consumption in the non deprived and deprived rat. *Psychopharmacology* 71, 1–6.

Cooper, S.J. and Kirkham, T.C. (1993) Opioid mechanisms in the control of food intake. In: Hertz, A. (ed.) *Handbook of Experimental Pharmacology*. Vol. 104. *Opioids II*. Springer-Verlag, Berlin, pp. 230–262.

Cooper, S.J., van der Hoek, G. and Kirkham, T.C. (1988) Bi-directional changes in sham feeding in the rat produced by benzodiazepine receptor ligands. *Physiology & Behavior* 42, 211–216.

D'Anci, K.E., Kanarek, R.B. and Marks-Kaufman, R. (1996) Duration of sucrose availability differentially alters morphine-induced analgesia in rats. *Pharmacology, Biochemistry, and Behavior* 54, 693–697.

Davis, J.D. and Levine, M.W. (1977) A model for the control of ingestion. *Psychological Review* 84, 379–412.

Devane, W.A., Hanus, L., Breuer, A., Pertwee, R.G., Stevenson, L.A., Griffin, G., Gibson, D., Mandekbaum, A., Etinger, A. and Mechoulam, R. (1992) Isolation and structure of a brain constituent that binds to the cannabinoid receptor. *Science* 258, 1946–1949.

Di Chiara, G. (1995) The role of dopamine in drug abuse viewed from the perspective of its role in motivation. *Drug and Alcohol Dependence* 38, 13–95.

Di Chiara, G. (2002) Nucleus accumbens shell and core dopamine: differential role in behavior and addiction. *Behavioral Brain Research* 137, 75–114.

Dickinson, A., Smith, J. and Mirenowicz, J. (2000) Dissociation of Pavlovian and instrumental incentive learning under dopamine antagonists. *Behavioral Neuroscience* 114, 468–483.

Doyle, T.G., Berridge, K.C. and Gosnell, B.A. (1993). Morphine enhances hedonic taste palatability in rats. *Pharmacology, Biochemistry, and Behavior* 46, 745–749.

Drewnowski, A., Krahn, D.D., Demitrack, M.A., Nairn, K. and Gosnell, B.A. (1992) Taste responses and preferences for sweet high-fat foods: evidence for opioid involvement. *Physiology & Behavior* 51, 371–379.

Dum, J., Gramsch, C. and Herz, A. (1983) Activation of hypothalamic β-endorphin pools by reward induced by highly palatable food. *Pharmacology, Biochemistry, and Behavior* 18, 443–447.

Ettenberg, A. (1989) Dopamine neuroleptics and reinforced behaviour. *Neuroscience and Biobehavioral Reviews* 13, 105–111.

Evans, S.M., Foltin, R.W. and Fischman, M.W. (1999) Food 'cravings' and the acute effects of alprazolam on food intake in women with premenstrual dysphoric disorder. *Appetite* 32, 331–349.

Everitt, B.J., Dickinson, A. and Robbins, T.W. (2001) The neuropsychological basis of addictive behaviour. *Brain Research Reviews* 36, 129–138.

Fedoroff, I.C., Polivy, J. and Herman, C.P. (1997) The effect of pre-exposure to food cues on the eating behaviour of restrained and unrestrained eaters. *Appetite* 28, 33–47.

Fedoroff, I.C., Polivy, J. and Herman, C.P. (2003) The specificity of restrained versus unrestrained eaters' responses to food cues: general desire to eat, or craving for the cued food? *Appetite* 41, 7–13.

Foltin, R.W., Ellis, S. and Schuster, C.R. (1985) Specific antagonism by Ro 15-1788 of benzodiazepine-induced increases in food intake in rhesus monkeys. *Pharmacology, Biochemistry, and Behavior* 23, 249–252.

Foltin, R.W., Fischman, M.W. and Byrne, M.F. (1988) Effects of smoked marijuana on food intake and body weight of humans living in a residential laboratory. *Appetite* 11, 1–14.

Fratta, W., Mereu, G., Chessa, P., Paglietti, E. and Gessa, G. (1976) Benzodiazepine induced voraciousness in cats and inhibition of amphetamine-induced anorexia. *Life Sciences* 18, 1156–1166.

Gallate, J.E. and McGregor, I.S. (1999) The motivation for beer in rats: effects of ritanserin, naloxone and SR 141716. *Psychopharmacology* 142, 302–308.

Gallate, J.E., Saharov, T., Mallet, P.E. and McGregor, I.S. (1999) Increased motivation for beer in rats following administration of a cannabinoid CB1 receptor agonist. *European Journal of Pharmacology* 370, 233–240.

Gaoni, Y. and Mechoulam, R. (1964) Isolation, structure and partial synthesis of an active constituent of hashish. *Journal of the American Chemical Society* 86, 1646–1647.

Gardner, E.L. and Vorel, S.R. (1998) Cannabinoid transmission and reward-related events. *Neurobiology of Disease* 5, 502–533.

Geary, N. and Smith, G.P. (1985) Pimozide decreases the positive reinforcing effect of sham fed sucrose in the rat. *Pharmacology, Biochemistry, and Behavior* 22, 787–790.

Genn, R.F., Higgs, S. and Cooper, S.J. (2003) The effects of 7-OH-DPAT, quinpirole and raclopride on licking for sucrose solutions in the non-deprived rat. *Behavioural Pharmacology* 14, 609–617.

Georges, F., Stinus, L., Bloch, B. and Le Moine, C. (1999) Chronic morphine exposure and spontaneous withdrawal are associated with modifications of dopamine receptor and neuropeptide gene expression in the rat striatum. *European Journal of Neuroscience* 11, 481–490.

Giraudo, S.Q., Grace, M.K., Welch, C.C., Billington, C.J. and Levine, A.S. (1993) Naloxone's anorectic effect is dependent upon the relative palatability of food. *Pharmacology, Biochemistry, and Behavior* 46, 917–921.

Glass, M.J., Grace, M.K., Cleary, J.P., Billington, C.J. and Levine, A.S. (2001) Naloxone's effect on meal microstructure of sucrose and cornstarch diets. *American Journal of Physiology* 281, R1605–R1612.

Gosnell, B.A., Levine, A.S. and Morley, J.E. (1983) *N*-Allylnormetazocine (SKF-10,047): the induction of feeding by a putative sigma agonist. *Pharmacology, Biochemistry, and Behavior* 19, 737–742.

Hajnal, A. and Norgren, R. (2001) Accumbens dopamine mechanisms in sucrose intake. *Brain Research* 904, 76–84.

Hajnal, A. and Norgren, R. (2002) Repeated access to sucrose augments dopamine turnover in the nucleus accumbens. *NeuroReport* 13, 2213–2216.

Hajnal, A., Smith, G.P. and Norgren, R. (2004) Oral sucrose stimulation increases accumbens dopamine in the rat. *American Journal of Physiology* 286, R31–R37.

Haney, M., Comer, S.D., Fischman, M.W. and Foltin, R.W. (1997) Alprazolam increases food intake in humans. *Psychopharmacology* 132, 311–314.

Hao, S., Avraham, Y., Mechoulam, R. and Berry, E.M. (2000) Low dose anandamide affects food intake, cognitive function, neurotransmitter and corticosterone levels in diet-restricted mice. *European Journal of Pharmacology* 392, 147–156.

Harvey, J., Wing, R.R. and Mullen, M. (1993) Effects on food cravings of a very low-calorie diet or a balanced low-calorie diet. *Appetite* 21, 105–115.

Hayward, M.D., Pintar, J.E. and Low, M.J. (2002) Selective reward deficit in mice lacking β-endorphin and enkephalin. *Journal of Neuroscience* 22, 8251–8258.

Hernandez, L. and Hoebel, B.G. (1988) Food reward and cocaine increase extracellular dopamine in the nucleus accumbens as measured by microdialysis. *Life Sciences* 42, 705–712.

Higgs, S. and Cooper, S.J. (1996) Effects of the benzodiazepine receptor inverse agonist Ro 15-4513 on the ingestion of sucrose and sodium saccharin solutions: a microstructural analysis of licking behavior. *Behavioral Neuroscience* 110, 559–566.

Higgs, S. and Cooper, S.J. (1997) Midazolam induced rapid changes in licking behaviour: evidence for involvement of endogenous opioid peptides. *Psychopharmacology* 131, 278–286.

Higgs, S. and Cooper, S.J. (1998a) Effects of benzodiazepine receptor ligands on the ingestion of sucrose, intralipid, and maltodextrin: an investigation using a microstructural analysis of licking behavior in a brief contact test. *Behavioral Neuroscience* 112, 447–457.

Higgs, S. and Cooper, S.J. (1998b) Evidence for early opioid modulation of licking responses to sucrose and intralipid: a microstructural analysis in the rat. *Psychopharmacology* 139, 342–355.

Higgs, S. and Cooper, S.J. (2000) The effect of the dopamine D2 antagonist raclopride on the pattern of licking microstructure induced by midazolam in the rat. *European Journal of Pharmacology* 409, 73–80.

Higgs, S., Williams, C.M. and Kirkham, T.C. (2003a) Cannabinoid influences on palatability: microstructural analysis of sucrose drinking after delta-9-THC, anandamide, 2-AG and SR141716. *Psychopharmacology* 165, 370–377.

Higgs, S., Street, M., Cooper, A.J. and Terry, P. (2003b) Effects of Δ^9-THC and diazepam on progressive ratio responding for food. *Behavioural Pharmacology* 14, S48.

Higgs, S., Roberts, D., Cooper, A.J. and Terry, P. (2004) Effects of benzodiazepine ligands on progressive ratio responding for food. *Journal of Psychopharmacology* 18, A25.

Holland, P.C., Petrovich, G.D. and Gallagher, M. (2002) The effects of amygdala lesions on conditioned stimulus-potentiated eating in rats. *Physiology & Behavior* 76, 117–129.

Holtzman, S.G. (1974) Behavioural effects of separate and combined administration of naloxone and D-amphetamine. *Journal of Pharmacology and Experimental Therapeutics* 189, 51–60.

Hsiao, S. and Smith, G.P. (1995) Raclopride reduces sucrose preference in rats. *Pharmacology, Biochemistry, and Behavior* 50, 121–125.

Jamshidi, N. and Taylor, D.A. (2001) Anandamide administration into the ventromedial hypothalamus stimulates appetite in rats. *British Journal of Pharmacology* 134, 1151–1154.

Kanarek, R.B. and Homoleski, B. (2000) Modulation of morphine-induced antinociception by palatable solutions in male and female rats. *Pharmacology, Biochemistry, and Behavior* 66, 653–659.

Kanarek, R.B., Przypek, J., D'Anci, K.E. and Marks-Kaufman, R. (1997) Dietary modulation of μ and κ opioid receptor-mediated analgesia. *Pharmacology, Biochemistry, and Behaviour* 58, 43–49.

Kelley, A.E. and Berridge, K.C. (2002) The neuroscience of natural rewards: relevance to addictive drugs. *Journal of Neuroscience* 22, 3306–3311.

Kelley, A.E., Bless, E.P. and Swanson, C.J. (1996) An investigation of the effects of opiate antagonists infused into the nucleus accumbens on feeding and sucrose drinking in rats. *Journal of Pharmacology and Experimental Therapeutics* 278, 1499–1507.

Kelley, A.E., Bakshi, V.P., Haber, S.N., Steininger, T.L., Will, T.J. and Zhang, M. (2002) Opioid modulation of taste hedonics within the ventral striatum. *Physiology & Behavior* 76, 365–377.

Kelley, A.E., Will, M.J., Steininger, T.L., Zhang, M. and Haber, S.N. (2003) Restricted daily consumption of a highly palatable food (chocolate Ensure®) alters striatal enkephalin gene expression. *European Journal of Neuroscience* 18, 2592–2598.

Kelly, T.H., Foltin, R.W. and King, L. (1992) Behavioral-response to diazepam in a residential laboratory. *Biological Psychiatry* 31, 808–822.

Kirkham, T.C. (1990) Enhanced anorectic potency of naloxone in rats sham feeding 30% sucrose: reversal by repeated naloxone administration. *Physiology & Behavior* 47, 419–426.

Kirkham, T.C. and Cooper, S.J. (1988a) Attenuation of sham feeding by naloxone is stereospecific – evidence for opioid mediation of orosensory reward. *Physiology & Behavior* 43, 845–847.

Kirkham, T.C. and Cooper, S.J. (1988b) Naloxone attenuation of sham feeding is modified by manipulation of sucrose concentration. *Physiology & Behavior* 44, 491–494.

Kirkham, T.C., Williams, C.M., Fezza, F. and Di Marzo, V. (2002) Endocannabinoid levels in rat limbic forebrain and hypothalamus in relation to fasting, feeding and satiation: stimulation of eating by 2-arachidonoyl glycerol. *British Journal of Pharmacology* 136, 550–557.

Koob, G.F. (1992) Drugs of abuse: anatomy, pharmacology, and function of reward pathways. *Trends in Pharmacological Sciences* 13, 177–184.

Leeb, K., Parker, L. and Eikelboom, R. (1991) Effects of pimozide on the hedonic properties of sucrose – analysis by the taste reactivity test. *Pharmacology, Biochemistry, and Behavior* 39, 895–901.

Levine, A.S. and Billington, C.J. (1989) Opioids: are they regulators of feeding? *Annals of the New York Academy of Sciences* 575, 194–209.

Leyton, M., Boileau, I., Benkelfat, C., Diksic, M., Baker, G. and Dagher, A. (2002) Amphetamine-induced increases in extracellular dopamine, drug wanting, and novelty seeking: a PET/[^{11}C]raclopride study in healthy men. *Neuropsychopharmacology* 27, 1027–1035.

Mansbach, R.S., Stanley, J.A. and Barrett, J.E. (1984) Ro 15-4513 and β-CCE selectively eliminate diazepam-induced feeding in the rabbit. *Pharmacology, Biochemistry, and Behavior* 20, 763–766.

Marks-Kaufman, R. and Kanarek, R.B. (1980) Morphine selectively influences macronutrient intake in the rat. *Pharmacology, Biochemistry, and Behavior* 12, 427–430.

Mattes, R.D., Engelman, K., Shaw, L.M. and Elsohly, M.A. (1994) Cannabinoids and appetite stimulation. *Pharmacology, Biochemistry, and Behavior* 49, 187–195.

Michener, W. and Rozin, P. (1994) Pharmacological versus sensory factors in the satiation of chocolate craving. *Physiology & Behavior* 56, 419–422.

Mitchell, J.E., Hatsukami, D., Eckert, E.D. and Pyle, R.L. (1985) Characteristics of 275 patients with bulimia. *American Journal of Psychiatry* 142, 482–485.

Morley, J.E., Levine, A.S., Kneip, J. and Grace, M. (1982) The role of κ opioid receptors in the initiation of feeding. *Life Sciences* 31, 2617–2626.

Mucha, R.F., Geier, A. and Pauli, P. (1999) Modulation of craving by cues having differential overlap with pharmacological effect: evidence for cue approach in smokers and social drinkers. *Psychopharmacology* 147, 306–313.

Parker, L.A. and Lopez, N. (1990) Pimozide enhances the aversiveness of quinine solution. *Pharmacology, Biochemistry, and Behavior* 36, 653–659.

Parker, L.A., Maier, S., Rennie, M. and Crebolder, J. (1992) Morphine and naltrexone-induced modification of palatability: analysis by the taste reactivity test. *Behavioural Neuroscience* 106, 999–1010.

Parker, S., Kamel, N. and Zellner, D. (2003) Food craving patterns in Egypt: comparisons with North America and Spain. *Appetite* 40, 193–195.

Parkinson, J.A., Dalley, J.W., Cardinal, R.N., Bamford, A., Fehnert, B., Lachenal, G., Rudarakanchana, N., Halkerston, K.M., Robbins, T.W. and Everitt, B.J. (2002) Nucleus accumbens dopamine depletion impairs both acquisition and performance of appetitive Pavlovian approach behaviour: implications for mesoaccumbens dopamine function. *Behavioural Brain Research* 137, 149–163.

Pecina, S. and Berridge, K.C. (1995) Central enhancement of taste pleasure by intraventricular morphine. *Neurobiology* 3, 269–280.

Pecina, S. and Berridge, K.C. (1996) Brainstem mediates diazepam enhancement of palatability and feeding: microinjections into fourth ventricle versus lateral ventricle. *Brain Research* 727, 22–30.

Pecina, S. and Berridge, K.C. (2000) Opioid site in nucleus accumbens shell mediates eating and hedonic liking for food: map based on microinjection fos plumes. *Brain Research* 863, 71–86.

Pecina, S., Berridge, K.C. and Parker, L.A. (1997) Pimozide does not shift palatability: separation of anhedonia from sensorimotor suppression by taste reactivity. *Pharmacology, Biochemistry, and Behavior* 58, 801–811.

Pecina, S., Cagniard, B., Berridge, K.C., Aldridge, J.W. and Zhuang, X. (2003) Hyper-dopaminergic mutant mice have higher 'wanting' but not 'liking' for sweet rewards. *Journal of Neuroscience* 23, 9395–9402.

Pelchat, M.L. (1997) Food cravings in young and elderly adults. *Appetite* 28, 103–113.

Pelchat, M.L. and Schaeffer, S. (2000) Dietary monotony and food cravings in young and elderly adults. *Physiology & Behavior* 68, 353–359.

Pertwee, R.G. (1997) Pharmacology of cannabinoid CB1 and CB2 receptors. *Pharmacology and Therapeutics* 74, 129–180.

Rideout, H.J. and Parker, L.A. (1996) Morphine enhancement of sucrose palatability: analysis by the taste reactivity test. *Pharmacology, Biochemistry, and Behavior* 53, 731–734.

Robinson, T.E. and Berridge, K.C. (1993) The neural basis of drug craving – an incentive sensitization theory of addiction. *Brain Research Reviews* 18, 247–291.

Robinson, T.E. and Berridge, K.C. (2003) Addiction. *Annual Review of Psychology* 95, 91–117.

Rockwood, G.A. and Reid, L.D. (1982) Naloxone modifies sugar-water intake in rats with open gastric fistulas. *Physiology & Behavior* 29, 1175–1178.

Rodin, J., Mancuso, J., Granger, J. and Nelback, E. (1991) Food cravings in relation to body mass index, restraint and estradiol levels: a repeated measures study in healthy women. *Appetite* 17, 177–185.

Roitman, M.F., Stuber, G.D., Phillips, P.E.M., Wightman, R.M. and Carelli, R. (2004) Dopamine operate as a subsecond modulator of food seeking. *Journal of Neuroscience* 24, 1265–1271.

Rolls, E.T., Rolls, B.J., Kelly, P.H., Shaw, S.G., Wood, R.J. and Dale, R. (1974) The relative attenuation of self stimulation, eating and drinking produced by dopamine receptor blockade. *Psychopharmacology* 38, 216–230.

Rozin, P., Levine, E. and Stoess, C. (1991) Chocolate craving and liking. *Appetite* 17, 199–212.

Salamone, J., Cousins, M. and Snyder, B. (1997) Behavioral functions of nucleus accumbens dopamine: empirical and conceptual problems with the anhedonia hypothesis. *Neuroscience and Biobehavioral Reviews* 21, 341–359.

Schneider, L.H., Gibbs, J. and Smith, G.P. (1986) D-2 selective receptor antagonists suppress sucrose sham feeding in the rat. *Brain Research Bulletin* 17, 605–611.

Schultz, W. (2002) Getting formal with dopamine and reward. *Neuron* 36, 241–263.

Schultz, W., Apicella, P. and Ljundberg, T. (1993) Responses of monkey dopamine neurons to reward and conditioned stimuli during successive steps of learning a delayed response task. *Journal of Neuroscience* 13, 900–913.

Sclafani, A. (1995) How food preferences are learned – laboratory animal models. *Proceedings of the Nutrition Society* 54, 419–427.

Shabir, S. and Kirkham, T.C. (1999) Diet-induced enhancement of naloxone sensitivity is independent of changes in body weight. *Pharmacology, Biochemistry, and Behavior* 62, 601–605.

Smith, G.P. (1995) Dopamine and food reward. In: Morrison, A.N. and Fluharty, S.J. (eds) *Progress in Psychobiology and Physiological Psychology*, Vol. 15. Academic Press, New York, pp. 254–261.

Smith, G.P. and Schneider, L.H. (1988) Relationships between mesolimbic dopamine function and eating behavior. *Annals of the New York Academy of Sciences* 537, 254–261.

Spangler, R., Wittkowski, K.M., Goddard, N.L., Avena, N.M., Hoebel, B.G. and Leibowitz, S.F. (2004) Opiate-like effects of sugar on gene expression in reward related areas of the brain. *Molecular Brain Research* 124, 134–142.

Teff, K.L., Young, S.N., Marchand, L. and Botez, M.I. (1989) Acute effect of protein or carbohydrate breakfasts on human cerebrospinal fluid monoamine precursor and metabolite levels. *Journal of Neurochemistry* 52, 235–241.

Ticku, M.K. (1991) Drug modulation of GABA-A mediated transmission. *Seminars in the Neurosciences* 3, 211–218.

Towell, A., Muscat, R. and Wilner, P. (1987) Effects of pimozide on sucrose consumption and preference. *Psychopharmacology* 92, 262–264.

Treit, D. and Berridge, K.C. (1990) A comparison of benzodiazepine, serotonin, and dopamine agents in the taste-reactivity paradigm. *Pharmacology, Biochemistry, and Behavior* 37, 451–456.

Treit, D., Berridge, K.C. and Schultz, C.E. (1987) The direct enhancement of palatability by chlordiazepoxide is antagonized by Ro 15-1788 and CGS 8216. *Pharmacology, Biochemistry, and Behavior* 26, 709–714.

Tuomisto, T., Hetherington, M.M., Morris, M.-F., Tuomisto, M., Turanmaa, V. and Lappalainen, R. (1999) Psychological and physiological characteristics of sweet food 'addiction'. *International Journal of Eating Disorders* 25, 169–175.

Uhl, G.R., Ryan, J.P. and Schwartz, J.P. (1988) Morphine alter prepropenkephalin gene expression. *Brain Research* 459, 391–397.

Viganò, D., Rubino, T., Di Chiara, G., Ascari, I., Massi, P. and Parolaro, D. (2003) μ-Opioid receptor signalling in morphine sensitization. *Neuroscience* 117, 921–929.

Volkow, N.D., Wang, G.J., Fowler, J.S., Logan, J., Jayne, M., Franceschi, D., Wong, C., Gatley, S.J., Gifford, A.N., Ding, Y.S. and Pappas, N. (2002) 'Non-hedonic' food motivation in humans involves dopamine in the dorsal striatum and methylphenidate amplifies this effect. *Synapse* 44, 175–180.

Volpicelli, J.R., Watson, N.T., King, A.C., Sherman, C.E. and O'Brien, C.P. (1995) Effect of naltrexone on alcohol 'high' in alcoholics. *American Journal of Psychiatry* 152, 613–615.

Weingarten, H.P. (1983) Conditioned cues elicit feeding in sated rats: a role for learning in meal initiation. *Science* 220, 431–433.

Weingarten, H.P. (1984) Meal initiation controlled by learned cues: basic behavioral properties. *Appetite* 5, 147–158.

Weingarten, H.P. and Elston, D. (1991) Food cravings in a college population. *Appetite* 17, 167–175.

Weinrieb, R.M. and O'Brien, C.P. (1997) Naltrexone in the treatment of alcoholism. *Annual Review of Medicine* 48, 477–487.

Welch, C.C., Kim, E.M., Grace, M.K., Billington, C.J. and Levine, A.S. (1996) Palatability-induced hyperphagia increases hypothalamic dynorphin peptide and mRNA levels. *Brain Research* 721, 126–131.

Wilkins, L. and Richter, C.P. (1940) A great craving for salt by a child with corticoadrenal insufficiency. *Journal of the American Medical Association* 114, 866–868.

Williams, C.M. and Kirkham, T.C. (1999) Anandamide induces overeating: mediation by central cannabinoid (CB1) receptors. *Psychopharmacology* 143, 315–317.

Williams, C.M. and Kirkham, T.C. (2002) Reversal of Δ^9-THC hyperphagia by SR141716 and naloxone but not dexfenfluramine. *Pharmacology, Biochemistry, and Behavior* 71, 341–348.

Williams, C.M., Rogers, P.J. and Kirkham, T.C. (1998) Hyperphagia in pre-fed rats following oral Δ^9-THC. *Physiology & Behavior* 65, 343–346.

Wilner, P., Papp, M., Phillips, G., Maleeh, M. and Muscat, R. (1990) Pimozide does not impair sweetness discrimination. *Psychopharmacology* 102, 278–282.

Wise, R.A. (1982) Neuroleptics and operant behavior: the anhedonia hypothesis. *Behavioral Brain Sciences* 5, 39–87.

Wise, R.A. (2004) Dopamine, learning and motivation. *Nature Reviews Neuroscience* 5, 483–494.

Wise, R.A. and Colle, L.M. (1984) Pimozide attenuates free feeding – best scores analysis reveals a motivational deficit. *Psychopharmacology* 84, 446–451.

Wise, R.A. and Raptis, L. (1986) Effects of naloxone and pimozide on initiation and maintenance measures of free feeding. *Brain Research* 368, 62–68.

Wise, R.A., Spindler, J., de Wit, H. and Gerber, G.J. (1978) Neuroleptic-induced 'anhedonia' in rats: pimozide blocks the reward quality of food. *Science* 201, 262–264.

Wyvell, C.L. and Berridge, K.C. (2000) Intra-accumbens amphetamine increases the conditioned incentive salience of sucrose reward: enhancement of reward 'wanting' without enhanced 'liking' or response reinforcement. *Journal of Neuroscience* 20, 8122–8130.

Wyvell, C.L. and Berridge, K.C. (2001) Increase incentive sensitisation by previous amphetamine exposure: increased cue triggered 'wanting' for sucrose reward. *Journal of Neuroscience* 21, 7831–7840.

Yeomans, M.R. and Gray, R.W. (1996) Selective effects of naltrexone on food pleasantness and intake. *Physiology & Behavior* 60, 439–446.

Yeomans, M.R. and Gray, R.W. (1997) Effects of naltrexone on food intake and changes in subjective appetite during eating: evidence for opioid involvement in the appetizer effect. *Physiology & Behavior* 62, 15–21.

Yeomans, M.R. and Gray, R.W. (2002) Opioid peptides and the control of human ingestive behaviour. *Neuroscience and Biobehavioral Reviews* 26, 713–728.

Yeomans, M.R. and Wright, P. (1991) Lower pleasantness of palatable foods in nalmefene-treated human volunteers. *Appetite* 16, 249–259.

Yeomans, M.R., Wright, P., Macleod, H.A. and Critchley, J.A.J.H. (1990) Effects of nalmefene on feeding in humans – dissociation of hunger and palatability. *Psychopharmacology* 100, 426–432.

Zellner, D., Garriga-Trillo, A., Rohm, E., Centeno, S. and Parker, S. (1999) Food liking and craving: a cross-cultural approach. *Appetite* 33, 61–70.

Zhang, M. and Kelley, A.E. (2000) Enhanced intake of high fat food following striatal μ-opioid stimulation: microinjection mapping and fos expression. *Neuroscience* 99, 267–277.

Zhang, M., Gosnell, B.A. and Kelley, A.E. (1998) Intake of high-fat food is selectively enhanced by μ-opioid receptor stimulation within the nucleus accumbens. *Journal of Pharmacology and Experimental Therapeutics* 284, 908–914.

Zhang, M., Balmadrid, C. and Kelley, A.E. (2003) Nucleus accumbens opioid, GABAergic, and dopaminergic modulation of palatable food motivation: contrasting effects revealed by a progressive ratio study in the rat. *Behavioral Neuroscience* 117, 202–211.

Zimmermann, U., Rechlin, T., Plakacewicz, G.J., Barocka, A., Wildt, L. and Kaschka, P. (1997) Effect of naltrexone on weight and food cravings induced by tricyclic antidepressants and lithium. *Biological Psychiatry* 41, 747–749.

9 Marketing Parameters and their Influence on Consumer Food Choice

KLAUS G. GRUNERT

MAPP – Centre for Research on Customer Relations in the Food Sector, Department of Marketing and Statistics, Aarhus School of Business, Haslegaardsvej 10, DK 8210 Aarhus V, Denmark

Introduction

In everyday life, when you say 'marketing' most people associate it with communication and persuasion. 'Marketing' is advertising, merchandising, sales promotions, samples, coupons and other measures aimed at increasing sales of a particular product. It is not uncommon to talk about 'marketing tricks', implying that these are measures to induce people to buy things which they neither need nor want.

In the academic treatment of marketing, the concept is somewhat broader. The American Marketing Association (AMA) defines marketing as 'The process of planning and executing the conception, pricing, promotion, and distribution of goods, services, and ideas to create exchanges that satisfy individual and organizational objectives'. The British Chartered Institute of Marketing defines it as 'the management process responsible for identifying, anticipating and satisfying customer requirements profitably'. Other definitions abound, but most of them have a common core: marketing deals with bringing about exchanges (Bagozzi, 1975), it designates processes for bringing about these exchanges which occur on the selling side of the exchange (if the exchange is goods or services for money), and it deals with processes which have the aim of making these exchanges profitable for the seller and satisfying for the buyer.

Marketing processes thus occur on the seller side, but deal with the buyer side. In order to bring about profitable exchanges, we need an understanding of what will make a potential buyer buy and what will make them satisfied with the purchase, so that they will come back for more exchanges in the future. This dual aspect of marketing has been coined in the concept of market orientation, which is meant to designate a business philosophy which tries to understand potential customers and then manage business processes in such a way that one is responsive to the understanding of potential customers one has generated (Kohli and Jaworski, 1990).

Marketing parameters are those parameters at the disposal of the seller that will have an impact on a potential buyer's probability of actually buying.

Historically, marketing theory is a descendant from economic theory, and in traditional economic theory there is only one parameter that affects demand: price. The relationship between price and demand can be analysed in a price response function. Marketing parameters as we know them today are a generalization of the price response function, taking into account that there are other parameters than price that are under control of a seller and that have an impact on demand. These other parameters became fully visible to everyone in the post-World War II period, when discretionary incomes rose and manufacturers answered by differentiating products and creating new forms of advertising.

The most well-known typology of marketing parameters is the famous 'four Ps' – product, price, place and promotion. It has become so popular that it even has entered some definitions of marketing, as the AMA example above shows. We should note, though, that numerous other proposals for typologies of marketing parameters have been advanced over the course of time.

In this chapter, we follow the classic distinction of four major marketing parameters and look at them in the context of food choice. In food marketing, as everywhere else, marketing parameters are defined as those parameters at the disposal of the seller that have an impact on the probability that a consumer will buy a certain food item. In a food context, the four major parameters are the product itself – usually defined as the physical product including its packaging and branding – all types of seller-controlled market communication relating to the product, the way the product is distributed and made available for consumer purchase, and the price of the product.

While we define marketing parameters as something that is under the control of the seller, we should note that it is by no means always clear who the seller is. The entity from which the consumer is buying food is usually a retailer, but the retailer does not autonomously control all marketing parameters (even though some would argue that we are on a route towards that state). The retailer is the end of a sometimes quite complicated value chain, where actors in primary agricultural production, in food processing, in distribution and a host of auxiliary actors work together in bringing about the final offering which is on the supermarket shelf. They jointly form marketing parameters, and they jointly have an impact on consumer buying, even though not all of them may think that way (Grunert et al., 2005). While consumer reactions may be central to the management processes characterizing retailers and major food processors, they may not be central at all in the thinking of some producers of agricultural commodities.

In the following, we go through the four major marketing parameters and discuss their possible impacts on consumer food choice.

Products, Product Quality and Branding

For most people, products are the basic ingredient that is traded in an exchange relationship. At least in the food sector, without a physical product, something that can be prepared and eaten, there is no exchange.

But when we look at the marketing literature, we find a term called 'product orientation', which designates a business philosophy that is regarded as inferior and, in the long run, unsuccessful. Theodore Levitt, who was one of the first to coin the term (Levitt, 1960), contrasted it with the term 'market orientation', which he regarded as the more promising business philosophy. This pair of terms, which has been central to marketing ever since, conveys one simple message: a successful business takes point of departure in consumers' needs, not in the physical products the business happens to deal in. In food, an implication would be that the starting point of business activities should be an analysis of the various needs consumers fulfil by eating, and not in the fact that one happens to be a slaughtering company.

The message is simplified and exaggerated in order to get it across. A slaughtering company will not become a confectionery producer overnight because some analysis of consumer needs indicates that this may be a good idea. We can even question the basic idea that production should follow consumer needs, because there seems to be ample evidence that consumer needs also follow production, at least in certain cases and up to a point. But the more moderate version of the message, namely that the product development of food producers should build on a thorough understanding of consumer needs and food choice, and that such an understanding will increase the likelihood of success of new products, has become widely accepted. Terms like 'consumer-led product development' (Grunert and Valli, 2001) or 'market-oriented product development' (Biemans and Harmsen, 1995) are widely used in the food industry.

The relationship between products and consumers is thus a reciprocal one. Products come about based on analyses of consumer behaviour, but once products are on the market they obviously have an impact on consumer behaviour.

A central term that we can use to analyse this reciprocal relationship between consumers and products is product quality. From the consumer point of view, quality is all that the consumer wants to get out of the product, and perceived quality, when traded off against price and other costs, will be a major determinant of food choice (Steenkamp, 1989). From the producer point of view, it is necessary to translate quality as perceived by the consumer into technical characteristics of the product, so that production processes can be designed in such a way that they will most likely result in product characteristics that consumers will perceive as high or desirable quality.

Food quality has, from the consumer perspective, four major aspects these days (Grunert, 2002). Sensory quality, and here especially taste, is perhaps the most central quality aspect. Health, both in terms of nutrition and safety, has become almost equally important in the minds of consumers. Convenience, not only in preparation, but also in buying, storing, eating and disposing of, is a quality aspect the importance of which has been rising. Finally, certain process characteristics such as organic production, animal welfare and free of genetically modified organisms (GMO) have been incorporated into the quality perception by some consumers.

Quite obviously, a product's quality can have an impact on consumer food choice only to the extent it is perceived. Only few qualities of a food product are what is termed search qualities, i.e. qualities which can be ascertained with certainty before the purchase. Taste and convenience are experience qualities (Nelson, 1970), i.e. qualities that can be experienced after, but not before the purchase; and healthiness is even a credence quality (Darby and Karni, 1973), i.e. a quality which remains intangible to the consumer after the purchase – after all, we do not expect to feel healthier just because we have had an extra serving of vegetables.

Since most aspects of the quality of a product are unknown to the consumer at the time of purchase, consumers form expectations about the quality. These expectations are formed based on quality cues (Steenkamp, 1990) – pieces of information that are being used to infer the quality of the product. Such quality cues can be part of the physical product, in which case we talk about intrinsic cues (Olson and Jacoby, 1972). For example, it is common to infer the expected taste and tenderness of a piece of meat from its visible fat and from its colour (Grunert *et al.*, 2004). In addition to that, the formation of quality expectations can be based on extrinsic cues, such as the shop in which the product is being bought, the price of the product, and of course the advertising of the product.

Packaging is a hybrid in this respect. Packaging can be part of the physical product and add extra quality to it: for example, by providing additional possibilities for storage and serving and by providing protection while taking the product home. In addition, packaging is a carrier of information, and may provide cues which consumers use to infer the quality of the product. Exclusive packaging is meant to raise expected quality, whereas degradable packaging may signal environmental friendliness and hence a desirable process characteristic (Bech-Larsen, 1996). Packaging usually also provides a range of cues related to healthiness. Most of these are in the form of verbal information, like lists of ingredients and best-by dates, but new developments aim at building sensors into packaging that can signal when a product is going over into a stage where human consumption is no longer recommended.

The perhaps most important quality cue is the brand (in cases where the products are branded). A brand is a symbol or name that identifies a product as being produced by a certain producer. Brands became prominent in the food sector about 100 years ago, when some producers wanted to signal to consumers that their products were of superior quality. When Danish dairy producers installed quality control measures that allowed them to produce a consistently high quality of butter, they introduced the Lurpak brand to signal this quality to consumers. In this way, they could avoid that their butter was mixed with other, inferior types of butter by wholesales and retailers, which was a prerequisite for them to obtain a price premium. Consumers who were satisfied with the quality experienced after the purchase could come back to retailers and ask for the same brand, which for them had become a signal of the superior quality. When brands become signals for superior quality in the minds of consumers, they can have a strong impact on consumer food choice, and when consumers become brand loyal, the brand attains brand equity (Barwise, 1993) for the producer. Obviously, a prerequisite for this to occur is that the quality which the brand signals actually is constant across products bearing that brand – otherwise the brand as a signal of quality will become useless, and use of the brand as a quality cue will gradually be unlearned by consumers (Erdem and Swait, 1998).

Branding has traditionally been the domain of food processors, but lately we have seen a development where retailers try to take over some of the branding function. This is a result of the structural development we have seen in the retail sector, which has led retailers not only to have more power facing food producers, but also to more head-on competition among themselves, which in turn has led to a need for clearer positioning in the minds of consumers. Retail brands are not strictly a new development, but have traditionally been interpreted by consumers mostly as signals of low price and basic quality. More recently many food retailers have tried to brand own products of higher quality, and try to teach consumers to reinterpret retailer brands as signals which also can mean higher quality.

As the discussion has shown, it is generally difficult to isolate the effect of the physical product on consumer food choice. Very rarely is the consumer confronted with a physical product, and only with a physical product, when making a choice. The product is 'packaged' in layers of information, which interact with the physical product in affecting consumer choice. This has been additionally reinforced by the increasing importance of product qualities which are by definition invisible at the time of purchase, like healthiness and process characteristics, and which require informational cues for the consumer to be able to form expectations about these qualities.

The experience qualities of the product, i.e. the sensory qualities and (if applicable) the degree of convenience, become amenable to experience after the purchase. Thus, consumers have a quality experience that they can compare with their quality expectations, and it is a common assumption in research on consumer satisfaction that the degree of satisfaction depends on whether expectations are confirmed or disconfirmed (Oliver, 1997). However, as we have shown, not all quality aspects are amenable to experience, and for those that are not – the expectations about, for example, healthiness – may just be carried over from the pre- to the post-purchase phase. In addition, we should also note that for those qualities that can be experienced, the experience will be determined by a host of factors in addition to the physical product. The most important factor here is how the product is used – a good food product can be ruined by bad preparation, and a good cook can prepare delicious meals even from mediocre materials.

The factors discussed on consumer quality perception before and after purchase are summarized in the total food quality model (Grunert, 2005), which is shown in Fig. 9.1.

Persuasion and Market Communication

Consumers are exposed daily to numerous stimuli urging them to buy or not to buy certain food products. Some of them are marketer-controlled, whereas others, while having similar effects, are not marketer-controlled – for example, food recommendations by family members, colleagues, dieticians and doctors. Here, we deal only with marketer-controlled information. We disregard communication emanating from packaging, which we have dealt with in the preceding section.

We can roughly distinguish six types of market communication that are (mostly) seller-controlled (Peter *et al.*, 1999). The most prominent is advertising,

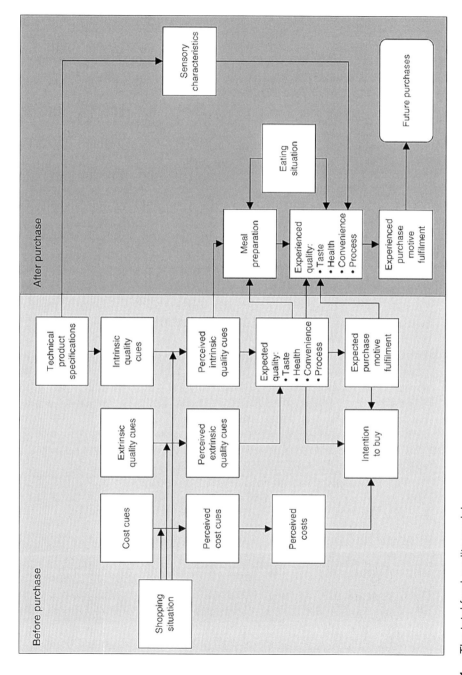

Fig. 9.1. The total food quality model.

usually defined as paid, non-personal information about the product, usually in mass media. Labels are symbols or other informational cues that are standardized across a range of products. In-store communication deals with displays, posters and other stimuli placed in the environment where the purchase is to take place. Personal selling involves direct personal interaction between buyer and seller and is, for food products, mostly restricted to special stores and sometimes special counters in supermarkets. Publicity is an unpaid form of communication, usually in the mass media, which, while not completely under marketer control, is many times prompted by press releases and other company measures. Publicity has been rising in importance as a tool in food marketing, because it can be used to communicate messages about the product which would be illegal to advertise, such as health claims of functional foods. Finally, sponsoring is a hybrid of advertising and publicity. The effects of sponsoring on consumer behaviour are largely unknown, in spite of the large sums that go into it.

The effects of market communication are usually analysed in terms of the classical effects hierarchy. It comes in many versions, but the generic one is that market communication first creates awareness, then comprehension, positive attitude and finally purchase. Most models for measuring advertising effects try to tap the various stages of the effect hierarchy, which obviously has close intellectual bounds to bottom-up models of attitude formation of the Ajzen/Fishbein type. We should also note that the classical effect hierarchy has been criticized by arguing that there may be cases, notably impulse purchases, where awareness can lead directly to purchase, and comprehension and attitude formation do not occur before but after the purchase.

Awareness presupposes exposure. Only communicational stimuli to which consumers are exposed can, obviously, have any impact on consumer behaviour. It is common to distinguish between accidental and intentional exposure (Peter *et al.*, 1999), depending on whether the consumer has made some effort to get into contact with the information, for example by ordering a catalogue, asking a shop attendant or visiting a website, or not. In the food area, the vast amount of market communication effects occurs in situations of accidental exposure. Consumers rarely make an effort to get information about new food products or their characteristics, with food freaks, gourmet magazines, cooking clubs and the like being the major exceptions. Under accidental exposure, there is a high likelihood that the information will never be consciously perceived by consumers. Much effort in market communication for food products therefore goes into getting consumers' conscious attention in a crowded environment. Unconscious scanning of the communication environment probably takes place, but its effect is expected to be limited to giving direction to the process of selective attention, which determines which of the environmental stimuli are selected for further conscious processing (Grunert, 1996).

In analysing the way advertising and other market communication stimuli bring about attitude change, the most popular class of theories has been dual processing models like the elaboration likelihood model (Petty and Cacioppo, 1986). When consumers are motivated and able to process the product-related information, the elaboration of this information will result in the generation of positive or negative cognitive responses, which result in a corresponding attitude change. When consumers are not motivated or not able to process the product-related information, they may process peripheral cues of the message, i.e. characteristics of the message that elicit affective responses, like the people appearing in an advertisement, the use of celebrity endorsers, humour and music. Such peripheral processing (as opposed to the product-focused central processing) can also lead to attitude changes with regard to the product advertised, although these attitude changes will be weaker and less stable. Since much exposure to food advertising is accidental, taking place in situations where motivation or ability to process the information is low, and since many food purchases are made habitually, we may assume that the processing of food advertising is characterized to a great extent by peripheral processing. This is in line with much current advertising practice, where the product-related information is not in focus.

Since attitude changes resulting from peripheral processing are weak and unstable, marketers will many times try to raise consumer involvement with the product in order to induce central processing. The means–end approach (Gutman, 1982) has been invoked in this context. The means–end approach to the analysis of consumer behaviour assumes that we can analyse the driving forces of consumer behaviour by looking at how consumers, subjectively, link perceived product characteristics to personal consequences and ultimately life values by so-called means–end chains. Means–end chains can be measured and analysed, and they can form the basis for the design of advertising strategy that has the aim to increase the extent of central processing. The MECCAS (means–end-chain conceptualization of advertising strategy) model for developing advertising messages recommends communicating whole chains – from product characteristics via personal consequences to life values – to consumers, since this will increase consumer involvement with the product in question and will hence increase the likelihood of central processing (Reynolds and Whitlark, 1995).

Figure 9.2 shows the result of a means–end analysis of a group of Danish consumers with below-average consumption of fish (Nielsen *et al.*, 1997). The analysis shows that these consumers believe that fish is difficult to prepare and to buy, that therefore it is a time-consuming dish which prevents one spending more time with the family and in this way detracts from a central life value. A communication campaign was then designed attempting to communicate the chain easy-to-prepare – more time with your family – good family life. At the same time, more convenience-oriented products were introduced in supermarkets. A pre–post measurement of the determinants of buying fresh fish, using the theory of planned behaviour as a framework, showed not only an increase in consumption of fresh fish, but also that the perceived control component had lost its impact on purchase intentions (Scholderer and Grunert, 2001).

While many food purchases are habitual and low involvement, others are not, and the recent increased interest in process characteristics has led to some food purchases becoming more involving for certain consumer segments. Those consumers who pay premiums for organic food, increased animal welfare or GMO-free products will have a higher degree of involvement with these

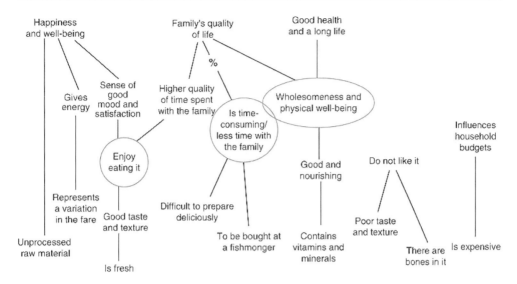

Fig. 9.2.   Results from means–end analysis of Danish consumers with below-average consumption of fresh fish.

purchases. Consumer attitudes in such cases can be quite stable and resistant to attempts to change them by communication. This was demonstrated in an experiment trying to change consumer attitudes towards the use of GMO in food production by various forms of communication (Scholderer and Frewer, 2003). Not only did consumer attitudes not change at all, the only effect of the persuasive communication was that consumers' likelihood to choose a GMO product instead of a conventional product in a choice situation fell. We have here an example of an attitude activation effect (Fazio, 1986): while the persuasive communication did not change consumers' attitudes, it did prime consumers' existing attitudes, made them more accessible and hence more behaviourally relevant.

Examples where professional advertising does not have the desired effect or even backfires are not rare. Consumers live in a cluttered communication environment and have developed effective means for screening out some information and interpreting other information in such ways that it fits their existing attitude structures. The role of advertising is biggest in inducing first trial purchases of new products, when consumers have no previous own experience to draw on.

Labelling deserves special mention, because it is so widely discussed (and in some areas also widely practised) with regard to food. For the consumer, labels are potential quality cues, and as for any other quality cues, their effect on consumer choice will depend on consumer perception of whether the label is predictive of any relevant quality aspect (Cox, 1967). Many labels are ignored or not used because consumers do not know what they stand for, or what they stand for is not regarded as relevant by consumers (e.g. labels guaranteeing certain hygiene standards in farming, which consumers assume are met under all circumstances). Other labels, like some forms of origin marking, are applied to so

many different products that consumers regard the underlying quality claim as
not credible. Some labels are indeed used by consumers, and in those cases a
number of studies indicate that misinterpretations of what the label stands for are
common (Laric and Sarel, 1981; Fotopoulos and Krystallis, 2001). Credible
labelling is especially important for credence qualities such as organic produce
(van Trijp *et al.*, 1997; Bech-Larsen and Grunert, 2001).

Price Perception and Price Impact

The price parameter affects consumer food choice in at least two different ways.
Most importantly, of course, the price indicates what the consumer has to give in
order to obtain the product, and thereby relates the product to the consumer's
and household's economic means. In addition to that, prices are sometimes
used as indicators of quality, and may enter consumer decision making as a
heuristic in different ways.

All price effects are contingent, though, on consumers actually knowing the
price they have to pay for a product. Interestingly enough, that seems often not
to be the case. A whole range of studies (e.g. Dickson and Sawyer, 1990;
Vanhuele and Drèze, 2002) has investigated consumer price awareness, by
employing variations of a basic technique that involves asking consumers about
the price of a product that they had just put into their shopping basket. The
results differ somewhat by method and there also seem to be cultural or national
differences, but the basic result is stable and clear: a sizeable percentage of
consumers buy products without knowing their price.

This does not necessarily imply that consumers do not care about price.
Several explanations can be advanced for this interesting phenomenon. First,
consumers may have a general idea about the price level of the product and
assume that the price has not changed (in which case they should be able,
though, to make a reasonably accurate guess about the price). Second, consumers may earlier have concluded that the price was reasonable, and they may
remember only this conclusion (in which case they would find it difficult to guess
the price). Third, they may assume that the shop in which they buy has low
prices, and that checking individual prices is therefore not necessary.

In addition to the question whether prices are indeed perceived, a good deal
of research has dealt with the question of how price information is processed
once it is perceived (Monroe, 1990). The basic price information processing
model in Fig. 9.3 summarizes the basic approach of this line of research. If the
price is perceived, consumers try to form an opinion on whether the price is
favourable or not; in other words, form an attitude towards the price. In most
cases, this involves comparing the perceived price to some kind of benchmark
price, which is termed the reference price (Winer, 1986; Gijsbrechts, 1993). With
frequently purchased food items, consumers may have a reference price for that
particular product, brand or variety. This will of course be based on price perception during previous purchases and other perceived price information. Helson's
adaptation level theory (Helson, 1964) has been a popular approach to explain

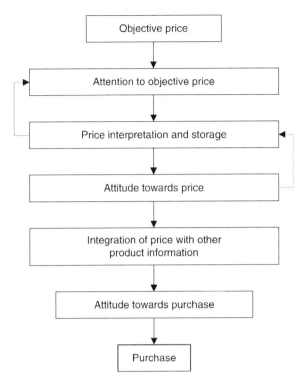

Fig. 9.3.   Price information processing model.

how the reference price is formed as a weighted average of previously perceived prices of the same product.

   With less frequently purchased products or products that are new on the market, the reference price that is used may refer to the product category, not the particular brand or variety. Qualitative research based on think-aloud protocols has shown that consumers try to construct reference prices even for products that they have never bought before and which are one of a kind, like buying a Maori souvenir when travelling as a tourist in New Zealand (Frances *et al.*, 2002).

   The tendency to form an evaluation of a price's favourableness by comparing it to a reference price can be exploited by sellers by providing explicit reference prices. Providing information about 'previous' prices, 'marked down from', competitors' prices or 'downtown' prices in airport shops are all attempts to provide price information which consumers can use as a reference price and which is likely to result in favourable price evaluations (Mayhew and Winer, 1992; Grewal *et al.*, 1998).

   There is no question that consumers sometimes use price as an indicator of quality, although much of the research investigating this question has been of questionable validity. When consumers in an experiment are provided with no other information about products they have to choose from than price, it is not astonishing that they use price as an indicator of quality, but it is not very informative either (Olson, 1979). More recent research has therefore concentrated on the role of price as a choice heuristic (Mitra, 1995). Choice heuristics are simplifying rules consumers employ to make choices in situations which are low involvement and/or time pressured, something which characterizes many food purchases. Choice heuristics usually involve using only one or a few pieces of information per product for making the choice, and price may be one of them. Price can be the only criterion, or it may be used to narrow down the choice set and then be supplemented by other criteria. Using price as a heuristic can take various forms. If consumers believe the products to choose from to be fairly homogeneous or believe that the differences that exist are not relevant, the heuristic may involve choosing the product with the lowest price. If relevant quality variations are assumed to exist, consumers may use price to find those products which are in the desired quality bracket. That can imply choosing a product with a medium price range (to obtain decent, but not top quality) or, in some cases, even to choose the most expensive product.

The maximum price a consumer is willing to pay for a given product is called the willingness to pay (WTP). WTP may be higher than the actual market price for a consumer who has bought the product, and can be anything between zero and the market price for those who did not. In well-functioning markets, economic theory expects the market price to approximate the average WTP in the market. For sellers, knowing consumers' WTP is a question of central importance in the context of new product development, and a variety of methods have been developed to measure WTP for products not yet on the market (Lee and Hatcher, 2001).

Distribution Channels and Modes of Shopping

Food products are distributed in various ways to consumers, and consumer shopping environments are characterized by an increasing degree of complexity. The bulk of food products are distributed via supermarkets and their bigger brothers, hypermarkets. In addition, there is a renaissance of smaller shops in the form of convenience stores. Speciality shops have been on the decline for many years, but have managed to survive and occasionally even grow in certain niche areas, often when integrated into bigger shopping malls. Farm-gate purchasing and box schemes play a role especially in the area of organic produce. Internet purchasing has been tried many times, and is working for some specialization areas like wine, but otherwise has not yet been a breakthrough success, with the possible exception of the UK (Grunert and Ramus, 2005).

Of course, manufacturers try to design distribution channels in such a way as to maximize reach of what they believe is their target group, but the big retailing chains have become such powerful actors these days that manufacturers no longer are the dominant player in the food distribution chain. Distribution channels therefore rather come about by a complex interplay of several forces.

The main construct that has been developed and used to explain consumer store choice has been store image (Pessemier, 1980; Chowdhury et al., 1988). Store image is simply the consumer's perception of the store, and is usually assumed to be multidimensional, with quality and variety of merchandise, price level, service, atmosphere and convenience being typical dimensions. Desirable store images can vary between consumers and also between situations for a given consumer (Thelen and Woodside, 1997), and store image can therefore be used as a positioning device by retailers.

In spite of much folklore about the effects of putting merchandise at various levels of height in the shelf, putting certain items by the cashier or putting basic food supplies like milk at the bottom of shop, so that shoppers have to walk through most of the aisles to get there, there is only very limited published research on the effect of store layout factors and effects of specific elements of merchandising and product placement. One of the few exceptions is a recent study by Esch *et al.* (2004), finding that impacts of displays on purchasing in the shop are stronger when the product category is bought on impulse, when the brand advertised is strong, and when the display design arouses emotion. Other aspects of the store environment that have received some research attention include shelf space allocated to a product, background music, and even use of scents (Peter *et al.*, 1999).

There have been some interesting attempts to apply Russel and Mehrabian's environmental psychology approach (Mehrabian and Russel, 1974) to retailing (although most applications have not been in the food area). The basic tenet of this approach, as illustrated in Fig. 9.4, is to characterize the store environment by two dimensions: sense modality variables, which deal with elements like colour and temperature, and information rate, where the latter deals with the quantity of information drawn from the store environment per unit of time. Consumers exhibit emotional reactions to this environment, and corresponding approach–avoidance behaviours, depending on the interaction of the two environmental variables and their own personality. In other words, the way in

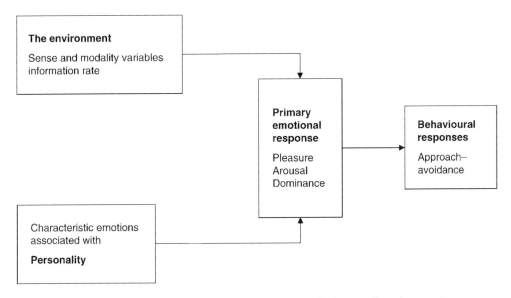

Fig. 9.4. The environmental psychology approach to analysing retail environments.

which a certain combination of music and a high information rate affects consumers will differ between consumer segments. This approach has been used in a number of retailing studies (Donovan and Rossiter, 1982; Bost, 1987; Gröppel and Bloch, 1990).

As already noted, food retailing via the Internet has not become a major factor yet. This may not necessarily be because consumers do not like the idea. A recent study (Ramus and Grunert, 2004) has shown that while some consumers reject the idea because they miss the fun and personal contact of traditional food shopping, others find Internet shopping by itself fun and exciting, and many appreciate the convenience that goes with shopping from home and getting the merchandise delivered there. The major hurdle here may therefore not be consumer behaviour, but the difficulties on the retailer's side. Internet selling involves that tasks which the consumer up to now had to handle herself – packing the products and taking them home – have to be taken over by retailers, involving a good deal of additional logistics and corresponding costs.

Market Orientation in the Food Industry

As noted in the introduction of this chapter, the core idea about marketing parameters is that producers orchestrate them in such a way that they maximize sales of their products, based on a thorough understanding of actual and potential customers. Businesses having this market-linked approach are said to be market-oriented. Market orientation in the food industry has traditionally not been very high, since the food industry was for decades more concerned with cost-effectiveness and high-volume production (Grunert *et al.*, 1996). With the importance attached to product differentiation and value adding these days, that has changed quite a bit, and the development of competencies in understanding consumers has been a priority for many food producers. Therefore the food industry today has a major interest in understanding the determinants of consumer food choice – including, but not limited to, marketing parameters.

References

Bagozzi, R.P. (1975) Marketing as exchange. *Journal of Marketing* 39, 32–39.

Barwise, P. (1993) Brand equity: Snark or boojum. *International Journal of Research in Marketing* 10, 93–104.

Bech-Larsen, T. (1996) Danish consumers' attitudes to the functional and environmental characteristics of food packaging. *Journal of Consumer Policy* 19, 339–363.

Bech-Larsen, T. and Grunert, K.G. (2001) Konsumentscheidungen bei Vertrauenseigenschaften: Eine Untersuchung am Beispiel des Kaufes von ökologischen Lebensmitteln in Deutschland und Dänemark. *Marketing ZFP* 23, 188–197.

Biemans, W.G. and Harmsen, H. (1995) Overcoming the barriers to market-oriented product development. *Journal of Marketing Practice: Applied Marketing Science* 1, 7–25.

Bost, E. (1987) *Ladenatmosphäre und Konsumentenverhalten.* Physica, Heidelberg, Germany.

Chowdhury, J., Reardon, J. and Srivastava, R. (1988) Alternative models of measuring store image: an empirical assessment of structured versus unstructured measures. *Journal of Marketing Theory and Practice* 6, 72–83.

Cox, D.F. (1967) The sorting rule model of the consumer product evaluation process. In: Cox, D.F. (ed.) *Risk Taking and Information Handling in Consumer Behavior*. Graduate School of Business Administration, Harvard University, Boston, Massachusetts, pp. 324–369.

Darby, M.R. and Karni, E. (1973) Free competition and the optimal amount of fraud. *Journal of Law and Economics* 16, 67–88.

Dickson, P.R. and Sawyer, A.G. (1990) The price knowledge and search of supermarket shoppers. *Journal of Marketing* 54, 42–53.

Donovan, R.J. and Rossiter, J.R. (1982) Store atmosphere: an environmental psychology approach. *Journal of Retailing* 58, 34–57.

Erdem, T. and Swait, J. (1998) Brand equity as a signaling phenomenon. *Journal of Consumer Psychology* 7, 131–158.

Esch, F.-R., Langner, T. and Redler, J. (2004) The impact of emotion, brand strength, and product category on the effectiveness of in-store advertising. In: *Proceedings of the 3rd International Conference on Research in Advertising*. Norwegian School of Management, BI, Oslo, pp. 24–28.

Fazio, R.H. (1986) How do attitudes guide behaviour? In: Sorrentim, R.M. and Higgins, E.T. (eds) *Handbook of Motivation and Cognition*. Wiley, New York, pp. 204–243.

Fotopoulos, C. and Krystallis, A. (2001) Are quality labels a real market advantage? A conjoint application on Greek PDO protected olive oil. *Journal of International Food and Agribusiness* 12, 1–22.

Frances, G., Juric, B. and Lawson, R. (2002) Schematic processing of the internal reference price. In: Fahrhangmehr, M. (ed.) *Marketing in a Changing World, Scope, Opportunities and Challenges, Proceedings of the 31st EMAC Conference* (CD-ROM). Universidade do Minho, Braga, Portugal.

Gijsbrechts, E. (1993) Prices and pricing research in consumer marketing: some recent developments. *International Journal of Research in Marketing* 10, 115–153.

Grewal, D., Monroe, K.B. and Krishnan, R. (1998) The effects of price-comparison advertising on buyers' perceptions of acquisition value, transaction value, and behavioral intentions. *Journal of Marketing* 62, 46–59.

Grunert, K.G. (1996) Automatic and strategic processes in advertising effects. *Journal of Marketing* 60, 88–101.

Grunert, K.G. (2002) Current issues in the understanding of consumer food choice. *Trends in Food Science and Technology* 13, 275–285.

Grunert, K.G. (2005) Consumer behaviour with regard to food innovations: quality perception and decision-making. In: Jongen, W.M.F. and Meulenberg, M.T.G. (eds) *Innovation in Agri-food Systems*. Wageningen University Press, Wageningen, The Netherlands, pp. 57–85.

Grunert, K.G. and Ramus, K. (2005) Consumers' willingness to buy food through the Internet: a review of the literature and a model for future research. *British Food Journal* 107, 381–403.

Grunert, K.G. and Valli, C. (2001) Designer made meat and dairy products: consumer-led product development. *Livestock Production Science* 72, 83–98.

Grunert, K.G., Larsen, H.H., Madsen, T.K. and Baadsgaard, A. (1996) *Market Orientation in Food and Agriculture*. Kluwer, Boston, Massachusetts.

Grunert, K.G., Bredahl, L. and Brunsø, K. (2004) Consumer perception of meat quality and implications for product development in the meat sector – a review. *Meat Science* 66, 259–272.

Grunert, K.G., Jeppesen, L.F., Jespersen, K.R., Sonne, A.-M., Hansen, K., Trondsen, T. and Young, J.A. (2005) Market orientation of value chains: a conceptual framework based on four case studies from the food industry. *European Journal of Marketing* 39, 428–455.

Gröppel, A. and Bloch, B. (1990) An investigation of experience-orientated consumers in retailing. *International Review of Retail, Distribution and Consumer Research* 1, 101–118.

Gutman, J. (1982) A means–end chain model based on consumer categorization processes. *Journal of Marketing* 46, 60–72.

Helson, H. (1964) *Adaption Level Theory*. Harper and Row, New York.

Kohli, A.K. and Jaworski, B.J. (1990) Market orientation: the construct, research propositions, and managerial implications. *Journal of Marketing* 54, 1–18.

Laric, M.V. and Sarel, D. (1981) Consumer (mis)perceptions and usage of third party certification marks. *Journal of Marketing* 45, 135–142.

Lee, K.H. and Hatcher, C.B. (2001) Willingness to pay for information: an analyst's guide. *Journal of Consumer Affairs* 35, 120–137.

Levitt, T. (1960) Marketing myopia. *Harvard Business Review* 38(July–August), 45–56.

Mayhew, G.E. and Winer, R.S. (1992) An empirical analysis of internal and external reference prices using scanner data. *Journal of Consumer Research* 19, 62–70.

Mehrabian, A. and Russel, J.A. (1974) *An Approach to Environmental Psychology*. MIT Press, Cambridge, Massachusetts.

Mitra, A. (1995) Price cue utilization in product evaluations: the moderating role of motivation and attribute information. *Journal of Business Research* 33, 187–195.

Monroe, K.B. (1990) *Pricing. Making Profitable Decisions*. McGraw-Hill, New York.

Nelson, P. (1970) Information and consumer behavior. *Journal of Political Economy* 78, 311–329.

Nielsen, N.A., Sørensen, E. and Grunert, K.G. (1997) Consumer motives for buying fresh or frozen plaice: a means end chain approach. In: Luten, J.B., Børresen, T. and Oehlenschläger, J. (eds) *Seafood from Producer to Consumer: Integrated Approach to Quality*. Elsevier, Amsterdam, pp. 31–43.

Oliver, R.L. (1997) *Satisfaction: A Behavioral Perspective on the Consumer*. McGraw-Hill, Boston, Massachusetts.

Olson, J.C. (1979) Price as an informational cue: effects on product evaluations. In: Woodside, A.G., Sheth, J.N. and Bennett, P.D. (eds) *Consumer and Industrial Buying Behavior*. Elsevier North-Holland, New York, pp. 267–286.

Olson, J.C. and Jacoby, J. (1972) Cue utilization in the quality perception process. Paper presented at the *Third Annual Conference of the Association for Consumer Research*, Chicago, Illinois, November.

Pessemier, E.D. (1980) Store image and positioning. *Journal of Retailing* 56, 94–106.

Peter, J.P., Olson, J.C. and Grunert, K.G. (1999) *Consumer Behaviour and Marketing Strategy – European Edition*. McGraw-Hill, Maidenhead, UK.

Petty, R.E. and Cacioppo, J.T. (1986) *Communication and Persuasion: Central and Peripheral Routes to Attitude Change*. Springer, New York.

Ramus, K. and Grunert, K.G. (2004) A study of the potential of grocery shopping on the Internet. Paper presented at the *33rd EMAC Conference*, University of Murcia, Mucia, Spain, 18–21 May.

Reynolds, T.J. and Whitlark, D.B. (1995) Applying laddering data to communications strategy and advertising practice. *Journal of Advertising Research* 35, 9–17.

Scholderer, J. and Frewer, L. (2003) The biotechnology communication paradox: experimental evidence and the need for a new strategy. *Journal of Consumer Policy* 26, 125–157.

Scholderer, J. and Grunert, K.G. (2001) Does generic advertising work? A systematic evaluation of the Danish campaign for fresh fish. *Aquaculture Economics and Management* 5, 253–272.

Steenkamp, J.-B.E.M. (1989) *Product Quality: An Investigation into the Concept and How it is Perceived by Consumers*. Van Gorcum, Assen, The Netherlands.

Steenkamp, J.-B.E.M. (1990) Conceptual model of the quality perception process. *Journal of Business Research* 21, 309–333.

Thelen, E.M. and Woodside, A.G. (1997) What evokes the brand or store? Consumer research on accessibility theory to modeling primary choice. *International Journal of Research in Marketing* 14, 125–145.

Van Trijp, H.C.M., Steenkamp, J.-B. and Candel, M.J.J.M. (1997) Quality labeling as instrument to create product equity: the case of IKB in the Netherlands. In: Wierenga, B., van Tilburg, A., Grunert, K.G., Steenkamp, J.-B. and Wedel, M. (eds) *Agricultural Marketing and Consumer Behaviour in a Changing World*. Kluwer, Dordrecht, The Netherlands, pp. 201–215.

Vanhuele, M. and Drèze, X. (2002) Measuring the price knowledge shoppers bring to the store. *Journal of Marketing* 66, 72–85.

Winer, R.S. (1986) A reference price model of brand choice for frequently purchased products. *Journal of Consumer Research* 13, 250–256.

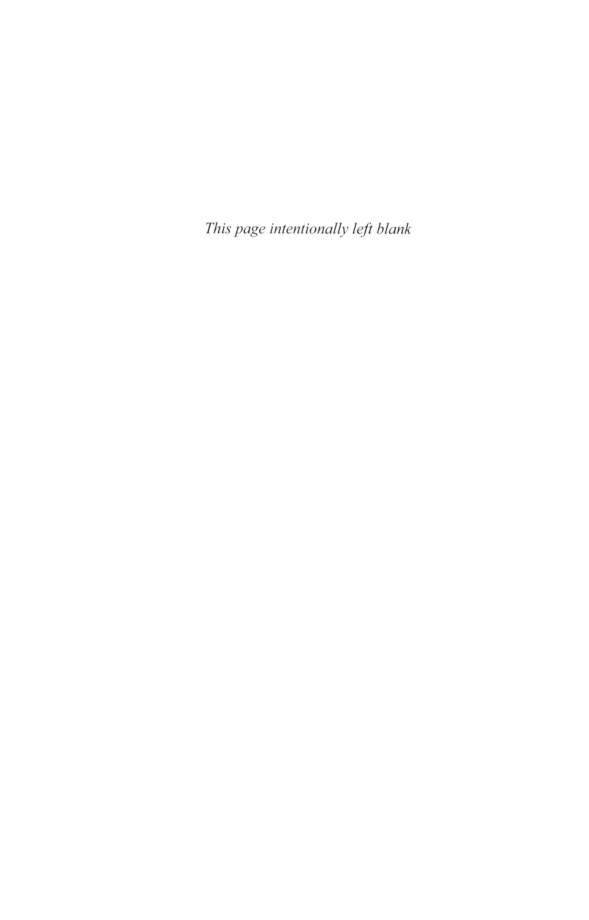

This page intentionally left blank

10 The Role of Context in Food Choice, Food Acceptance and Food Consumption

HERBERT L. MEISELMAN

Natick Soldier Center, Natick, MA 01760-5020, USA

Introduction

This chapter tries, quite literally, to both put eating into context and put context into eating by adding contextual variables and considerations to the overall treatment of food choice, food acceptance and food consumption. The goal of the chapter is to achieve a much broader, more naturalistic view of what controls eating. In research on contextual variables, many of us have come to believe that context has as much influence as product considerations even though it is still rarely included in research on food choice. That is beginning to change as we see papers dealing with contextual topics appearing more frequently at conferences and in journals. Nevertheless, the fields supporting both product development and health sciences are still dominated by those with a product orientation and or a patient orientation. The former include food technologists and the product companies, and the latter include nutritionists, dieticians and physiologists.

Both product research and patient (or human) research are still usually carried out in laboratories, despite consistent findings that laboratory research produces different results from research carried out in naturalistic settings. The reason for this is at least twofold. First, most researchers are strictly trained in the laboratory tradition, and naturalistic settings require modified methods and different concerns about control on the part of the researcher. Second, many investigators feel that, 'Contextual influences are a nuisance, because they complicate the simplification process that is so successful in scientific analysis . . . This facilitates identification of causes but entails the risk of stripping away contextual features that are essential to the phenomenon under study' (Rozin and Tuorila, 1993, p. 12). This chapter tries to achieve a better balance among consideration of the product, the person and the environment. The treatment of contextual variables follows the distinction between laboratory and natural settings in order to emphasize the differences in results obtained in different contexts.

Defining Context and Categorizing Contextual Variables

At present there is no standardized terminology for context or classes of contextual variables. The words context, situation, location and environment are used interchangeably in many discussions of context. The word 'location' might be the most specific of these, often referring to a physical setting, whereas the other three words refer to much more than physical location. Although in some cases the difference between laboratory tests and natural tests is obvious, in some cases the difference might be more subtle. A natural eating environment is one that exists in nature without modification, such as the home, restaurant or cafeteria. One can make slight changes to the natural eating situation for test purposes; for example, add or substitute a food item in a cafeteria. Non-natural settings include laboratories and questionnaire studies done outside eating establishments, for example in the classroom. Defining a laboratory is more difficult because investigators like to think that some laboratories are more natural than others. A laboratory is any eating situation designed by researchers for the purpose of collecting data which is not normally an eating situation. Natural eating environments contain a very wide range and number of variables; many of these variables cannot be duplicated in the laboratory, nor can the interaction of these variables. The easiest way, and perhaps the only way to study different contexts, is to use natural contexts.

In general terms, context is defined as 'the interrelated conditions in which something exists or occurs' (Merriam's Dictionary, 2002). This very broad definition gives the reader an idea of how broad and undefined context might be. Within the field of sensory and consumer research on food there have been attempts to define context. Rozin and Turorila (1993) begin their paper with the statement, 'Food acceptance cannot be understood without consideration of context' (p. 11). They define context in terms of a reference event, any phenomenon involving a product, such as taking a bite of a food, or planning a menu. They then state, 'The context will be taken to mean that set of events and experiences that are not part of the reference event but have some relationship to it' (pp. 11–12). This is a very broad definition of context, because many people would argue that many parts, perhaps all parts, of one's eating world are interconnected. How much you ate for breakfast might affect your appetite for lunch, and what you ate for breakfast today might affect your choice tomorrow, and so on. Rozin and Tuorila distinguish two classes of contextual influences, simultaneous and temporal (past and future), which will be discussed below.

Before discussing contextual variables Rozin and Tuorila (1993) consider the unit of consideration, distinguishing bite, dish, meal and pattern over time. These terms indicate growing degrees of complexity and growing breadth of temporal and spatial importance. Bites are usually eaten in a small time in a single space, while diets cover much more time and much broader space. The unit of context implies an increasing numbers of variables, with the variables from the smaller unit (such as the bite) being included in the larger number of variables in the larger units (such as the meal). Thus, food flavour is important for bites, and also for meals, while dietary frequency is less important at the bite level and more important at the meal level. Meiselman (1994) notes that the unit of context is related to different applications of food choice research: the bite is related to sensory evaluation and product development; the meal is related to food service/catering; and the dietary pattern is related to health.

At the 1987 Conference on Food Acceptability in Reading, UK (Thomson, 1988), Meiselman *et al.* (1988) defined environmental or situational factors as 'the numerous variables in our eating environment which make it easier or harder for us to begin, continue, or complete a meal' (p. 78). The authors' perspective in that paper was strongly related to the relationship between food acceptance and food consumption, and the important role of context within that relationship (see Marriott, 1995). For example, the presence of friends or family might enhance meal continuation or completion.

Bell and Meiselman (1995) state that 'Choice in eating situations is determined by the combination of the state of the eating/provisioning environment prior to and during the choice experience, and the state of the individual prior and during the choice experience' (p. 292). The authors see the interaction of the individual and the environment as critical in determining the outcome of food eating occasions. The same individual in different environments might produce different outcomes, and different individuals in the same environment might have different outcomes. Bell and Meiselman propose two categories of contextual variables: those antecedent to food choice, and those simultaneous with food choice. Examples of the former are prior expectations and prior habits, and examples of the latter are social facilitation and effort to obtain food. This temporal distinction is similar to that proposed by Tuorila and Rozin.

By 1996, the chapter titles in the book *Food Choice, Acceptance and Consumption* (Meiselman and MacFie, 1996) suggest that something was changing in the preoccupation with products and product attributes. Chapters included 'The socio-cultural context of eating and food choice' (Rozin), 'The contextual basis for food acceptance, food choice, and food intake: the food, the situation and the individual' (Meiselman), 'Marketing and consumer behaviour with respect to foods' (van Trijp and Meulenberg), 'Economic influences and food choice' (Bonke) and 'Attitudes and beliefs in food habits' (Shepherd and Raats). Many of these topics clearly represent the context in which a product is used rather than the product itself. In the first chapter, Cardello (1994) gives a modified sensory- and product-oriented approach to what determines food acceptance, with the emphasis on sensory attributes and sensory liking, both of which are moderated by 'physiological status' and 'learning/memory/context/expectations' (Fig. 1.1, p. 3). He acknowledges that food acceptance contributes, 'along with social, situational, and marketplace factors, to the choice and consumption of food' (p. 4). In that book, Meiselman (1994b) proposes that contextual variables can be organized under three headings (food, individual, situation), and notes the similarity of this approach to the marketing emphasis on product, person and place.

More recently, Wansink (2004) presents a different categorization of environmental influences, the eating environment and the food environment, and, more than other reviews, attempts to organize environmental factors and explain possible mechanisms for their effects. The food environment deals with factors related to the way food is presented such as portion size, while the eating environment deals with 'ambient factors' that are independent of the food such as social inter-action. Wansink lists four factors in the eating environment (atmospherics, effort, socialization, distractions) and five factors in the food environment (salience, structure and variety, size, stockpiling, and shape of containers). Wansink's organization of contextual factors adds to other attempts, but we still need an agreed-upon organization and terminology to assist in communicating about context.

A number of technical journals deal with environment, but none appears to address the concern with the interaction of people, products and situations. The scopes of several major journals are presented below, taken directly from their pages. *The Journal of Environmental Psychology* emphasizes the 'study of the transactions and interrelationships between people and their sociophysical surroundings', while *The Journal of Environmental Medicine* focuses 'on the adverse effects on humans of external physical, chemical and biological factors in the general environment, primarily from a medical stand-point'. *The Journal of Occupational and Environmental Medicine* presents 'clinically oriented research articles . . . that can be readily applied in the indus-trial or commercial employment setting'. In addition, a number of sociological journals address environment, but usually concerns about protecting the nat-ural environment, and address context from the perspective of social context. None of these journals appears to address the interaction of people, products and places.

Contextual variables

Studies that have investigated the effects of contextual variables on food acceptance, food choice and food consumption are presented in two groups: studies in natural eating environments and studies in laboratories and other non-natural eating environments. A natural eating environment is a place where people normally eat; for example, home, cafeteria, restaurant, hospital, street market or other setting.

First I discuss several variables that I believe are critical in distinguishing different eating contexts. For some time I have tried to identify which variables are critical in distinguishing different testing environments or different contexts. The following list is not based on strict criteria, but rather based on my own experience.

1. *Choice*. Different environments give the consumer more or less choice. The least choice is probably in the laboratory, where experimental subjects, once they volunteer for a study, have no choice of whether to try the samples and no choice of whether to offer an opinion of a product. Subjects are expected to conform to expectations of investigators, are expected to sample products, and respond using scientific techniques. I present data below indicat-ing that having a choice or not having a choice might produce different product perceptions.

2. *Meal context.* When studying foods and beverages, it is important to remember that most food is consumed as part of a meal. Yet many food products are tested individually rather than as meal components. Again, data indicate that a meal context affects product perceptions.

3. *Social context.* Products are often tested in isolation; that is, panellists are not permitted to speak with one another or are tested individually. Yet meals are often social occasions, and data indicate that product perceptions might vary with and without other people present, and the amount consumed varies with and without other people present.

4. *Enhanced physical environment.* Most natural meals are consumed in relatively pleasant surroundings with attractive dinnerware and other niceties. Laboratories usually strip away these physical environmental enhancements. Does the immediate physical environment make a difference in food perception and food intake?

5. *Confounding of people and contexts.* One difficulty in studying the effects of different environments is that different people are associated with different locations: students are found in universities, elderly in elderly housing, etc. People and locations are not independent; they are confounded. When one moves from elderly housing to university cafeterias, are differences in results due to the location or to the people or to both? I return to this issue below.

King *et al.* (2004) combined these variables in a sequence of sensory evaluation studies to determine whether these contextual variables affect scores from product testing and affect the ability of consumers to discriminate products. These results are presented below (see 'Combining variables in the same study to investigate product acceptance').

Another approach to context has been through the concept of appropriateness. Schutz (1988) argues that appropriateness is a more predictive measure than liking to predict acceptability in given situations. Appropriateness is usually measured by rating the appropriateness of different uses, attributes and situations of products. Seven-point scales from very inappropriate to very appropriate have been used. These can include time of day (noon), occasion (birthday), where served (kitchen), physiological states (food-deprived), how used (snack), psychological characteristics (depressed), person served (waiter), physical characteristics (cold) and sensory characteristics (sweet). Others have experimentally manipulated appropriateness by asking subjects to construct meals for different activities in different physical locations, for example 'eating while in the student refectory' (Marshall and Bell, 2003).

Variables studies in natural environments

Effort

The first study I conducted with contextual variables in a natural eating situation addressed effort to obtain food. I was interested in this variable because our experience at Natick suggested that effort to obtain food was critical in the under-consumption of food by soldiers in training exercises out of doors

(Marriott, 1995; Hirsch et al., 2005). In an earlier laboratory study, Engell et al. (1996) had demonstrated that male subjects in a taste test drank more water when the water was on the table (444 g water) than when it was 7 m away (197 g) or 13 m away (187 g). Also, an earlier set of studies had found that more accessible foods in cafeterias and buffets were eaten more (Nisbett, 1968; Stunkard, 1968; Myers et al., 1980). Myers et al. (1980) observed staff, students and visitors at a hospital cafeteria for 6 days near the check-out pay point. They varied the accessibility of high- and low-calorie desserts, and observed that most customers (about 70%) did not choose dessert. Of those who did choose dessert, most (about 55%) picked the dessert in the more accessible location in front rather than in back. People seemed more willing to overcome inaccessibility for high-calorie desserts than for low-calorie desserts.

I did two effort studies with my colleagues at Bournemouth University, UK, using the student cafeteria/refectory (Meiselman et al., 1994). In study 1, we first obtained 1 week of baseline measurement in which we sampled item selection, item acceptance scores and weighed intake for a group of students. All measurements were taken by student volunteers, who approached students in the cafeteria and asked them if they would like to 'rate the canteen'. Students rated the foods after their meal, which also gave us their food choices, and then they returned their tray to the kitchen where we weighed the food waste out of sight of the diners. During the effort week we moved the chocolate confection from its place at the check-out and pay point to a separate line about 35 m away. To obtain chocolate, students had to select and pay for their regular meal, then go to a second line where they selected and paid for their chocolate. We expected their choice and intake of chocolate to drop, and we expected their ratings of chocolate to increase because it was more difficult to obtain. We were surprised at the results: chocolate selection and intake dropped to almost zero, while the hedonic scores of chocolate during baseline and during the effort condition showed no difference. While students stopped consuming chocolate, their overall intake did not decline, because they substituted other accessory foods (fruit, etc.) rather than adding more main meal items (meat, vegetable, potato).

Based on this first study we tried a second, longer and more complex effort study. In the second study, we moved potato crisps (also known as potato chips) about 70 m away during the effort condition. Instead of collecting data every day of the week (Monday–Friday) we collected data on Tuesdays and Thursdays only, for 2 weeks of baseline, 3 weeks of effort, and 3 weeks of recovery when the crisps were returned to their original location. During effort, crisp consumption dropped dramatically, and students substituted other starch items such as potato and rice. Acceptance ratings of crisps did not vary over the three conditions of baseline, effort and recovery. By the end of the 3-week recovery period, crisp consumption had only partially recovered (Table 10.1).

We were very impressed by the large effects shown by the effort variable, and we realized that contextual variables might produce larger effects than typically seen with product variables or consumer variables. This has shown to be the case in subsequent research. We also began to realize that variables such as effort could be of great practical use when people want to restrict their intake or enhance their intake. Rather than develop 'lighter' foods or practise different

Table 10.1.   Effort studies in a student cafeteria. (Adapted from Meiselman *et al.*, 1994.)

Move chocolate 35 m

- Consumption drops to zero
- Students substitute other accessory foods

Move potato crisps 70 m

- Crisp consumption drops dramatically
- Students substitute other starch
- Crisp consumption does not quickly recover
- Crisp ratings did not vary

Table 10.2.   The effect of queuing on food preferences. (Adapted from Edwards, 1984.)

Delay	Chicken	Potatoes		Carrots
		Roast	Boiled	
No delay	7.28	6.42	6.27	6.76
3 min	6.94	6.16	4.50	6.11
6 min	6.75	5.05	3.67	6.14
9 min	6.50	4.44	3.42	6.20
	$n = 62$	$n = 98$	$n = 32$	$n = 50$

forms of self-control, dieters could use the effort principle to simply make their food more difficult to obtain. Conversely, hospitalized or elderly patients might be advised to make their foods easier to obtain to enhance intake.

Another way to make food more difficult to obtain is to increase waiting time. While this is known to be a major problem in food service, there is little published research. Edwards (1984) found that the acceptance rating of different foods declined with longer waits, sometimes going from acceptable (rating > 5) to unacceptable (rating < 5) on the 9-point scale (Table 10.2).

Cost

Using the same student cafeteria at Bournemouth University, the cost of food was manipulated. This has been tried in laboratory settings (for example, with auction methods) but rarely have published studies been able to manipulate actual cost in a natural eating environment. Cost studies sometimes fund the purchases by giving the subjects an initial amount of money to spend. Marketing studies sometimes ask how much people are willing to pay for an item, but that approach lacks the behavioural data we wanted to obtain. Our goal was twofold: to examine the effects of cost on food choice and acceptance, and to examine the impact of cost on healthy diet choice. At the time of the cost study, all food in the student cafeteria was item-priced; we offered a set price meal consisting of meat, vegetable and starch (potato or rice), which was priced less than the three items priced separately. Other item-priced food was available, and students did not have to choose the test set meal. In naturalistic testing one usually depends on the consumer to select the item offered; this is very different from the laboratory where the subject usually has no choice.

In the cost study, hedonic ratings of the same food selected separately and selected as part of a set meal differed. Overall meal ratings on a 9-point scale were higher when people selected their own meal (7.21) than when someone else selected a set meal (6.71); the same effect showed for vegetables with higher ratings for self-selection (7.00) than set meal selection (6.15). Most interestingly, selection of vegetables increased with set meals. We had demonstrated that students will eat more vegetables when the price of eating vegetables is lowered by inclusion in a set meal. In the laboratory, other methods have been used to study product cost, for example the Vickrey auction method, in which paid subjects use money given to them to bid on products (Lange *et al.*, 2002).

Décor

The décor study was carried out in the training restaurant at Bournemouth University. This restaurant is operated by students, with paying customers from the local area reserving seats for lunch. One hundred and forty-two customers ate lunch in one of two conditions: with traditional British décor with white table-cloths, etc., or in an Italian decor with red-checked table-cloths, Chianti bottles, etc. Data were collected on item selection, item acceptance and ethnicity ratings. Restaurant patrons selected more pasta and more desserts on Italian days (spaghetti 11%, 21%; macaroni 6%, 23%) than on British days, and less fish (30%, 12%) and veal (25%, 19%). Further, the patrons rated their meal as more Italian on Italian days (Bell *et al.*, 1994).

Music

Milliman (1986) varied music tempo in a restaurant. Slower music was associated with a slower rate of eating and higher bar bills. Customers stayed at the table longer with slower music, suggesting that music might operate like the presence of other people, extending duration in the eating environment (Table 10.3). North *et al.* (2003) reported that customers spend more money on food, but not drink, with classical music as opposed to no music or pop music (Table 10.4). They did

Table 10.3. Effect of fast and slow music on eating duration and expenditure. (Adapted from Milliman, 1986.)

Variable	Slow music	Fast music	Significance
Service time (min)	29	27	> 0.05
Customer at table (min)	56	45	0.01
Food purchased ($)	55.81	55.12	> 0.05
Bar purchased ($)	30.47	21.62	0.01
Estimated gross margin ($)	55.82	48.82	0.05

Table 10.4. Classical music and expenditure. (Adapted from North *et al.*, 2003.)

Variable	Expenditure (£)		
	Classical music	Pop music	No music
Total drink	8.36	7.55	8.03
Total food	24.13[ab]	21.92[a]	21.70[b]
Total spend	32.52[ab]	29.46[a]	29.73[b]

Numbers with the same superscript letters (a,b) are not significantly different; numbers with different letters are different.

not measure eating duration. Milliman had reported higher bar bills with slow music as compared with fast music.

The influence of other people – social facilitation

For a broader treatment of sociability and eating, the reader is referred to Sobal (2000) who covers social facilitation, as well as commensality and interaction: 'Social facilitation is the positive enhancement of performance when others are present' (p. 121). Herman *et al.* (2003) have also recently reviewed this area. A number of studies have been reported in natural eating environments. Krantz (1979) reported that cafeteria customers purchased more food when accompanied than when alone, and Klesges *et al.* (1984) found that people eating alone in both fast-food and more formal restaurants ate less than those eating with others.

De Castro and de Castro (1987) paid subjects to keep a diet diary for 1 week. Every time the person ate or drank they were to fill out their diary indicating what they ate, the amount and preparation of the food, the time and their hunger level, and the number of people present. Fewer meals were reported eaten alone (1.61 meals/day) than were reported eaten with other people (2.12 meals/day); further, the meals eaten alone were smaller on average (1715 kJ, 410 kcal) than the social meals (2473 kJ, 591 kcal). De Castro *et al.* (1990) extended the phenomenon of social facilitation to a broad range of eating situations. In diary data, dinner energy > lunch energy > breakfast energy, and the number of people reported at these meals is in the same order of dinner > lunch > breakfast. Restaurant meals are reported to be bigger than meals at home, and the number of people reported present at restaurant meals is larger than those at home meals. Meals consumed with alcohol are reported to be larger than meals without alcohol, and the reported number of people present is in the same direction. Thus, there appears to be a strong correlation between amount consumed and number of people present under a wide variety of conditions.

While a number of variables have been used to explain the social facilitation effect, there has been continued interest in the variable of eating duration. De Castro's work suggested that eating duration might underlie social facilitation (De Castro *et al.*, 1990; De Castro and Brewer, 1992). Data from several studies have shown that people eating with others stay longer in a variety of eating establishments. Sommer and Steele (1997) studied meal duration in a coffee shop and in a restaurant. Mathey *et al.* (2000) observed longer meals in a cosy setting (35 min) rather than a non-cosy setting (27 min) where subjects ate alone in an undecorated space. And Feunekes *et al.* (1995) concluded based on correlational data that increased duration was responsible for social facilitation. Bell and Pliner (2003) studied eating duration in three natural eating situations. They observed that people spent more time eating when more people were present at their table in fast-food restaurants, worksite cafeterias and moderately priced restaurants. Group sizes ranged from one to eight in the cafeteria and restaurant, and from one to seven in the fast-food restaurant. When the number of people present increased from one to five, eating duration increased from 11 to 22 min in fast-food restaurants, from 13 to 44 min in cafeterias, and from 28 to 59 min in restaurants. These are large increases, accounting for the correlation of 0.49 between group size and eating duration. In follow-up research, Pliner *et al.* (2003) independently varied group size and eating duration in a laboratory lunch. Meal duration was 12 or 36 min, and the number of people at the table was one, two or four. They found that the facilitation of eating was entirely due to eating duration. There was no social facilitation based on group size alone. This initial finding needs further replication and study, but duration might be like effort, a basic and potent contextual variable controlling how much we eat. Like effort, duration might also have applied potential, with people being able to influence food intake with changes in meal duration, produced through social facilitation or other non-social means.

Edwards and Hartwell (2004) have applied the social facilitation phenomenon to the problem of under-consumption in hospitals. Many hospital patients enter the hospital undernourished, and leave the hospital more undernourished. Edwards and Hartwell provided food to patients in the bed, by the bed, or at a table in the centre of a multi-patient room. Food intake was the same in the bed and by the bed, but higher at the table with other people. The authors did not report duration of eating at the three locations (Table 10.5).

Positive and negative cues

In many eating environments, what people say can have an influence on food choices and food appreciation. Some research in this area falls under the subheading of social modelling below; social modelling refers to the impact of the actions of influential people on the behaviour of others. We have also studied

Table 10.5. Social facilitation: the effects of eating locations in hospital. (Adapted from Edwards and Hartwell, 2004.)

Variable	Meals at the table	Meals by the bed	Meals in the bed
Energy (kcal)	1632	1348	1363
Protein (g)	59.2	48.2	44.2
Fat (g)	60.6	52.6	63.5
Carbohydrate (g)	226.4	181.2	163.9

verbal social influence in a natural eating environment, in this case the training restaurant at Bournemouth University (Edwards and Meiselman, 2005). In the training restaurant, neighbourhood people pay for a three-course lunch in a formal British setting with white table-cloths and uniformed waiters. The wait-staff are students. We designed both positive and negative verbal conditions and measured what customers selected and how highly they rated their food. Customers are used to being asked questions by the student waiters so this probably did not seem out of place in the training restaurant. In the positive condition the waiter said, 'To assist in your selection, could I just say that the "target dish" [name] has been particularly popular this week (yesterday/last week)'. In the negative condition the waiter changed the comment to '. . . has not been particularly popular . . .'. There was a strong effect on selection, with double the percentage of people selecting the target dish with the positive comment (41%) or no comment (40%) as compared with the negative comment (19%). However, there were no significant effects on the hedonic scores on a 9-point scale for the no comment condition (7.5), positive condition (7.9) and negative condition (7.8). It appears that people were deterred from selecting the negative target dish, but once they did select it, they made up their own mind about liking it, independent of the advice of the waiter.

Lighting level, the presence of art, chair comfort and many other variables could be investigated for their effect on mood, and through mood, their effect on food-related behaviour. There is virtually an unlimited number of variables which could be identified in food eating environments, and studied for their effects and their interactions. Within the food service sector many of these variables are the subject of folklore and proscriptions on what to do and what not to do; it would be worthwhile to test many of these variables, for both their practical advice and for the light the results would shed on how food choice and food intake are controlled by the environment. Each variable might have a small or even negligible effect, but the summed effects of many variables, or the interactive effects, might be larger. Many of these contextual variables might have easy and potent application to a range of health issues such as under-nutrition in hospitals and other institutions, and overeating in some other environments.

Conducting studies in natural eating environments

I have suggested for some time that more studies be conducted in natural eating environments (Meiselman, 1992a,b, 1993). While there has been an increase in such studies, the great preponderance of eating research continues to take place in laboratories. The reasons for this are several. First, many researchers are trained in the traditional approach to research in which variables are varied one or two at a time while all else is held constant. The problem with this in eating is that eating might be controlled by hundreds of variables. How will we ever study these one at a time? Second, there is an assumption that naturalistic studies are difficult to set up. This is not the case, although it might take some effort on the first one or two. Since the natural setting already exists, and the customers already exist, the main effort is getting access to it through the manager. This is usually made easy by the promise of data for the management, data that can often be put to use to improve service or reduce costs. Third, another bias is that naturalistic testing is expensive. The opposite is often the case, because the naturalistic situation already exists, the subjects do not have to recruited and paid, and the data collectors often work within the situation. If a study involves a new food product, the cost of that product might be an additional expense. Fourth, one leaves the naturalistic eating situation alone, without any controls. This reduces the difficulty and cost of naturalistic research. It is tempting to try to control the selection of foods or the costs or the waiting lines or any number of things, but it is best to leave everything alone. This is difficult for researchers trained to control the situation. These conditions naturally lead to some degree of variation during the data collection period. The weather might change every day; the customers might change every day; the chef might change; the food might change – but if the data show consistent trends through this variation, then these trends must be very robust.

Variables studied in other environments

The presence of other people – social modelling

In an earlier study, Engell et al. (1996) combined effort and social modelling in a laboratory meal taste test study. Male subjects were served either alone or with a confederate who was working with the experimenter. The confederate drank either one small cup (55 g) or ten small cups (550 g) of water, which was either on the table or across the room (7 m). Subjects drank more from the table (307 g of water) than from across the room (226 g), and subjects drank more when the confederate drank more (334 g) than when the confederate drank less (234 g) or when the subjects were alone (233 g). Interestingly, there was no social facilitation of eating although group size was either one or two (with confederate). Clendenen et al. (1994) had observed that, with group sizes of one, two or four, whether dining companions were friends or strangers limited social facilitation of eating, but did not affect eating duration. The authors studied groups of one, two or four female subjects at tables for four in a decorated laboratory. Groups ate more, almost double, than singles, but groups of four did not eat more than groups of two. Groups composed of friends ate substantially more than groups composed of strangers. Groups of two took longer to eat (1715 s) than groups of four (1487 s), who took longer than lone diners (766 s). Groups of friends did not take longer to eat than groups of strangers. There appear to be limits to the social facilitation effect. Sobal (2000) discusses commensality, i.e. with whom we choose to eat.

Meals and Mealtime

While some authors have claimed that 'the meal' is the basic unit of eating (Pliner and Rozin, 2000), defining the word 'meal' has proved to be rather difficult, because the definition is usually affected by the orientation of the speaker (see Meiselman, 2004). For discussion of meanings of the word 'meal' the reader is referred to Meiselman (2000) and *Appetite* (1999, volume 32, issue 1). Considering how fundamental and important meals are to eating, research in meal context has not been widely reported.

Whether appropriate mealtimes affect food ratings in questionnaire and taste test situations has produced variable results. To some degree, different foods are eaten at breakfast than at lunch. For example, Marshall (1995) reported that national UK data showed that almost all cereal was consumed at breakfast (96%) but only 44% of eggs and 53% of bacon. Birch *et al.* (1984) examined hedonic ratings of breakfast and non-breakfast foods in taste tests at both morning (08.00–10.00 hours) and non-breakfast (15.30–17.30 hours) times. They found foods were more acceptable when tasted at the appropriate time. In questionnaires people usually assign higher ratings to appropriate foods at appropriate times (e.g. breakfast foods at breakfast). But Kramer *et al.* (1992) concluded from a series of three taste test studies that, 'Serving food at times considered inappropriate had little impact on food intake or hedonic ratings' (p. 12). Subjects rated breakfast foods more highly but ate more of lunch foods. The reader interested in a broader treatment of meals is referred to the interdisciplinary text on *Dimensions of The Meal* (Meiselman, 2000a). The reader is also referred to the extraordinary data set on meals compiled for the Nordic countries, and available in the English book, *Eating Patterns: A Day in the Lives of Nordic Peoples* (Kjaernes, 2001).

There has been very little published research on the combinations of foods which compose meals. Assumptions of how meals are composed are risky given the actual meal compositions reported. The large data set from four Nordic countries (Makela, 2002) shows that other than a main dish and a beverage (95%), only some meals contain a staple such as potato (60%), vegetable (49%), trimmings (27–47%) and bread (10–37%). Further, while 92% of Nordic respondents reported eating at least one hot meal per day, only 56% reported eating a traditional proper meal. Earlier research studied how much each meal component contributes to overall meal acceptance (Rogozenski and Moskowitz, 1982; Turner and Collison, 1988) and Hedderley and Meiselman (1995) extended that research to naturally occurring student cafeteria meals. All of the research has shown that the main dish contributes about half of overall meal acceptance; Hedderley and Meiselman showed that this proportion increased for sandwich and pizza meals where the main dish dominates. Some earlier research by Moskowitz studied meal issues such as component compatibility (Moskowitz and Klarman, 1977) and the effect of spacing on meal acceptance (time since last serving; Balintfy *et al.*, 1975). Meal context remains a little researched area for those interested in food choice, acceptance and consumption. Studies on combining several variables reported below suggest that meal context might be a main controlling variable and deserves more attention.

Variety and Monotony in the Laboratory and in the Field

Variety and monotony have been studied as factors in food choice for some time. Two recent papers call into question the traditional laboratory approach to studying variety and monotony. Meiselman *et al.* (2000a,b) provided a free lunch meal to volunteer employees at Natick Laboratories. The monotony group received the same meal (meat, vegetable, potato) for 5 days, while the variety group received the same meal as the monotony group on Monday and Friday, but three different meals on Tuesday, Wednesday and Thursday. Both food ratings and intake declined for the monotony group, while food ratings stayed the same for the variety group and intake actually increased slightly. This study represents the traditional, laboratory approach to studying monotony where subjects have no choice of condition (monotony–variety) or diet.

Kramer *et al.* (2001) considered another way of approaching monotony/variety. Natick Laboratories has extensive field data on soldiers eating army rations for prolonged periods of time (see Marriott, 1995). They analysed whether soldiers selected the same thing repetitively or selected a variety of things. Interestingly, the majority of soldiers selected a highly varied diet. There is a monotonic decreasing function relating frequency of consumption to number of times consumed; that is, most soldiers ate each menu item once, the next largest number ate each item twice, and so on. However, those who selected items more than once gave the item slightly (but significantly) higher hedonic scores. This was true for two different test sites, and for both all foods overall and for main dishes analysed separately. The difference in value between those eating items and those choosing it more than once varied from 0.3 to 0.8 scale points. These data present a more agreeable answer on monotony: people who select items frequently out of choice like those items more than people selecting the item less often. Monotony, as defined in the laboratory, could be affected by the issue of choice; people who do not select a monotonous diet might not like it, while those selecting it might be happier with the food repetition.

Combining variables in the same study to investigate product acceptance

Recently King *et al.* (2004) studied a number of contextual variables in a planned sequence of six tests to determine whether traditional laboratory sensory testing produced the same discrimination between tests samples and the same hedonic scores as tests containing various contextual variables. All of the tests used two versions each of iced tea, salad and pizza. Test 1 was a traditional central location test (CLT) with small portions of foods tested individually. Each test added a new variable to the test design, so that by Test 5 all variables were present. Test 2 changed the food from small portions served individually to full portions served as a meal. Test 3 added social contact and interaction from the typical non-social CLT. Test 4 changed the social meal testing from a plain laboratory room to an enhanced attractive physical setting. Test 5 gave the subjects a choice of two beverages, two salads and two pizzas. Test 6 moved from the laboratory to a neighbourhood restaurant. Each test had about 100 participants except for 35 in the restaurant.

The addition of contextual variables produced differences in product discrimination but not in all tests and not for all products. The overall effect was an enhancement of hedonic score with contextual variables, but this did not work for the pizza. It is not clear whether context works differently for pizza and other fast foods, or whether contextual variables work differently for different product categories. Hedderley and Meiselman (1995) found that in pizza meals the overall meal acceptability is determined almost entirely by the pizza product alone, the other meal components having very little influence on overall meal appreciation. This might account for the findings that pizza performed differently in King et al.'s (2004) study. An alternative view is that the pizza product in fact varied from test to test, although care was taken to ensure product stability (Table 10.6).

There were differences in product acceptance across the six tests. Salad acceptance increased from 7.0 to scores of 7.1–7.7. Iced tea acceptance increased dramatically from 5.9 in the traditional CLT to scores of 6.8–7.3 in all other tests. Pizza acceptance was the same in the CLT, the meal context and in the restaurant, but decreased with addition of socialization (Test 3), enhanced physical environment (Test 4) and choice (Test 5). Thus, addition of contextual variables added from half to a full scale point in most cases, except for pizza. Comparison of different versions of each product also changed with the addition of contextual variables. This was most marked with the addition of socialization in Test 3. Testing products in a controlled laboratory setting probably underestimates eventual product acceptance when the product is tested in the real world with more contextual cues present.

Another test of the effect of context on product acceptance was carried out by Hersleth et al. (2003). Eight Chardonnay wines differing in three product characteristics were served either in a sensory laboratory or a reception room, with or without food. Products were rated on a 9-point scale by 55 consumers/wine users, each of whom completed all four sessions. The reception room had groups of eight in an enhanced social setting. Context effects were as large as product effects. The presence of food and the enhanced reception room raised hedonic scores by 0.3–0.5 scale points (as did the product factors, one of which reduced liking). The presence of food was a more effective enhancer in the reception room than in the laboratory.

King et al. (2006) have recently attempted a partial replication of their laboratory–field study working with a national food service company in the USA. In a

Table 10.6. Mean values for the overall meal and meal components across tests. (Adapted from King et al., 2004.)

Meal component	Test 1, traditional ($n = 104$)	Test 2, meal ($n = 93$)	Test 3, social ($n = 106$)	Test 4, environment ($n = 106$)	Test 5, choice ($n = 101$)	Test 6, restaurant ($n = 35$)	P value
Overall	–	7.5[a]	7.3[a]	7.3[a]	7.3[a]	7.5[a]	
Salad	7.0[c]	7.5[abc]	7.6[ab]	7.1[bc]	7.7[a]	7.4[abc]	0.0021
Pizza	7.2[ab]	7.2[ab]	6.5[c]	6.9[abc]	6.7[bc]	7.4[a]	0.0032
Tea	5.9[b]	7.0[b]	6.8[a]	7.2[a]	7.1[a]	7.3[a]	< 0.0001

Numbers with the same superscript letters (a,b,c) are not significantly different; numbers with different letters are different.

series of three studies, products were compared in: (i) a laboratory CLT with a pre-recruited sample; (ii) a product test in a restaurant with a pre-recruited sample; and (iii) a national sample drawn from the same chain restaurants in other locations. The results showed the same pattern as the earlier study (King *et al.*, 2004): the laboratory CLT produced lower scores than either on-site study. And the restaurant product test produced lower scores than the actual restaurant sampling with real customers. Approximately half a scale point divided each pair of tests (CLT < restaurant test < restaurant meal). This is further confirmation that laboratory testing underestimates product acceptance in a natural setting. And once again, giving consumers a choice and providing a meal context appeared to influence results.

Comparing the same product in different environments

Context has been studied in two basically different ways. First, as described above, individual contextual variables have been identified and studied in controlled testing, either in natural eating environments or in laboratory settings. Another approach to studying context is to keep the food product constant and vary the environment in which the product is studied. We have conducted a series of food tests in naturalistic settings. The results have shown uniform differences. These studies on acceptance of food in different contexts are paralleled by earlier work on consumption in different locations. Coll *et al.* (1979) observed food choice patterns near the check-out point at nine different sites including a fast-food establishment, cafeteria and sandwich bar, and a faculty club. They observed that people ate much more in restaurant settings than in snack settings, leading them to conclude: 'The major influence on how much people choose to eat is where they eat . . .' (p. 797).

In the first study on acceptance in different locations (Meiselman *et al.*, 2000a,b), we brought packaged army rations to Bournemouth University and served them on china plates in both the student refectory and the training restaurant, both of which had paying customers choosing from a selective menu. Diners did not have to select the test meal. But for those diners who did select the test meal, the diners in the restaurant rated their meal approximately 1 scale point higher on the 9-point scale (7.06) than the students (6.17), and every product except one rated lower in the student refectory. A second study at the University of East Carolina, USA, compared three different locations: a training restaurant with paying customers eating a no choice lunch, students in their cafeteria with choice, and students in a sensory laboratory with no choice. The restaurant and dining hall customers both paid for their meal. Results again showed a difference, with a 1.4 scale point spread between restaurant (6.67) and cafeteria (5.28), with the laboratory falling in between (5.79), although still almost 1 scale point below the restaurant.

In neither of the above studies was it possible to examine demographics to understand the problem of confounding of subjects and locations as discussed above. Edwards *et al.* (2003) conducted a larger-scale study of ten locations using an identical chicken and rice product which was centrally prepared and distributed to the different sites. Customers were both paying and non-paying, and most customers had a choice of food. The demographics of the groups were quite wide, with one group of young people (age 13–17 years) and several groups of older people (65+ years), groups of both males and females, and both smokers and non-smokers. The hedonic scores again ranged over 1 scale point from the army camp (6.63) and university staff refectory (6.64), private boarding school (6.66) and freshman buffet (6.69) to the restaurant (7.58) and the 4-star restaurant (7.63). When data were rearranged by age group, there was a regular increase in hedonic score with age, except that the age group 46–65 years was transposed with the oldest group (65+ years) for the highest scores. The range from lowest to highest scores by age was approximately 0.8 points, about the same as the spread by location. The same population groups were tested in the different environments; for example, the university staff members were tested in their cafeteria/refectory as well as in a private house party, and were also included in the training restaurant sample. Students were tested at freshman week and in the student refectory. The same groups produced different hedonic scores when tested in different environments (Table 10.7).

The results of these tests are uniform. Institutional settings show reliably lower acceptance scores when identical products are tested in different locations; conversely, restaurant settings show reliably higher scores, usually about 1 scale point higher. It is important to keep in mind that most foods are rated within the range 5.5–8.5 on the 9-point hedonic scale. A 1 point difference is a large difference, and can often determine whether a company decides to further develop a prototype product or commercially produce a test product. Our current hypothesis (Edwards *et al.*, 2003) is that consumer expectations produce at least part of these location effects. When we compared what people expected (Cardello, 1994; Cardello *et al.*, 1996) and what actually occurred in the different settings, the two data sets agreed. Customers enter different eating

Table 10.7. Ratings of overall acceptability on different locations. (Adapted from Edwards *et al.*, 2003.)

Location/situation	Mean rating	*N*
Army camp	6.63	43
University staff refectory	6.64	36
Private boarding school	6.66	88
Freshers' week buffet	6.69	83
Private party	6.99	77
Elderly residential home	7.05[ab]	43
Student refectory	7.09[ab]	33
Elderly day-care centre	7.09[ab]	33
Restaurant patrons	7.58[b]	19
4-star restaurant	7.63[b]	32

Numbers with the same superscript letters (a,b) are not significantly different; numbers with different letters are different.

establishments with different expectations, and they rate their food accordingly. Thus, it would appear to be difficult to change these impressions by changing the products, because the product is probably not controlling the expectation, especially in the short term.

Conclusions

1. A number of variables have been demonstrated to contribute to the contextual or environmental effect in eating. This list includes effort to obtain food, the number of people present, eating duration, positive or negative verbal feedback, cost, time of day and mealtime.

2. Many further variables need to be identified and investigated. A difficult challenge ahead lies in determining how these factors integrate into an eating experience.

3. The effects of contextual variables can be large; context effects are as large as, and often even larger than, product effects. A major reason for considering contextual variables is the large size of their effects.

4. Contextual variables can show dramatic effects on eating amount, including the cessation of eating (e.g. from effort) and large increases in eating (from socialization and duration).

5. Contextual variables can also show large effects on product appreciation, producing enhancements of food acceptability of 1 scale point or more on the 9-point scale. These differences are often the difference between whether a product will be further developed and commercialized or abandoned.

6. Contextual variables are easy to observe/manipulate in natural eating environments, demonstrating the robustness of these effects across a wide range of conditions.

7. Instead of manipulating contextual variables in natural eating environments or laboratories, contextual variables can also be demonstrated by comparing reactions to the same food in different eating situations. Studies in natural eating situations reliably show that institutional food is rated lower than restaurant food. This finding has important implications for major feeders such as hospitals and schools, the military and airlines.

8. Laboratory ratings of food acceptability are also reliably lower than for food served in enhanced environments or in restaurants. Since so much of the food industry depends on laboratory testing of food acceptability, it is important to realize that such testing underestimates the acceptability of that food in a natural context.

9. A number of variables appear to contribute to the differences between laboratory-based studies and field studies, or, in general, between different eating locations. These variables include: (i) presenting food in a meal context rather than as individual meal components; (ii) socialization during the meal and the concomitant variable of eating duration; (iii) whether diners choose their food or are presented their food without making a choice such as in the laboratory; and (iv) the confounding between people and locations; the fact that different people are found in different eating locations. These variables have been studied together in recent contextual research.

References

Balintfy, J.L., Sinha, P., Moskowitz, H.R. and Rogozenski, J.G. (1975) The time dependence of food preferences. *Food Product and Development* (November), 33–36, 96.

Bell, R. and Meiselman, H.L. (1995) The role of eating environment environments in determining food choice. In: Marshall, D. (ed.) *Food Choice and the Consumer*. Blackie Academic & Professional, Glasgow, UK, pp. 292–310.

Bell, R., Meiselman, H.L., Pierson, B. and Reeve, W. (1994) The effects of adding an Italian theme to a restaurant on the perceived ethnicity, acceptability and selection of the foods by British customers. *Appetite* 22, 11–24.

Bell, R. and Pliner, P.L. (2003) Time to eat: the relationship between the number of people eating and meal duration in three lunch settings. *Appetite* 41, 215–218.

Birch, L.L., Billman, J. and Richards, S.S. (1984) Time of day influences food acceptability. *Appetite* 5, 109–116.

Cardello, A.V. (1994) Consumer expectations and their role in food acceptance. In: MacFie, H.J.H. and Thomson, D.M.H. (eds) *Measurement of Food Preferences*. Blackie Academic & Professional, London, pp. 253–297.

Cardello, A.V., Bell, R. and Kramer, F.M. (1996) Attitudes of consumers toward military and other institutional foods. *Food Quality and Preference* 7, 7–20.

Clendenen, V.I., Herman, C.P. and Polivy, J. (1994) Social facilitation of eating among friends and strangers. *Appetite* 23, 1–13.

Coll, M., Myers, A. and Stunkard, A.J. (1979) Obesity and food choices in public places. *Archives of General Psychiatry* 36, 795–797.

De Castro, J.M. and Brewer, E. (1992) The amount eaten in meals by humans is a power function of the number of people present. *Physiology and Behavior* 51, 121–125.

De Castro, J.M. and de Castro, E.S. (1987) Spontaneous meal patterns of humans: influence of the presence of other people. *American Journal of Clinical Nutrition* 50, 237–247.

De Castro, J.M., Brewer, E.M., Elmore, D.K. and Orozoco, S. (1990) Social facilitation of the spontaneous meal size of humans occurs regardless of time, place, alcohol and snacks. *Appetite* 15, 89–101.

Edwards, J.S.A. (1984) The effects of queuing on food preferences. *International Journal of Hospitality Management* 3, 83–85.

Edwards, J.S.A. and Hartwell, H.J. (2004) A comparison of energy intake between eating positions in a NHS hospital – a pilot study. *Appetite* 43, 323–325.

Edwards, J.S.A. and Meiselman, H.L. (2005) The influence of positive and negative cues on restaurant choice and food acceptance. *International Journal of Contemporary Hospitality Management* 17, 332–344.

Edwards, J.S.A., Meiselman, H.L., Edwards, A. and Lesher, L. (2003) The influence of eating location on the acceptability of identically prepared foods. *Food Quality and Preference* 14, 647–652.

Engell, D., Kramer, M., Malafi, T., Salomon, M. and Lesher, L. (1996) Effects of effort and social modeling on drinking in humans. *Appetite* 26, 129–138.

Feunekes, G.I., de Graaf, C. and van Staveren, W.A. (1995) Social facilitation of food intake is mediated by meal duration. *Physiology & Behaviour* 58, 551–558.

Hedderley, D. and Meiselman, H.L. (1995) Modeling meal acceptability in a free choice environment. *Food Quality and Preference* 6, 15–26.

Herman, C.P., Roth, D. and Polivy, J. (2003) Effects of the presence of others on food intake: a normative interpretation. *Psychological Bulletin* 129, 873–886.

Hersleth, M., Mevik, B.-H., Naes, T. and Guinard, J.-X. (2003) Effect of contextual variables on liking for wine – use of robust design methodology. *Food Quality and Preference* 14, 615–622.

Hirsch, E., Kramer, F.M. and Meiselman, H.L. (2005) Effects of food attributes and feeding environment on acceptance, consumption and body weight: lessons learned in a twenty year program of military ration research (Part 2). *Appetite* 44, 33–45.

King, S.C., Weber, A.J., Meiselman, H.L. and Lv, N. (2004) The effect of meal situation, social interaction, physical environment and choice on food acceptability. *Food Quality and Preference* 15, 645–653.

King, S.C., Meiselman, H.L., Hottenstein, A.W., Work, T.M. and Cronk, V. (2006) The effect of contextual variables on food acceptability: a confirmatory study. *Food Quality and Preference* (in press).

Kjaernes, U. (ed.) (2001) *Eating Patterns: A Day in the Lives of Nordic Peoples.* Report No. 7-2001. National Institute, Lysaker, Norway.

Klesges, R.C., Bartsch, D., Norwood, J.D., Kautzman, D. and Haugrud, S. (1984) The effects of selected social and environmental variables on the eating behavior of adults in the natural environment. *International Journal of Eating Disorders* 3, 35–41.

Kramer, F.M., Rock, K. and Engell, D. (1992) Effects of time of day and appropriateness on food intake and hedonic ratings at morning and midday. *Appetite* 18, 1–13.

Kramer, F.M., Lesher, L.L. and Meiselman, H.L. (2001) Monotony and choice: repeated serving of the same item to soldiers under field conditions. *Appetite* 36, 239–240.

Krantz, D.S. (1979) A naturalistic study of social influence on meal size among moderately obese and nonobese subjects. *Psychosomatic Medicine* 41, 19–27.

Lange, C., Martin, C., Chabanet, C., Combris, P. and Issanchou, S. (2002) Impact of the information provided to consumers on willingness to pay for champagne: comparison with hedonic scores. *Food Quality and Preference* 13, 597–608.

MacFie, H.J.H. and Thomson, D.M.H. (eds) (1994) *Measurement of Food Preferences.* Blackie Academic & Professional, London.

Makela, J. (2001) The meal format. In: Kjaernes, U. (ed.) *Eating Patterns: A Day in the Lives of Nordic Peoples.* Report No. 7-2001. National Institute for Consumer Research, Lysaker, Norway, pp. 125–258.

Marriott, B.M. (ed.) (1995) *Not Eating Enough.* National Academy Press, Washington, DC.

Marshall, D. (1995) Eating at home: meals and food choice. In: Marshall, D. (ed.) *Food Choice and the Consumer.* Blackie Academic & Professional, Glasgow, UK, pp. 264–291.

Marshall, D. and Bell, R. (2003) Meal construction: exploring the relationship between eating occasion and location. *Food Quality and Preference* 14, 53–64.

Mathey, M.-F.A.M., Zandstra, E.H., de Graaf, C. and van Staveren, W. (2000) Social and physiological factors affecting food intake in elderly subjects: an experimental comparative study. *Food Quality and Preference* 11, 397–403.

Meiselman, H.L. (1992a) Methodology and theory in human eating research. *Appetite* 19, 49–55.

Meiselman, H.L. (1992b) Obstacles to studying real people eating real meals in real situations: reply to commentaries. *Appetite* 19, 84–86.

Meiselman, H.L. (1993) Critical evaluation of sensory techniques. *Food Quality and Preference* 4, 33–40.

Meiselman, H.L. (1994) Bridging the gap between sensory evaluation and market research. *Trends in Food Science and Technology* 5, 396–398.

Meiselman, H.L. (ed.) (2000) *Dimensions of the Meal*. Aspen Publishers, Gaithersburg, Maryland.

Meiselman, H.L. (2004) Introduction to meals. Pangborn Workshop: What to Eat: a multidiscipline view of meals. *Food Quality and Preference* 15, 901–902.

Meiselman, H.L. and MacFie, H.J.H. (eds) (1996) *Food Choice Acceptance and Consumption*. Blackie Academic & Professional, Glasgow, UK.

Meiselman, H.L., Hirsch, E.S. and Popper, R.D. (1988) Sensory hedonic and situational factors in food acceptance. In: Thomson, D.M.H. (ed.) *Food Acceptability*. Elsevier Applied Science, London, pp. 77–88.

Meiselman, H.L., Hedderley, D., Staddon, S.L., Pierson, B.J. and Symonds, C.R. (1994) Effect of effort on meal selection and meal acceptability in a student cafeteria. *Appetite* 23, 43–55.

Meiselman, H.L., de Graaf, C. and Lesher, L. (2000a) The effects of variety and monotony on food acceptance and intake at a mid-day meal. *Physiology & Behaviour* 70, 119–125.

Meiselman, H.L., Johnson, J.L., Reeve, W. and Crouch, J.E. (2000b) Demonstrations of the influence of the eating environment on food acceptance. *Appetite* 35, 231–237.

Milliman, R.E. (1986) The influence of background music on the behaviour of restaurant patrons. *Journal of Consumer Research* 13, 286–289.

Moskowitz, H.R. and Klarman, L. (1977) Food compatibilities and menu planning. *Journal of the Institute of Canadian Science and Technology Alimenta* 10, 257–264.

Myers, A., Stunkard, A. and Coll, M. (1980) Food accessibility and food choice. *Archives of General Psychiatry* 37, 1133–1135.

Nisbett, R.E. (1968) Determinants of food intake in obesity. *Science* 159, 1254–1255.

North, A.C., Shilcock, A. and Hargreaves, D.J. (2003) The effect of musical style on restaurant customers' spending. *Environment and Behaviour* 35, 712–718.

Pliner, P. and Rozin, P. (2000) The psychology of the meal. In: Meiselman, H.L. (ed.) *Dimensions of the Meal*. Aspen Publishers, Gaithersburg, Maryland, pp. 19–46.

Pliner, P., Bell, R., Kinchla, M. and Hirsch, E.S. (2003) Time to eat? The impact of time facilitation and social facilitation on food intake. Paper presented at *5th Pangborn Sensory Science Symposium*, Boston, Massachusetts, 20–24 July 2003.

Rogozenski, J.E. and Moskowitz, H.R. (1982) A system for the preference evaluation of cyclic menus. *Journal of Food Service Systems* 2, 139–161.

Rozin, P. and Tuorila, H. (1993) Simultaneous and temporal contextual influences on food acceptance. *Food Quality and Preference* 4, 11–20.

Schutz, H.G. (1988) Beyond preference: appropriateness as a measure of contextual acceptance of foods. In: Thomson, D.M.H. (ed.) *Food Acceptability*. Elsevier Applied Science, London, pp. 115–134.

Sobal, J. (2000) Sociability and meals: facilitation, commensality and interaction. In: Meiselman, H.L. (ed.) *Dimensions of the Meal*. Aspen Publishers, Gaithersburg, Maryland, pp. 119–133.

Sommer, R. and Steele, J. (1997) Social effects on duration in restaurants. *Appetite* 29, 25–30.

Stunkard, A.J. (1968) Environment and obesity: recent advances in our understanding of regulation of food intake in man. *Federation Proceedings* 27, 1367–1373.

Thomson, D.M.H. (ed.) (1988) *Food Acceptability*. Elsevier Applied Science, London.

Turner, M. and Collison, R. (1988) Consumer acceptance of meals and meal components. *Food Quality and Preference* 1, 21–24.

Wansink, B. (2004) Environmental factors that increase the food intake and consumption volume of unknowing consumers. *Annual Reviews in Nutrition* 24, 455–479.

This page intentionally left blank

11 The Impact of the Media on Food Choice

JACQUIE REILLY

Public Health and Health Policy, University of Glasgow, 1 Lilybank Gardens, Glasgow G12 8RZ, UK

Introduction

An important question for health promotion, government and indeed the food industry is how the public understands media messages about the safety of foodstuffs and whether this impacts on the purchase, preparation and consumption of food (Miller and Reilly, 1994, 1995a,b; Reilly and Miller, 1997; MacIntryre *et al.*, 1998).

This chapter looks specifically at food 'risks' and public understandings of risk messages as assessed in work carried out at the Media Research Unit at Glasgow University. It has been argued that the effects of the media on public attitudes and behaviour are mainly negative. But such a view of the 'malign' influence of the media assumes that the media's impact is straightforward and direct (Eldridge and Reilly, 2003). Consumers and especially children are perceived as vulnerable and thought to be at risk from media messages. The problem with such as view is that people do not passively absorb all media messages but rather they interpret and contextualize new information (Miller and Reilly, 1994). It can be argued that they do so in relation to a range of factors, including their own past history and experience, and deploy a range of assumptions on, for example, the credibility of information sources, before deciding what information to believe or reject (Reilly, 1998). This chapter discusses how the nature, content and route of provision of media information may affect perceptions of risks and impact on food choices. The main risks highlighted will be those around salmonella in eggs, bovine spongiform encephalopathy (BSE) and genetically modified (GM) foods.

Methods

The first component of the research involved the analysis of media outputs on food risks from 1986 to 1998, which included both television and newspaper accounts.

The result is a large archive on media coverage of food risks in Britain for that period. Certainly the influence of the media on public opinion cannot be predicted or assessed by a reading of media content alone, but access to a substantial archive does allow for the analysis of how stories appear and, more crucially, disappear from media agendas (Kitzinger and Reilly, 1997; Reilly, 1999, 2001).

Focus groups were convened across the UK to investigate how media messages were received, understood and acted upon by the public. These were carried out at different stages between 1992 and 1998. We studied 'pre-existing' social groups (people who knew each other through work, friendships or family connections) in order to preserve the 'elements of the social culture within which people actually receive media messages' (Eldridge *et al.*, 1996). The sampling of the groups was purposive, and was designed to ensure the inclusion of a range of sociodemographic characteristics rather than to generate a representative sample of the general population (Reilly, 1997; MacIntyre *et al.*, 1998; Philo and Reilly, 1998). We report here on a number of different aspects of the findings from the focus groups.

Within each focus group session respondents were asked to fill in a questionnaire (on biographical details and use of media products) as well as participate in a 'news game' (effectively writing their own news bulletin with the aid of still photographs taken from television programmes and newspapers relating to food). They then took part in a discussion about different food issues.

The groups were 56% female and 44% male and ranged in age from 16 to 73 years. Seventy-nine per cent of the respondents read a daily newspaper and watched at least one television news programme regularly. More of the respondents read a tabloid newspaper (67%) on a regular basis. Regional tabloid newspapers were bought by a high percentage of respondents within each country: England (72%), Wales (65%), Northern Ireland (73%) and Scotland (71%). The majority of television news programmes watched were the early evening bulletins (74%). *BBC News* was preferred by more people than *ITN News* or Channel 5 bulletins while a smaller number watched *Newsnight* (10%) or *Channel 4 News* (16%) regularly. Only 7% had ever purchased magazines specifically about food.

The 'News Game' Exercises

Respondents were given a set of photographs and asked to construct a news item about food. The photographs included images of government and opposition spokespeople, government officials, scientists, pressure group representatives, food industry officials, food producers, retailers and consumers. There were also pictures of different foodstuffs included such as eggs, meat, cheese, etc. and different food outlets. The exercises were used to show that respondents were familiar with the basic language and structure of news and that they did have good recall and understanding of a number of specific concerns about food.

More than half of the stories written centred specifically on BSE. All of these were 'negative', in the sense that they were always critical of government, farmers or the food industry and concerned with a seeming lack of attention to 'victims'.

Examples of the types of stories written were:

> Today the government announced that they were going to award the farmers of the UK a subsidy to help them overcome the hardships occurred since the BSE crisis of 1996. Roger Tallis, a farmer's spokesman, claimed that the subsidy was not enough to cover the hardships suffered by the industry. Ronnie Richardson, whose wife died from CJD [Creutzfeldt-Jakob disease] said the victims deserved more compensation than the farmers. Frank Dobson, Health Secretary, commented that the question of compensation cannot be addressed until such times as the report from the BSE inquiry is completed.
>
> (Local café workers, Inverness)

> Despite the BSE crisis having emerged 10 years ago, history may show that successive agricultural and government policies have been ineffectual in establishing confidence in British beef. The public seem to have to rely on consumer and food programmes for update and information on the situation. Food safety is forefront in the public's mind and many feel they are not being kept sufficiently informed. The more cynical observers among us tend to believe that money is the primary factor in this.
>
> (Sports centre employees, Coleraine)

> Families of the victims of CJD, the human form of BSE, were today in Parliament to tell the BSE inquiry their stories. While it has been 10 years since we were first told there was no risk from BSE and that infected meat would not get into the food chain, it has become clear that some people are getting this horrific disease who should not. Family lawyers said that it was the government's responsibility to compensate the victims because it was their fault that BSE had been allowed to so infect the British food chain. They went on to say that it would be a travesty of justice if nothing were done about the victims of the BSE fiasco as the government had finally come out and admitted there may be a link between the two diseases.
>
> (Chefs, Swansea)

Stories written around genetic modification were based mainly on the fact that some products were on supermarket shelves and criticisms that the risks potentially associated with them had not been taken into proper consideration:

> Food that we consider to be naturally 'healthy' is being genetically engineered for a longer shelf-life and cosmetic purposes, the long-term effects of which are not made available to the general public. Consumer watchdogs are concerned that the industry is veering towards profit rather than nutritional values of fresh food.
>
> (Unemployed, Wishaw)

> Genetically modified foods are now on our supermarket shelves. While the government have claimed that they are entirely safe to eat, consumer groups are concerned that yet again we are being put at risk from foods which have not been proven to be entirely safe. Following on from the problems with BSE in British beef it is clear that measures are going to have to be taken to ensure that the public are not being forced to purchase any of these products without their full consent. This means they should be clearly labelled at least and, more importantly, that research is carried out to reassure the public that there are no risks. The government have

promised that it is taking consumer concerns very seriously, but until something
more happens it seems that the public are simply not buying the stuff.

(Nurses, Belfast)

A small number of stories were written specifically about salmonella or food poisoning in general. These tended to centre on the need for 'proper' hygiene and
cooking practices:

> Following a spate of recent food poisoning episodes of salmonella nation-wide,
> more advice is being given to consumers on how to ensure they say safe. An
> announcement made by Frank Dobson, Health Secretary, today stated that the
> public should be more vigilant in the preparation and cooking of certain foods.
> Top of his list came eggs and poultry which he said should always be thoroughly
> cooked, particularly when being served to children and old people. For the rest of
> us it seems that using common sense and not taking unnecessary risks by under-
> cooking or improperly storing food is the main way of ensuring levels go down.
>
> (Ancillary nursing staff, mixed, Bedford)

> A report today said that food poisoning levels are on the increase in Britain because
> of the growth of small outlets such as cafes and food-vans. Consumers should take
> care when deciding where to buy fast-food from, and make sure that anything they
> do buy is properly cooked.
>
> (16-year-olds, mixed, Oxford)

There were a small number of stories that took a generalized look at food issues,
incorporating a number of different 'risks' and, more specifically, the need to
look into the costs of organic farming:

> Surveys have shown that most food products on sale in supermarkets carry an
> element of risk because of additives, preservatives or, in the case of red meat,
> irresponsible methods of production. Frank Dobson, Health Secretary, and the
> Minister of Agriculture have recently met to discuss long-term plans to introduce
> healthier and safer food. Outcries have come from the general public about the cost
> of organically grown food. The two Ministers are hoping to obtain government
> funding to assist food producers with the aim of keeping prices realistic.
>
> (Crisis care workers, mixed, London)

Responses to Different Food Risks

The story of food safety as a public issue in Britain illustrates the important role
different organizations play in helping to either discourage or encourage
debate on food safety issues. It is certainly the case that most food safety
'scares' arose at a particular juncture in history for particular reasons. It is also
the case that their rise and fall from the media can occur for a number of different
reasons. There are a number of 'news values' which may be relevant to the
appearance of food in the news sections (as opposed to food or health sections)
of newspapers, television and radio. These are 'scientific advances', 'divisions
amongst experts', 'matters of state', 'division in the government' and 'government suppression' (Kitzinger and Reilly, 1997; Eldridge and Reilly, 2003).

These criteria for newsworthiness have been in place for a number of the high-profile risk stories such as salmonella, BSE or GM food.

Salmonella in eggs

On 3 December 1988 the then Junior Health Minister, Edwina Currie, told *ITN News*:

> we do warn people now that most of the egg production of this country, sadly, is now infected with salmonella. If however, they've used a good source of eggs, a good shop that they know, and they're content, then there seems no reason for them to stop. But we would advise against using raw egg – mayonnaise and dressings and bloody mary's and that sort of thing. They are not a good idea anymore.
>
> (ITV, 3 December 1988)

The remarks triggered a crisis. Within days egg sales had fallen by up to 50% (House of Commons Agriculture Committee, 1989) and the egg industry was in disarray. To understand why salmonella in eggs came upon the public scene it is necessary to explore a number of issues.

The emergence into the public sphere of *Salmonella enteritidis* PT4 as a potential health threat reflected the political stance being taken on its existence and on the treatment of other food risks (Reilly, 1999). Throughout 1988 mass media coverage of food-borne risks had been varied, if not remarkably extensive, and covered salmonella in pepperoni sticks, bean sprouts and frozen or chilled chicken, paratyphoid from frozen curry meals, meningitis from Greek goats' cheese, and listeria in pre-packed salads and cheese. Added to this were the more readily recognizable stories about outbreaks in, for example, restaurants, takeaways, hospitals, overseas holiday resorts and one in the House of Lords (May 1988). From January to the end of November 1988 there were a total of 263 national press and television stories about these issues. Seventy-four per cent of the stories were framed around individual consumers' and food outlets' hygiene and cooking practices.

The issue became relevant in policy circles because the number of cases of *S. enteritidis* reported in England and Wales had increased between 1981 (1087) and 1987 (4962; Public Health Laboratory Service annual report data). By the end of 1988 over 12,522 cases had been reported, a third of all known salmonella cases. *S. enteritidis* PT4 had come to light first with the publication of research by the American Centers for Disease Control (CDC) in April 1988 (*Dispatches*, Channel 4, 25 October 1989). The CDC study claimed that salmonella was occurring in eggs, not only on contaminated eggshells but within the eggs themselves. The advice from the USA was that for complete safety from salmonella food poisoning, eggs should be boiled for a minimum of 7 min, poached for 5 min, or fried for 3 min on each side. This view was met with scepticism on the part of British health experts who claimed that the particular strain of salmonella in question, *S. enteritidis* PT4, was not commonly found in eggs in Britain. According to one Department of Health and Social Services spokesman, 'there was no reason for any new advice about preparing eggs and chicken, beyond observing normal hygiene and ensuring both are thoroughly cooked' (*The Times*, 16 April 1988). But enough concern was felt for the Department of Health and the Ministry of Agriculture, Fisheries and Food (MAFF) to set up a joint government working party to investigate the rise in cases. In August 1988 the Department of Health issued a warning to hospitals about the risk of eating raw eggs (but not to the public and producers until November). Figures released by the department, based on data from the Public Health Laboratory Service, showed that some 21 cases of salmonella in 1988 had been linked to eggs (*Guardian*, 27 August 1988). More evidence of the problems with *S. enteritidis* PT4 appeared in a paper in *The Lancet* in September 1988. Then, on 2 December, Plymouth Health Authority took action and banned eggs from all of their hospitals. It was at this point that Edwina Currie made the issue public.

Instantly, a number of different interest groups, namely the Department of Health, MAFF and the egg industry, were forced to become involved in an issue of public concern with which they were not ready to deal. What Edwina Currie had unleashed, however unintentionally, was a number of problems associated with drawing public attention to a potential health risk which cuts across commercial interests. A number of very different positions were taken on this issue, as is clear from television news following Currie's statement.

Advice to consumers from the Department of Health was that while eggs were a public health problem, individual eggs were unlikely to be infected. Precautions to be taken included stopping eating raw eggs or foods made with raw egg. While it was admitted there was a risk, it was seen as an 'acceptable' risk for healthy people to eat soft eggs. Those deemed vulnerable (i.e. the elderly, young children, pregnant women and those with lowered immunity levels) were advised to eat eggs that had been cooked until they were hard (*ITN News*, ITV, 5 December 1988).

The egg production industry demanded that something be done to restore public confidence in eggs, claiming that the Minister's remarks were costing them £5 million per week and that the threat of bankruptcy loomed as many producers began to lose orders. The issue of blame became paramount. While it was a mark of government concern that a new voluntary code of practice for the egg industry was to be introduced, in the early stages of what would become known as the 'eggs crisis' blame was firmly put in the lap of the Minister who had brought the issue to light. MAFF blamed Edwina Currie, claiming that she had been 'factually incorrect' in her statement which had been made without consulting them. The egg producers threatened legal action against Edwina Currie and demanded a full retraction and/or her resignation for the damage she had done to the industry. But Currie refused to retract her words and was eventually forced to resign 2 weeks after making her statement following immense pressure.

With awareness raised, the government had to respond very quickly to the problem. A committee was set up to investigate the salmonella affair. In addition, a damage limitation strategy was necessary as the main protagonists were at pains to ensure that public confidence in the egg was restored. Agriculture Minister John MacGregor's department announced they would give half a million pounds to instigate a government advertising campaign to counter the scare. But a row developed as neither department could agree on how the advert should be worded. MAFF wanted it to say that eggs were safe to eat while the Department of Health would not agree to such complete assurances of safety. The phrasing of the 200-word statement was finally agreed and appeared to include the interests of both departments. It was generally criticized by the egg industry as being no more than a 'health warning' because it offered information on how to cook eggs 'safely'. With a national average drop of 60% in sales, a surplus of 20 million unused eggs daily, 100,000 chickens being killed and the threat of job losses, the industry demanded compensation. The government announced a £19 million package on 19 December but still no answers were given about the actual safety of eggs. It seemed that the scientific experts themselves were as divided as the politicians over the extent of the salmonella problem in eggs. In the end it was left to the Chief Medical Officer to admit to the underlying uncertainties by saying that while Britain was suffering an 'epidemic' increase of *S. enteritidis* PT4 there was no clear scientific evidence to say that eggs were infected.

With Edwina Currie's resignation and the compensation package offered to the producers, the political battle moved inside Whitehall and out of the public gaze. The affair may not have resurfaced but for media reporting in January 1989 of the House of Commons Agriculture Committee's investigation, which gave the public a chance to hear the full story. The debates around *S. enteritidis* were reopened as representatives of MAFF, the Department of Health and the egg industry went to the committee armed with statistics which appeared to support their differing viewpoints. Contradictory evidence abounded but all parties seemed to agree on the fact that what Edwina Currie had said was wrong. The public profile of these proceedings was also heightened by Edwina Currie's refusal to appear before the committee to give evidence. Following three letters to her she eventually agreed to appear. She did not retract her statement and certainly did nothing to help clear up the question of the safety of eggs, saying that she had nothing new to add to the investigation. In fact, it was in an interview on Channel 4's documentary programme *Dispatches* on 25 October 1989 that Mrs Currie said, for the first time, not that she had been wrong, but rather that she had 'got the words wrong'. Up to this point she had refused to withdraw the remark 'most of the egg production'; she now claimed that she did not intend to say 'most eggs', she should have said 'many' or 'some' or 'a few'. Almost 9 months after the initial statement, it seemed still that no-one knew the precise answer.

While the committee collected evidence, food safety was undoubtedly high on the political and media agendas. The end of *S. enteritidis* as a high-profile public issue came with the publication of the Agriculture Select Committee's report on the affair in February 1989 (House of Commons Agriculture Committee, 1989). The report criticized Edwina Currie but also put the affair down to a failure of government. They recommended that to deal with the complexity of the salmonella problem there needed to be more research and resources, the development of procedures for tracing food outbreaks, compensation for the slaughter of infected breeding and laying flocks, assurances that catering establishments used pasteurized eggs in all uncooked egg dishes, and a properly funded campaign to promote better hygiene in the home.

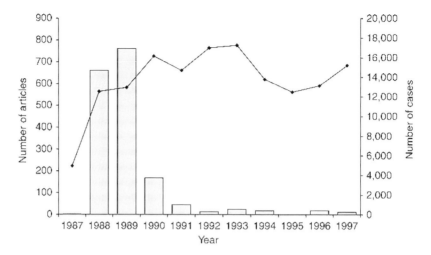

Fig. 11.1. *Salmonella enteritidis* PT4 in England and Wales: the number of cases of infection (—♦—; data published on the Public Health Laboratory Service website, http://www.phls.org.uk/) and the number of articles (▢) in the UK national press, 1987–1997.

Following this, media interest in the story completely dissipated as a resolution to the affair was seen to have been reached, both at the political level and with the constant reminders to consumers of how to cook eggs 'properly'. Egg sales also began to rise again slowly and were up to around 75% of earlier levels by early 1989 (Mintel, 1990). From 244 newspaper stories in January 1989, there were only 20 in the whole of April of that year. The issue was never again to enjoy such a profile in the British media. Interestingly, while media interest has undoubtedly diminished since 1988/9, according to Public Health Laboratory Service figures, cases of *S. enteritidis* were higher in 1997 than they were in 1988, accounting for 71% (22,806) of all salmonella cases reported, while the PT4 strain accounted for 47% of all enteritidis cases (data published on Public Health Laboratory Service website, http://www.phls.org.uk/; Fig. 11.1).

It is also interesting to note that the same warning about how to cook eggs was broadcast on television news programmes on 9 April 1998 with nothing like the same impact it had caused 10 years before. Why was this the case? There is a sense in which the salmonella affair was less a food 'scare' and more a political 'scare'. What seemed most important at the time was the role played by both the Department of Health and MAFF, and the battle played out to assess who should be handling food safety.

Public understandings

While very high profile for a short space of time, our research found that instead of discussions of political conflicts within media formats, salmonella poisoning was seen most clearly as a cooking or storage problem. There was no real sense in which it was perceived as being a problem of industrialized agriculture.

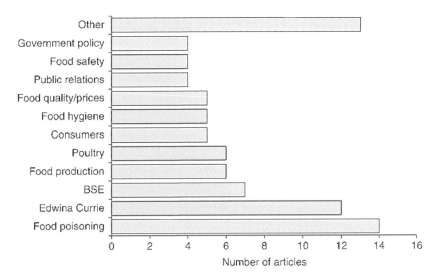

Fig. 11.2. Themes of feature articles on salmonella and eggs, 1995–1997 (BSE, bovine spongiform encephalopathy).

This overall attitude fitted into the way salmonella stories had previously been presented by the media and health education/food safety materials (Fig. 11.2).

Respondents in our groups felt that there was a lot of information available that stressed how they could minimize the risks from salmonella poisoning, but that much of this was basic 'common sense':

> It's about common sense, isn't it? Everyone knows that you have to cook food thoroughly and store it properly to ensure it's safe. . . I always check the food pages in my magazines – they're really good for giving out helpful information on good practices and how to make sure you don't poison anybody.
>
> (Female, East Kilbride)

It was also consistently stressed that there were very practical ways of ensuring that you did not become infected with salmonella:

> You don't eat soft eggs and undercooked chicken, that's the rule. I remember that from the *Food and Drink* programme and it has always just stuck with me.
>
> (Male, Bristol)

> I used to take quite a lot of raw egg, especially when I was training for running, but I wouldn't do that anymore. I make sure everything is thoroughly cooked and won't let the kids touch mayonnaise or anything like that.
>
> (Male, Bedford)

> I think we all know we have to be careful, and while you can be vigilant at home it's harder to do that when you're eating out. So, I'm really careful when I go out, I won't have anything with eggs in just in case the place hasn't been storing them properly or they're out of date.
>
> (Female, Coventry)

It was commonly stated that 'it was your own fault' if you ate out-of-date eggs, sandwiches or other related foodstuffs and the same applied if people ate from what was seen as unhygienic premises (mostly fast-food outlets such as snack vans).

It was interesting that while respondents all remembered the Edwina Currie egg story, none was aware that advice relating to the cooking of eggs remained the same as it did in 1988 or that the same warning (about cooking and storing of eggs) was reissued in April 1998 given the rise in cases of the PT4 strain. While there was a great deal of surprise at this information, there was no major level of concern from any of the groups. This was mirrored by the lack of media coverage at the time. As can be seen From Fig. 11.1, while the number of cases of salmonella increased, media coverage remained low and actually declined markedly.

Factors determining public responses to salmonella

Most respondents had been eating eggs for a long time and had never been poisoned, or at least did not relate such poisoning to eggs:

> I didn't know that at all, but then I follow that advice anyway, always have. I think I remember the cook eggs for seven minutes advice from the medical officer guy at the time because I have kids, and you they're one of the risk groups aren't they. . . but I don't worry unduly about salmonella because as I said, we're very careful about cooking chicken and eggs.
>
> (Male, Omagh)

> I wouldn't really be bothered too much if the media came out and said there were problems with eggs. I mean they did it before and nothing happened, I mean I've been eating eggs all my life and have never been poisoned by one.
>
> (Female, South Uist)

It was interesting that this was particularly the case for 'older' groups who are one of the main risk categories in relation to food poisoning. Asked how they would react if the media highlighted a potential problem with salmonella, most respondents said that they would take advice offered by the chief medical officer or scientific advisor. They made it clear that they would not accept information from politicians (from any party) on food safety issues as politicians were most commonly seen as having an agenda that was not in consumers' interests.

> I would have to say the chief medical officer, I mean that's what he's there for, isn't it? I don't think they should let the politicians come on and tell us what's safe or not because let's face it, nobody believes a word any of them say, do they?
>
> (Female, Dover)

> It's up to the public health people and the scientists to tell us what's right and wrong with food and what precautions to take. If you let the political people do it then there's always the thought that they're trying to cover something up, or make sure the farmers don't lose any money.
>
> (Male, Aberdeen)

> It's all about money, about making sure that markets don't collapse. I think that there aren't enough people about taking the consumers' side in all these issues, it was like that with the Edwina Currie story. All I can remember is seeing loads of farmers and politicians shouting about how much it was all going to cost.
>
> (Male, Dundee)

Salmonella was discussed in relation to eggs and foodstuffs associated with them (mayonnaise, etc.) and chicken. It was also commonly discussed in relation to *Escherichia coli* (particularly within the Scottish groups). Concerning those who mentioned *E. coli*, it was interesting that people removed from the problem (not actually affected) discussed *E. coli* as a hygiene/contamination problem in the same way they discussed salmonella. The two separate issues were seen as being 'the same type of thing'.

In contrast, those most affected – i.e. a group in Wishaw where the outbreak occurred – discussed it in relation to poor production standards (still a hygiene issue but one occurring in a different institutional context). This group of people were remarkably supportive of the butcher's shop involved in the outbreak and claimed that the owner had become a 'scapegoat' for what was in reality a bigger problem. One respondent in this group who had been hospitalized by the out-break and spent a number of days in intensive care was adamant about his support for the butcher and had not stopped eating cold meats once he was out of hospital. An anecdote from this respondent was that when he was removed from intensive care into a general ward the first meal provided for him was a cold-meat salad, which the rest of the group found very amusing. What this poisoning outbreak had done for these respondents was to (in their words) 'politicize' them about food. They stated that had *E. coli* not occurred in their town none of them would have paid half as much attention to information on BSE. This point reinforces other research findings which suggest that personal experience is one of the most important features of determining how people may react to particular risk information.

The most influential sources of information in relation to salmonella were women's magazines, which were seen to be sensible, 'non-hysterical advice', and cookery programmes. It was suggested that if these programmes all used eggs in their recipes commonly people would be more likely to assume that they were indeed a safe source of food. Delia Smith was referenced extensively as was *Ready, Steady, Cook*, which was seen as offering advice as well as recipe ideas. Because actual chefs were using particular foodstuffs respondents were more likely to be reassured of their safety.

> If you see the like of Ainsley or whoever cooking these things then you think, right, it must be alright then. I mean they're hardly going to be using risky foods in their shows because if anything bad happened it would ruin their reputation.
>
> (Male, East Kilbride)

> I go by the women's magazines and I watch loads of cookery programmes, so I think I have a fairly good idea about what to do and what not to do. I think these things are really useful because it's a simpler clearer way of finding out things than watching the news, which is all negative. I mean, I find much more helpful to actually see people preparing food and getting hints on how to make sure there aren't any risks.
>
> (Female, Lurgan)

> Its really funny on that *Ready, Steady, Cook* programme because you see the chefs sometimes fluffing it up by using a chopping board to cut a vegetable when they've just used it for meat – and that Fern comes over and says, 'Now now, you know

that's not allowed'. I think that's quite good because it is funny but you will remember that you aren't supposed to do that.

(Female, Portsmouth)

This is potentially a very important point in relation to the communication of risk information, particularly since these programmes were cited as being useful in helping people to decide whether to continue to eat beef following the outbreak of BSE.

Bovine spongiform encephalopathy or 'mad cow disease'

The BSE story has perhaps been the most dramatic 'risk crisis' in Britain so far. It has been an extremely long-running and complex saga. The handling of the BSE issue and its implications for human health has been subject to controversy throughout its history. This issue involves 'risks' associated with modern agricultural policy, the effects of intensive farming, and the role of government in ensuring the safety of animal and human health.

In April 1985 a vet was called out to see a cow in Ashford, Kent. The animal was panicky and aggressive, began drooling and falling over. The vet assumed the cause was a brain tumour, put the animal down and thought nothing more of it. That is, until he was called back to the same farm to see a second cow with the same symptoms. More cases followed. He discovered that the brains of the animals had a spongy texture similar to those of sheep infected with scrapie. He called in the local MAFF vet, and in November 1986 the Central Veterinary Laboratory in Surrey confirmed what was thought to be the world's first case of spongiform brain disease in cattle.

MAFF took complete control over all aspects of BSE. It was not until June 1986 (7 months after the first diagnosis) that MAFF informed ministers of the new outbreak and a further 10 months elapsed before the government moved to have the threat assessed. MAFF also attempted to keep the nature of the disease to itself for as long as possible. When MAFF finally announced the existence of the new disease in October 1987 it did so in the Short Communications section of *The Veterinary Record* (journal of the British Veterinary Association). The government also kept tight control of information on BSE and journalists were given very little information. The very strictness of the official government line meant that those who disagreed with it had to find ways of communicating their ideas. So, willing alternative experts could easily be found and used as a balance to what little official information was being offered. This allowed the debate to widen and introduced a conflict at the level of science over the behaviour of the BSE agent and its potential consequences for animal and human life.

At the centre of this whole issue was the role of science. Had more been known about the BSE agent, clearer statements about diagnosis and treatment could have been made. But what quickly became obvious was that until scientific uncertainties about mad cow disease were cleared up, reassurances about the safety of British beef were not entirely convincing, and no firm resolution to the problem could be reached. The main debate centred on the science of BSE and whether, through contamination via infected bovine products, it could be passed to humans. There has always been a theoretical risk that BSE could pass in this way. However, while many 'experts' on the subject have admitted to the possibility (however unlikely or remote they believed it to be), politicians did not, publicly at least. The message that was always highlighted by government was: 'There is no risk to humans'.

BSE remained in the public sphere because controversy surrounded the subject. In April 1988 the UK government set up a committee (Southwood) to assess the significance of the new disease. The committee reported that: 'the risk of transmission of BSE to humans appears remote and it is unlikely that BSE will have any implications for human health'. But they also added,

> if our assessments of these likelihoods are incorrect, the implications would be extremely serious . . . with the long incubation period of spongiform encephalopathies in humans, it may be a decade or more before complete reassurances can be given.
>
> (Southwood *et al.*, 1989)

In the government press conference held to highlight the report it was stated: 'the report concludes that the risk of transmission of BSE to humans appears remote and it is therefore most unlikely that BSE will have any implications for human health' (*BBC News*, 27 February 1989).

The Southwood committee had wanted 75% compensation for those farmers with infected cattle (fearing they might sell them, send them to market quickly, or destroy and bury them privately). But the government disagreed, and the farmers had to settle for 50%. In July 1988, John MacGregor, then Minister of Agriculture, stopped brains and offal being fed to cattle and sheep. Inevitably, the next question to be asked (by the health department and opposition party) was about human food. While animals were no longer eating specified offal, there was no such legislation for humans. Pre-clinical BSE cattle were still going into the national food chain as if they were healthy animals. Brains, spinal cord, spleen, thymus, tonsils, intestines and bits of spinal tissue in 'mechanically recovered meat' were being used in a variety of products such as burgers, meat pies, pates, lasagne, soups and stock cubes, and baby foods. In early 1989, the official government view was that the removal of offal from human food was completely unnecessary. By March 1989 MacGregor was asked to ban human consumption of any organs known to harbour infectious agents. In May of that year, Hugh Fraser, from the Institute of Animal Health and one of the most senior researchers at the time, said on Radio 4's *Face the Facts* programme that he no longer ate bovine offal, and that it would be prudent if suspect tissues were removed from human consumption. This was finally done in November 1989.

Other factors ensured that BSE would remain a high-profile issue. There was already a well developed interest in food safety because of salmonella and listeria, which were high-profile public issues throughout 1988/89. By 1989, other countries began to be interested in the disease (Australia had already banned British beef cattle exports in July 1988). Germany, Italy and France banned British beef imports. The issue, in British terms, became political and economic. European countries claimed they were protecting the public health. John Gummer, the next Minister of Agriculture, treated this as powerful vested interests playing at protectionism. In Britain, local councils began banning British beef from the menus of 2000 schools. Then the death of a domestic cat from a spongiform encephalopathy caused alarm, opening the debate on transmission and bringing the potential threat to humans a little closer to home. Early on in the crisis John Gummer took a close interest in the presentations of MAFF. He became the pre-eminent spokesman on BSE and Ministry vets were therefore not at the forefront of any public relations efforts. By 1990 BSE was the biggest story on the news. The government was forced into action. As part of a move to try to restore public confidence in beef they instituted a 'Beef is Safe' campaign. One of the most memorable aspects of the media campaign was Gummer's attempt at banishing 'mad cow hysteria' by feeding a beef-burger to his young daughter. Surprisingly enough, it did not work, and concern mounted.

Yet the BSE story could not be sustained on a day-to-day level in news terms. Government inaction can cause uproar but that will die down when officials are seen to be doing something about it. This was clear when we see how BSE began to disappear from the media agenda once Britain had some success in stopping European bans on beef in 1990. While media coverage of BSE all but disappeared after 1990/1, the disease (as with salmonella levels) did not go away (Fig. 11.3).

Although there was a certain amount of media interest in the intervening years, it was not until March 1996 that a full-scale attack on this assessment of risk was heard. The fading interest had nothing to do with a change in MAFF activity, nor any kind of scientific resolution, nor a decline in the spread of BSE. Rather, coverage reduced because there was a resolution of sorts on a political level. A compromise solution was instituted that reinstated beef imports to Europe so long as they were certified to come from BSE-free herds. However, the central issue of human transmission was not resolved by the European

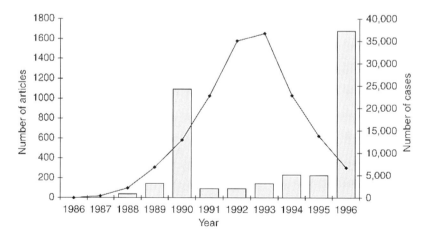

Fig. 11.3. Bovine spongiform encephalopathy: number of cases of infection in the UK (—♦—; data published on the Public Health Laboratory Service website, http://www.phls.org.uk/) and the number of articles (▪) in UK national newspapers, 1986–1996.

Community decision. In spite of, or perhaps because of, the outstanding scientific uncertainty, the decline in coverage towards the end of 1990 was sustained for the next 5 years, with only the occasional minor peak.

BSE retained the potential to re-emerge as a high-profile media story but required further scientific evidence or renewed official action. At this stage, MAFF efforts to control the issue were actually quite effective. But also because MAFF attempted to keep such tight control over information on BSE and Creutzfeldt-Jakob disease (CJD), alternative media sources were found, and 'experts' as such created. Behind the scenes, sources used by the media would be scientists, researchers and organizations such as the British Veterinary Association. In this way questions that were not being asked at other levels could be addressed. The highlighting, for example, of conditions and practices within slaughter houses changed the issue from whether bovine offal was being removed to how effectively or safely this was being done. An Environmental Health Office (EHO) document sent to MAFF in February 1990 had pointed out that poor practices were evident (*Guardian*, 28 April 1991). They received no reply from the Ministry. It was only in 1995 (6 years after implementation) that MAFF took steps to tighten controls on slaughter house practices. Had the media not brought research into poor hygiene and clear breaches of regulation into the open, then work e.g. by the EHO might have gone unnoticed.

The general low level of media interest in Britain during 1991–1995 was due, in part, to the feeling that BSE had exhausted its news value. There were also very few new events to maintain a momentum of media concern. While a number of journalists remained intensely interested in BSE, they fell foul of editorial decision making and the demands of news. As one journalist we interviewed said:

> Scientists continually said 'we don't have the data, we need further research'
> . . . so we tended not to write about it . . . It just doesn't make very good copy,
> to simply say 'we don't know, we need further research', 'we can't answer that'.
> However honest that is, it doesn't play very well in terms of headlines.
>
> (Broadsheet journalist, interviewed 1995)

At the same time the lack of policy activity meant that editors lost interest in the subject because 'nothing was happening'. This reaction frustrated some journalists, because, as one broadsheet specialist pointed out: 'Of course that was the whole point, *nothing was happening* to destroy this thing; but in newspaper terms I wouldn't be given the space to say that *every day* or *every week*'. Simultaneously, MAFF caution over what could be said in public minimized the chance that official sources would make controversial statements. For example, official experts who were taking precautions were not prepared to say that in public:

> as far as we know at the moment there doesn't seem to be a risk to humans. While
> I personally don't believe that there ever will be, we just don't know at the minute,
> but that's science for you. [JR: 'So, do you eat bovine offals at all?'] Well, no
> I don't actually. But I could never say that in public because I shudder to think what
> the media would make of it. And I don't think that it would be very sensible
> professionally given the highly emotive nature of the subject.
>
> (Official expert, interviewed 1995)

While clear pronouncements about safety were being made to the public, new CJD cases had started to appear in 1994, when there were six, and continued in 1995. The most important aspect of them was that they were similar both in clinical symptoms and in the pathological damage that appeared in the brain. John Pattison, head of the Spongiform Encephalopathy Advisory Committee (SEAC), suggested that projected cases of BSE in humans, calculated on current information, could represent a major public health problem.

By the end of 1995 ten new cases of CJD had appeared in younger people (under 42 years). Under Pattison's headship SEAC decided that the news had to be made public. The announcement led to an explosion of media coverage, even exceeding the previous peak of interest in 1990. While public health interests were finally brought into play, government failure to deal with BSE adequately earlier was all the more strongly criticized and European interventions were dramatically strengthened in 1996 with demands for a worldwide ban on British beef and a major culling policy.

Going public with information on a new strain of CJD changed the nature of the BSE debate. Health interests were brought into play. While SEAC made recommendations that the 'risk' to humans from food would probably be small if there were better controls on offal, and more rigorous enforcement of those controls, Prime Minister John Major was seen on television saying that beef was 'entirely safe' and that this 'had been confirmed by British scientists' (*PM*, 23 April 1996).

There is a sense in which lessons have been learned from BSE. Government is now seen to be at some level more open. For example, data from the BSE inquiry, set up to investigate how it happened, are accessible to the public. Confidence in British beef is seen to be returning. But all of this has come at a cost.

Factors determining public responses to bovine spongiform encephalopathy

Reactions to BSE within our groups were conditioned by a number of factors. Initially respondents discussed their reactions to the announcement in 1996 of a potential link between BSE and CJD. It was clear that respondents felt strongly about the issue of BSE, specifically about how it had been handled and the number of years they had been 'kept in the dark' about the potential risks.

Discussion on BSE centred on the loss of trust in government experienced by people and how attitudes to food had been radically altered by the BSE crisis:

> Well, they let it happen didn't they? All they wanted was to make sure everybody kept on buying meat without a single regard for our safety. The whole thing was a complete fiasco and I hope someone actually pays for that.
>
> (Male, Inverness)

> Nothing will ever be the same again I think, we are now in a post-BSE world and that means that what you may have ignored or not thought much about before has become central. . . and I don't just mean about the actual food, I think this issue highlighted quite radically how our political institutions work and who they are most concerned about, and what came out is that it isn't us.
>
> (Female, Bristol)

I never really thought that much about what I ate before BSE, but there comes a time when you have to take on board the fact that not everyone's interest are going to be served by the political system, and the public are certainly not very high on British governments' priority lists. It's a trust thing, you think they're there to keep us safe as far as possible, and then you learn that what they are there for is to keep the food industry and farming safe.

(Male, London)

If they hadn't have said there was no risk at all for all those years then I don't think it would have been so bad. I mean, was there really a need to keep the potential problems covered up like that? How stupid do the government think we are? And that's the thing, they think we're stupid and don't trust us to make sensible decisions. Well all that BSE has done has shown me that I can't trust these people to ensure that what I'm eating is safe and that they've treated the whole nation like fools.

(Male, Coleraine)

While there was commonly a clear attitude that what BSE was about was a failure of government, the issue of continued consumption highlighted the contradictions between believing something and changing actual eating practices. There were very different attitudes to the level of risk associated with eating beef. This is not to say that respondents had stopped eating beef or beef products. Levels of concern about actually consuming beef differed radically. Some respondents stated that they had removed certain foodstuffs from their diet, most notably burgers, sausages and pies. This was particularly the case for those respondents who had children. But, on the whole, while the belief that a link between BSE and CJD was held to be true, more complex reasons were at play in relation to whether individuals continued to buy beef:

I still eat beef yes, I don't eat burgers anymore but that's mainly because I didn't know what was in them. The kids aren't allowed to eat them either but I don't have a problem with steak because I don't think you can get it from that. [JR: 'Why not?'] It was on that documentary about BSE a while back, the one that was on for about three weeks. One of the scientists said that the risk was miniscule from steak and I just thought well, I'll keep eating it then.

(Male, Edinburgh)

Well, I haven't stopped eating anything at all, I was one of those ones who was out buying the fillet steak when it was all being sold off cheap . . . I do think there is a link between the two diseases but I've always been a big meat eater and I suppose I'll have taken the risk loads of times, there's no point stopping now.

(Female, Lurgan)

It's banned from our house, all of it, except that is Scottish beef, I will eat that. I think I wanted to stop altogether but that's dead hard when you really like something so I decided to check out the things that were seen as being safe, and the papers were always talking about how Scottish beef was safest so I decided to move to that.

(Male, Perth)

I didn't really think about stopping because we were always told that there wasn't a problem here [Northern Ireland] because of the computerized system we have in place to check where animals are coming from and going to. When I went to England though I wouldn't eat it, no chance, it's not worth the risk.

(Male, Belfast)

It became clear that this was the first issue in which there were clear differences between groups, particularly in relation to their geographical location. Where people came from was a particularly important factor in determining whether they were concerned about the risks associated with BSE. The groups in Northern Ireland all said that 'their beef' was by far the safest and claimed that they felt safe continuing to eat it. Asked why they thought their meat was 'safer', these respondents stated that both media (particularly local media) and advertising in shops selling meat were the main reasons:

We don't have BSE here, its all English and Scottish stuff that's the problem. We know that because it's always on the news, that we have a proper system in place which can say where all the animals have come from.

(Male, Omagh)

You see it advertised everywhere, this is Northern Irish beef, it's in all the butchers and supermarkets. So, you don't really think there's a problem as long as you know that it's definitely from here.

(Female, Belfast)

They tell you on the news that if you ask the butcher he should be able to say what farm the meat has come from and that it's BSE-free. You can't ask for more than that now.

(Male, Coleraine)

Very few of the people in the groups had stopped eating beef altogether. One nurse in Belfast stated that he had stopped because of CJD. His concern centred on the nature of the disease and it was this which made him decide to stop. As he said:

I just thought, no that's a really horrible disease. No cure, people have a nightmare time, I've seen them. I thought what if you can get this from eating burgers or whatever, it's just not worth it. So I just thought, no, I'm not taking that risk. It's funny, I'm not usually squeamish but this just made me feel really odd, like, I could give this to myself and I definitely don't want CJD I can tell you.

(Male, Belfast)

It was interesting that the rest of this group found his reasoning amusing and made comments on the risk associated with CJD as opposed to other life-style habits:

You're an eejit, do you know that? You do more risky things to yourself every day. I mean you smoke like a trooper and, let's face it, you're always in the pub. What on earth makes you think you're going to get CJD, I mean hardly anyone gets it, it's really rare, even the one associated with meat.

(Female, Belfast)

I don't know, I can't really explain it really. I just know that I have seen people with CJD and it's horrible.

(Same male)

While in Scotland respondents argued that 'their' beef should have the same mark of safety as Northern Ireland had, here respondents discussed BSE in much the same way as in both Wales and England. Most of the respondents said that while they had not actually stopped eating beef they had become more careful about choosing particular products and particularly more aware of where it came from.

What did become clear in all groups in association with BSE was that individuals initially blamed the media for creating a 'scare', but following the 1996 announcement the media was more likely to be used as a trusted source of information by respondents (Reilly, 1999).

Genetically modified foods

Following on from BSE, the debate over GM foods was next to become high-profile. We carried out focus groups in early 1998 where none of the respondents knew anything about genetic modification. It was clear that they had not picked up any information appearing within media formats on the subject. In these groups there was very little discussion of this issue, and when respondents attempted to talk about it there was a general sense of confusion in relation to the issues involved:

> I have no idea about that kind of thing at all, sorry.
>
> (Male, Edinburgh)

> Is it a big media story then? I haven't seen anything about it, I would've remembered if I had.
>
> (Female, Carlisle)

> I know it's something to do with genes, about putting genes from one thing into another, but that's it, I'm afraid.
>
> (Female, Milton Keynes)

> I haven't the faintest idea, and I don't think I want to know to be honest.
>
> (Male, Bristol)

> I've read a bit about it, about us not wanting the stuff on the supermarket shelves. I think its coming from Europe isn't it, they don't want the stuff.
>
> (Female, East Kilbride)

None of the respondents knew whether there were any products already being sold to them and wouldn't know what to look out for were they to check. When asked where they might go to get information if they were concerned, most of the respondents in these groups stated that they would contact a consumer group. At this stage though there was no real concern about genetic modification and no real interest by any respondents in learning more about the issues:

> I've too much to do to be bothered about something I haven't even heard of. It'll probably all blow over.
>
> (Female, Carlisle)

> I'm not concerned about that stuff, it's all too up in the air and I don't really understand anything about it. If there is a problem with it I'm sure we'll hear about it soon enough, we always do.
>
> (Male, Aberdeen)

I think we've had about enough about food scares for the present. We're all still
getting over the BSE thing.

(Female, Nottingham)

These were reasonable responses given the level and content of media coverage
before 1998. It was from 1998 that increasing mainstream media interest in the
costs and benefits of GM foods appeared. Malcolm Walker's refusal to stock GM
soya in Iceland stores (March 1998) and Monsanto taking out full-page adverts
in the national press (June 1998) about the GM food it produces caused much
debate. There was also Prince Charles commenting on the potential problems of
growing genetically engineered crops in June (his views on this issue having
been made public from as early as 1995), the arrest of campaigners for attempting to destroy such crops (August 1998) and the reporting of new EU laws on the
labelling of foods using GM ingredients (September 1998).

GM food began receiving increasing media coverage specifically from 1996
for a number of reasons. First, they are here – the crops are being grown and the
products are on supermarket shelves. This is an important factor in whether
issues will be covered as mainstream media formats which deal, on the whole, in
'news' (i.e. something which has happened) rather than speculation (i.e. something which may happen in the future).

Second, there were growing and concerted attempts by pressure groups
(both environmental and consumer) to get GM food and crops on to the political
agenda via the media (and more recently, efforts by industry to clearly get their
perspective across in the face of perceived public mistrust over GM products). A
clear disparity between public and both industry and official perceptions of relevant issues relating to GM food and crops was emerging which came to the fore
in mass media coverage.

Third, for a number of reasons Britain's reputation as a quality food producer had been tarnished. In the post-BSE era trust in both industry and political
institutions was seen by the media to have been seriously damaged. BSE was
one of the biggest and long-running high-profile media issues and serious analo-
gies between that and the potential risks and uncertainties surrounding GM food
and crops were inevitably going to be highlighted.

While the mass media began paying increasing attention to GM foods,
coverage on the whole did remain selective. Newspaper coverage, for example,
remained predominantly report-based. Sixty-four per cent of coverage was
report-based 'news-led' (i.e. based on scientific discoveries, agricultural, business
news, law and regulation). These were found most commonly in the agriculture,
science and business news pages of newspapers. The vast majority of coverage
appeared in broadsheet newspapers with tabloid coverage making up only 10%
of items. (If we look specifically at the low-range tabloids such as the *Sun*,
the *Mirror* and the *Daily Star*, this figure goes down to only 3%.)

Newspapers are not the ideal format for huge features on the future of science
in the 20th century. A new discovery may be reported, but there is seldom time
to research the subject more fully. In general, under pressure of deadlines, journalists will give priority to official/scientific sources. In saying that, in relation to
genetic modification there has been an increasing amount of space for longer

articles, feature and editorial articles where issues can be critically discussed and assessed. These constituted 23% of newspaper stories in 1998 (these types of stories constituted 15% of coverage in 1995). This increase was due primarily to the appearance of GM products on supermarket shelves and because of the legal and agricultural changes that had occurred because of GM crops. It was also because there had been a growing debate in general on food issues such as BSE and *E. coli*. While there were a number of papers which were questioning the risks and benefits associated with GM food before March 1996 (most notably in the *Guardian*, the *Independent* and the *Observer*), the vast majority of feature coverage centred on the uncertainties associated with these technologies and problems perceived with a lack of proper regulation.

One point to mention here is the fact that coverage has largely been determined by the nature of the sources used. GM food (until 1999) was an issue that had no central 'official' spokespeople (whereas with BSE there were official sources seen to dismiss risks). This meant that the debate developed with the opposing interests of pressure groups and industry, producers and supermarkets at the fore. At the same time newspapers took particular lines on advances, particularly in editorial pieces where the views of the public are aired (this is most clearly seen in the *Guardian* and the *Observer* in particular, where a lot of debate on whether 'we' need or want GM foods has taken place).

The development of the debate in this way has impacted at different levels. For example, it seems that the companies producing GM products did not sufficiently take into account 'negative' media coverage around consumer groups and EU concerns over maize and soya that had been building up in newspapers since July 1996. By October of that year headlines were reading like this: 'Controversy around new GM crops may have caught biotech companies by surprise' (*Financial Times*, 15 October 1996). Yet the controversy and uncertainties around the use of GM foods had not come out of the blue. As far back as 1990 negative media coverage about approval for use of a GM brewer's yeast was in part blamed for the fact that the product was not put on the market.

In 1997 the debates began to become more centred on particular subjects. Labelling became the central issue (taking up 40% of coverage in that year). As more products entered into the food market it was becoming clear that opposition to these products was becoming more organized (differences in the type of coverage between the entry on the market of tomato purée in 1996 as opposed to soybeans and tinned tomatoes where the labelling of products and needs of consumer choice had become central to media debates; it is worth noting that consumer and food pressure groups were three times more likely to be interviewed for reports than industry officials and five times more likely than government officials). From January to June 1997 GM food and crops were becoming a political issue and as such received extensive coverage on the political pages of the major newspapers. The introduction of EU laws over labelling and patenting dominated this type of coverage. Following the introduction of EU approval for the labelling of genetically altered products in June, media coverage returned to the science, agricultural and consumer pages.

On television, news reports are – as in newspapers – short articles which are event-driven. BBC and ITV news programmes do not have the time for in-depth coverage and so items were more likely to be found on either Channel 4 news or *Newsnight*, with television news items constituting only 10% of all coverage (both television and newspaper) from 1995 to 1998. Channel 5 had a consumer-led remit which may have affected what issues they covered. They recently broadcast a series of programmes entitled *The Clone Zone* dealing with genetics (both in factual and fictional formats). On the remaining four channels documentary/consumer/agricultural/cookery programmes have dealt with GM food and crops to some extent. The plethora of cookery programmes on network television (on average between 15 and 20 hours per week) very rarely mention food production issues, sticking closely to the cookery format. Food programmes such as *Food and Drink*, *Watchdog*, *Foodfile* and *The Food Chain* have covered GM foods, centring on general issues around the food production system and consumer interests (specifically about products like tomatoes and GM soybeans). Yet they remain one-off items or programmes as there is such a wide remit for these types of programme. The same can be said for agricultural programmes such as *Landward* and *Countryfile*, and science programmes such *Big Science*, *Equinox*, *Heart of the Matter* and *Tomorrow's World*. In the main, documentaries are still more likely to cover human genetics (70% of documentaries during 1995–1998 were about human genetic issues specifically) although the number of documentaries on GM food and crops trebled in 1998 compared with 1995. These have centred on the food production system in general, GM crops and GM soybeans (*Watchdog*: 'The Big Dinner' (BBC1, 28 May 1998); *World in Action*: 'Eat up your Genes' (ITV, 10 August 1998); *Private Investigations* (GM crops; BBC2, 2 September 1998)).

In general there is a sense in which mass media formats have failed to address some of the fundamental and more complex questions present in contemporary debates (it is easier to get more information via the Internet, for example). It is obvious that media coverage of GM food and crops is selective. This can be explained by the nature of media coverage as a whole and specifically by source competition (who gets on and who is available for comment) and 'newsworthiness' (the contemporary nature of the issue and the need for television and newspapers to be 'news-led'). News momentum and the organization of news beats and media outlets determine what will be reported at different times. Press and television news are on the whole not adapted to sustaining high-level or sustained coverage of issues, and media interest is not capable of being maintained in the face of ongoing scientific uncertainty or speculation. However, consumer choice, health confidence, the control of scientific advances and uncertainties surrounding new technologies have all taken a higher-profile image within mainstream media formats since 1998.

Responses to genetically modified foods following heightened media coverage

We returned to these groups in late 1998 and early 1999, and there were a number of very significant changes relating to discussions of genetic modification. Respondents quite openly discussed the issues (whereas there was very little conversation about it before). The issues stressed were those which had begun to be defined in the mass media, such as choice, labelling and public confidence. The respondents stated that they had begun looking at media coverage mainly because 'you couldn't really get away from it' (particularly in 1999).

In general terms, the issue of genetic modification was not commonly understood by respondents in any of the groups (apart from the general practitioners in Dundee). Discussions centred not on the science, but on the role of choice, 'naturalness' and economics:

> I have no idea what it's about but it doesn't sound right to me, it's not natural, and there's no need for it in this day and age.
>
> (Female, Llangollen)

> It's all about money again, these big companies can do this modification and can see how to make lots of money from it.
>
> (Male, Swansea)

> I don't like the idea of it, and I won't be buying any of the stuff they produce in this way . . . at least with this I have the choice to do that. We never had that with BSE.
>
> (Female, Swindon)

> You can see the same thing happening again as with BSE, they're not prepared to regulate big companies properly before they're sure this stuff is safe, and that's not on.
>
> (Male, London)

> Why do they need to do this, we have perfectly good tomatoes as it is, and I don't want them to last longer than they already do, it's not natural . . . and I don't think they can prove yet whether it will do any harm.
>
> (Female, Bedford)

> They have to be careful because it could end up being like BSE, you know, the problems being seen to exist far too late to do anything about it.
>
> (Male, South Uist)

In all discussions GM food was linked with BSE. The problems which had been highlighted with the BSE crisis could be seen to happen again with this issue. Because of a lack of understanding of the scientific processes relating to the technology (as respondents themselves stated), discussion centred on the role of uncertainty and potential risks. This involved the role of science and its links to business, government and farmers, all of whom were perceived as being capable of putting market interests before public health. They were seen as having done so before with BSE.

The implication here is that it will in the future be difficult to separate these two debates. There were frequent references to being in a 'post-BSE' society and these were used to highlight concerns around GM food. There were a number of contradictions within these discussions in relation to the role of consumer choice and perceived safety measures.

The most frequent arguments around genetic modification centred on the ability to choose freely whether to eat these products and the perceived lack of government action in ensuring they were either properly tested or removed until proven safe. It was interesting that the same respondents discussed their resentment and indignation in relation to the 'beef-on-the-bone' ban which was seen as taking away the ability to choose. The most likely explanation for this contradiction is that there was a marked difference between the debates on BSE and GM food at the level of what was seen as reliable knowledge.

At the centre of this was how much information was seen to have been given out. In 1998/9 BSE was perceived as being a 'known entity' as it were, and armed with what was described as 'the full story' individuals believed that they then had the right to make up their own minds about food consumption, and to make their own risk assessments. It was constantly stated that if people were given the full facts and left to make up their own minds (in what was understood to be scientifically uncertain areas) then there would not be so many potential crises.

Conclusion

The findings confirmed that the respondents were knowledgeable about media formats and the debates highlighted by these three major food scares. It was also clear that much of their information had come from the mass media (although in a lot of cases they initially did not appreciate how much they did know and how much they had actually picked up from the media). As such, the media can make people think about what they eat: the data described on sales and the reported consumption of certain food products make it clear that media reporting of some food risks can cause dramatic shifts in buying and eating behaviour.

Media influence on public belief or action is, however, dependent on a number of factors and our respondents seemed actively to negotiate their understandings of the safety of foods and the role the media played in highlighting potential risks. Certainly developing and targeting specific messages via the mass media is important in risk communication. At the same time the communicators need to have a better understanding of how people themselves negotiate information as well as a firmer grasp of both what people believe or reject and the reasons why.

References

Eldridge, J. and Reilly, J. (2003) Risk and relativity: BSE and the British media. In: Pidgeon, N., Kasperson, R. and Slovic, P. (eds) The Social Amplification of Risk. Cambridge University Press, Cambridge, UK, pp. 138–155.

Eldridge, J., Kitzinger, J. and Williams, K. (1996) Mass Media Power in Britain. Oxford University Press, Oxford, UK.

House of Commons Agriculture Committee (1989) First Report: Salmonella in Eggs, Vol. 1. HMSO, London.

Kitzinger, J. and Reilly, J. (1997) The rise and fall of risk reporting: media coverage of human genetic research, 'false memory syndrome' and 'mad cow disease'. European Journal of Communication 12, 319–350.

MacIntyre, S., Reilly, J., Miller D. and Eldridge, J. (1998) Food choice, food scares and health: the role of the media. In: Murcott, A. (ed.) The Nation's Diet: The Social Science of Food Choice. Longman, London, pp. 228–249.

Miller, D. and Reilly, J. (1994) Food and the media: reporting health scares. In: Henson, S. and Gregory, S. (eds) *The Politics of Food, 1994*. Department of Agricultural Economics, Reading University, Reading, UK.

Miller, D. and Reilly, J. (1995a) Food and the media: explaining health scares. In: Feichtinger, E. and Kohler, B. (eds) *Current Research into Eating Practices: Contributions of the Social Sciences*. Umschan Zeitscher-Verlag, Frankfurt am Main, Germany.

Miller, D. and Reilly, J. (1995b) Making an issue of food safety: the media, pressure groups and the public sphere. In: Maurer, D. and Sobal, J. (eds) *Food, Eating and Nutrition as Social Problems: Constructivist Perspectives*. Aldine De Gruyter, New York, pp. 305–336.

Mintel (1990) *Eggs: Market Intelligence*. Mintel, London.

Philo, P. and Reilly J. (1998) *Information Sources and their Influence on Public Understandings of Food Hazards*. Final Report (FS1845) to Ministry of Agriculture, Fisheries and Food, London.

Reilly, J. (1997) *The Impact of the Re-emergence of BSE on Public Beliefs and Behaviour*. Final Report (L211252058) to Economic and Social Research Council, Swindon, UK.

Reilly, J. (1998) Just another food scare? Changes in public understandings of BSE. In: Philo, P. (ed.) *Message Received*. Longman, London, pp. 129–145.

Reilly, J. (1999) The salmonella-in-eggs crisis in Britain. In: Applebaum, M. (ed.) *Alimentation, Peurs et Risques: Ouvrage sous la Direction*. Observatoire Cidil de L'harmonie Alimentaire, Paris.

Reilly, J. (2001) *Dishing up Death: Is our Food Poisoning Us?* South Street Press, Reading, UK.

Reilly, J. and Miller, D. (1997) Scaremonger or scapegoat? The role of the media in the emergence of food as a social issue. In: Caplan, P. (ed.) *Food, Identity and Health*. Routledge, London, pp. 234–251.

Southwood, R., Epstein, M.A., Martin, W.B. and Walton, J. (1989) *Report of the Working Party on Bovine Spongiform Encephalopathy (The Southwood Report)*. Department of Health and Ministry of Agriculture, Fisheries and Food, London.

This page intentionally left blank

12 The Impact of Advertising on Food Choice: the Social Context of Advertising

MARTIN CARAHER[1] AND JANE LANDON[2]

[1]Centre for Food Policy, Department of Health Management and Food Policy, Institute of Health Sciences, City University, Northampton Square, London EC1 0HB, UK; [2]National Heart Forum, Tavistock House South, Tavistock Square, London WC1H 9LG, UK

Introduction

Advertising and its impact on food choice is an issue of vast discussion and debate. Among the reasons for this are the global rise in obesity and the linking of food advertising, especially that directed at children, to such rises by health advocates (Robinson, 1998; World Health Organization (WHO)/Food and Agriculture Organization (FAO), 2003; House of Commons Health Committee, 2004; WHO, 2004). Both the food and the advertising industries dispute the validity of this claim. For example, while television viewing is associated with obesity, it is difficult to separate the potential effect of television advertising from other aspects of television viewing (e.g. programme content or sedentary behaviour). Thus we have a polarized debate with tensions over the role, function and the impact of advertising. The public health nutrition movement tends to see unfettered advertising as a means of promoting unhealthy eating practices and calls for its control and even banning. Food industry and advertising advocates portray it as a necessary part of modern consumer society and emphasize its potential in promoting healthy eating. As Fine et al. (1996) note, certain sections of the food industry view any proposals to limit advertising and marketing as pushes against market growth and limitations on personal freedom, while the public health lobby views it as a force to be contained and controlled in the pursuit of health. These concerns from the food sector have recently been questioned by the publication of two reports from investment bankers/financial analysts pointing out that regulation of foods high in sugar/fat and advertising aimed at children is almost inevitable in the current global epidemic of obesity (UBS Warburg, 2002; JP Morgan, 2006).

The role, controls and the social milieu of advertising contribute to the strength of the impact of advertising on food choice and behaviour. This location of advertising within the social norms and rules of society mutes or contributes to the enhanced impact of advertising. In addition, the indicators used to gauge the impact of advertising are often indirect ones such as obesity rates in the case of the health sector and sales in the case of food manufacturers and producers. In the midst of these debates the mechanisms that advertising uses to impact food choice are not well understood or discussed. It also needs to be recognized that advertising is but one part of what is called the marketing mix, which is generally taken to be composed of the '4Ps': product, price, place and promotion (Kotler et al., 2002).

   This chapter sets out the mechanisms that inform advertising practice followed by a discussion on the social context of advertising, examining the evidence and claims for and against restrictions on advertising, before moving on to looking at some ways that advertising practice is monitored and controlled and concluding with a discussion of the implications for practice and policy. The focus is on children and television advertising, as in this area there are concerns about the role of advertising in children's health and calls for better/stricter regulation. The spotlight is on television advertising as this medium still sets the standard against which other media are judged and still accounts for the largest single advertising spend. Most of the discussion is within the context of the developed world, as it is here that there are well developed media and regulatory frameworks; this is not to imply that the situation is any less grave in the developing world as a recent WHO (2004) report makes clear, but the problems related to food are different with the burden of disease also different.

The Psychology of Advertising: How Does it Work?

Advertising theory has progressed from the days of Vance Packard when the consumer was seen as the passive recipient of knowledge and targeted messages. Now the consumer is seen as an active participant in the process if only because they have the power to make the choice from a myriad of options, options perhaps previously not available. It is generally agreed that there are three aims of advertising:

1. To retain existing users of a product, goods, service or behaviour.
2. To encourage users of other similar products, goods or services to switch to the one advertised.
3. To entice new users to purchase the products, goods or services being advertised.

With reference to children the advertising industry maintains that the function of advertising is to encourage children to switch brands, not to eat greater quantities from a widening range of products, and to act as a means of communication. Some of this approach is based on the supposition that children are relatively passive consumers not in charge of their own food spending. There are two psychological avenues through which advertising can be channelled, central and peripheral routes. Central route persuasion is the approach most often used by public health nutrition and social marketing campaigns based on a rational appeal to the consumer on the basis of factual information. This approach is often chosen due to a lack of resources, no actual product to promote and the lack of a marketing plan. For these reasons they tend to be one-off or have to be capable of standing alone with distinct single-issue messages. Public health nutrition campaign messages are often exhortations to healthy behaviours based on a logical thought process, with appeals to healthy eating behaviour on the principle of danger or damage to health. In practice, due to a lack of resources, the medium of communication is the written leaflet or booklet rather than television advertising (Caraher and Baker, 2001). For these reasons they cannot easily draw on one of the central premises of advertising and psychology, which is repetition and the reinforcement of messages.

Peripheral routes are the approaches most favoured by the food and advertising industries and are based on the principles of feelings and identification being as important in the decision-making process as logical processes. Peripheral persuasion techniques seek though exposure and reinforcement of cultural norms to influence behaviour (de Mooij, 1998). This leads to change in behaviour and with enough resources advertisers can influence cultural norms or even create them where none existed previously. Peripheral approaches are less likely to be about the food itself and more to do with the values, images, branding, value for money and social values surrounding the food. For example, we know from research that the key determinants influencing the choice of foods in the school setting relate to taste, convenience and price (Caraher *et al.*, 2003). So any advertising for food in the school setting would emphasize price as a central persuasion technique; but given that the options open to children may be limited, the major focus would be on the affective aspects of food choice, such as the benefits of eating with friends or promoting the feeling of belonging.

Conner and Armitage (2002) point out that central routes, at least in theory, are likely to be more effective and less expensive than peripheral routes, yet in practice peripheral routes are seen to be more efficient. Among the reasons for this are that central route persuasion relies on the individual making decisions based on cognitive processes. These are judged to be largely process-based: the provision of information changing attitudes and in turn changing behaviour. In reality the process of decision making is much more complex than this and nowhere more so than when food is involved, where culture, taste and personal aesthetics all come into play. Peripheral route persuasion, contrary to what the name implies, directly taps into behaviour via impulses.

What many public health campaigns fail to realize or acknowledge is that food choice and behaviour are not, *per se*, logical processes but are based on peripheral processes and personal preferences and habits, and decisions about food choice are not based solely on the salutogenic properties of food. Also the rewards system for healthy eating is often based on messages of long-term or delayed gratification and often is accompanied by a personal cost in the form of the adoption or avoidance of a behaviour. In contrast, the food industry can offer immediate gratification – in the here and now, with minimal personal cost – as long as you can afford it. Parallel lessons have been in the area of smoking control, where exhortations to children not to smoke in return for long-term health benefits were found to make little impact. The focus of public health campaigns was found to be better spent on creating a situation where smoking was 'uncool' and appealing to affective issues of belonging and feelings about the behaviour as opposed to the health outcomes. (Note that the messages and approach may be different for smokers in middle age, who see the costs/benefits as being closer to them and not long-term or distant as do children.)

As a general psychological principle, it is easier to influence the attitudes of consumers who do not feel personally involved than those who are and to reinforce behaviours that already exist as opposed to asking or persuading people to adopt new behaviours or quit existing ones. For example, it would be easier to convince those who already eat fruit to expand their range of fruit intake than to persuade those who do not eat fruit to begin. It is also important to recognize that advertising is only part of the whole marketing process. If you advertise a new brand of chocolate, then it is essential you make sure that it appears in the shops, when and where consumers demand it. With many health promotion messages in public health campaigns this control of the marketing process is not an option. So if a public health campaign advocates increased intake of fruit through their substitution for energy-dense products such as chocolate or crisps, then you need to ensure the product is available, attractive and is priced competitively with the alternatives, or limit the range of alternatives. Public health advertising campaigns can be very effective in increasing knowledge, influencing attitudes and even creating demand, but they ultimately fail if the individual cannot access the product or change behaviour with minimum disruption. The classic example is the UK AIDS/HIV advertising campaign from the late 1980s, where the television campaign achieved increases in awareness and knowledge of AIDS/HIV in the general population over an extremely short period of time, referred to colloquially as the 'tombstones and iceberg ads'. The campaign was judged by many to be a failure as it did not achieve a significant reduction in risky behaviour. As Ind (1993) points out, this shows a lack of understanding of the role and place of advertising within the marketing process; the failure here was a lack of marketing and condom availability. Condoms could have been made readily available, but they were not for a myriad of political reasons, which is a feature limiting the marketing of many public health campaigns (Garfield, 1994).

Vaughan (1980) and Jones (1998), in the model of planning for advertising, see a hierarchy of effect in psychological terms of the engagement with advertising. The involvement is based on the three interrelated processes of:

- learning;
- feeling; and
- doing.

The central persuasion process described above is based on the principle of learning (logic), leading to feeling (affective processes) and this to doing (see Fig. 12.1). What advertisers have learned is that you can start with any of the processes. Psychological reinforcement comes from the affective aspects of a behaviour; this could be the taste or appearance of a food or snack or the

	Think	Feel
High involvement	Quadrant 1.	Quadrant 2.
	Based on information/logical approach	Affective (psychological)
	Learn feel do	Feel learn do
Low involvement	Quadrant 3.	Quadrant 4.
	Habitual	Satisfaction (social)
	Do learn feel	Do feel learn

Fig. 12.1. Psychological processes in advertising showing the type of engagement.

situation in which it is consumed. This latter aspect can be seen in the work of Chapman and MacLean (1993), who found that adolescents knew that 'junk' food eaten in fast-food restaurants was unhealthy but associated it with friends, fun, independence and being away from home. Home-cooked food, on the other hand, was recognized as healthy but seen as boring, being with family and unexciting. So on balance adolescents in the Chapman and MacLean study did not made decisions about fast-food restaurant food on the basis of the healthiness or otherwise of the food; the social aspects of eating such as being with friends and away from parental authority weighed as more important than the information-led approach to decision making.

The ultimate purpose of any advertising is to stimulate action in the consumer, so advertising has to be placed in the hierarchy of marketing and demand alongside other the factors of place, price and appeal.

Many of the models informing public health practice are based on the logical approach of thinking and a high involvement with this process (Egger *et al.*, 1999; Conner and Armitage, 2002). This equates with quadrant 1 in Fig. 12.1. The various aspects of the table can be summarized as follows:

- Quadrant 1 applies to big purchase items or major buys such as clothes and toys or where to spend your money, e.g. McDonalds as value for money or Starbucks as saying something about you as a consumer.
- Quadrant 2 applies to branded items which make a statement about you. So Coke or Pepsi?
- Quadrant 3 applies to everyday commodities such as snacks. Apple or orange/Mars bar or Kit-Kat?
- Quadrant 4 applies to the pleasures in life, so adolescents deciding that they want to eat at McDonalds as a means of spending time with friends.

The use of peripheral routes is crucial with young children and adolescents. Of course the approaches outlined in quadrants 2, 3 and 4 could be used to promote positive aspects of eating, so ensuring that young children eat fruit at break time in an atmosphere conducive to making it a positive experience and supplemented by positive advertising or imagery. An example of such an approach, although at the micro-level of the school, is the 'Food Dudes' initiative: this uses cartoon characters to promote positive images of eating fruit and vegetables (Horne *et al.*, 1998).

The Debates and Evidence on Advertising to Children

The key debates related to advertising policy and children revolve around the following:

- The rights of children.
- The rights of an industry to promote its products, ideas and communications.
- The place of advertising in a child's life – whether it is seen as a normal part of growing up or an aspect requiring control and regulation.
- The impact of advertising on the attitudes, behaviour and health of children including 'pester power'.
- The role of the state in public health protection and promotion.

A report from JP Morgan (2003) on food manufacturing concludes that:

- The rise in obesity raises serious concerns and threats for the food industry.
- Food manufacturers face the risk of increased regulation and litigation.
- The food industry will have to review its marketing practices and adapt itself to address these concerns.
- The soft drinks and snacks sectors are in particular danger as they are identified by academic research as contributory factors to obesity.
- Global concerns with obesity create an opportunity for players focused on healthy segments of the industry and with food portfolios that are focused on the health side.

Similar conclusions were reached by UBS Warburg (2002). Both reports point to the potential to promote and advertise the 'not so healthy + healthy' foods' category as opposed to the current emphasis on unhealthy foods. This may well involve public–private partnerships between the food industry and public health nutrition (Ollila, 2003).

The WHO/FAO (2003) report on chronic diseases reported consistent strong relationships between television viewing and obesity in children and that this may relate to the food advertising to which they are exposed (see also Taras and Gage, 1995; Lewis and Hill, 1998). Children are increasingly becoming consumers both directly and indirectly, responsible for stocking the family shelves and influencing purchases through 'pester power' as well as being consumers with their own buying power and access to money (Lindstrom with Seybold, 2003). In an international study across seven countries, Lindstrom with Seybold showed that children are increasingly becoming consumers in their own right as well as influencing household purchases. This introduces a debate as to the extent that young children should be protected or allowed to partake as consumers and be subject to advertising without constraints. Descriptive research on the type of foods promoted in countries across the globe consistently shows that, for children, food products are the most heavily advertised, followed by toys. Food types can be classified under five categories (Lewis and Hill, 1998):

1. Cereals (i.e. breakfast).
2. Snacks, sweet.
3. Snacks, savoury.

4. Convenience foods.
5. Fast-food outlets.

These five categories display a bias towards unhealthy energy-dense foods. In most national food pyramids or dietary guidelines, snack and convenience foods and carbonated/sugary beverages are classified under the 'eat least' heading, yet these are the foods most likely to receive most air time and spend on television advertising. In the year 2000, £596 million was spent on advertising food in the UK, with another £284 million on drinks; this was part of the total of £17,000 million spent on advertising (Advertising Association, 2001). Of this a disproportionate amount went on snacks, sweets and fatty foods. In 1994, according to Consumers International (1996), 15% of all food advertising in the UK went on chocolate confectionery, while only 0.5% was spent on promoting fresh fruit, vegetables and nuts. The groups of children most likely to be exposed to advertisements from the five categories are those from low-income groups, resulting in a double jeopardy effect of not having enough resources to buy food and feeling culturally isolated because of this lack of purchasing power.

Figure 12.2 shows an inverse relationship between the foods recommended and their exposure during children's television. On the left is a food pyramid showing recommended proportions of food groups in a child's diet and on the right actual advertising content. The shaded area in the figure represents the fatty and sugary foods that should be 'eaten sparingly' (Coalition on Food Advertising to Children, 2003; Dalmeny *et al.*, 2003). Television

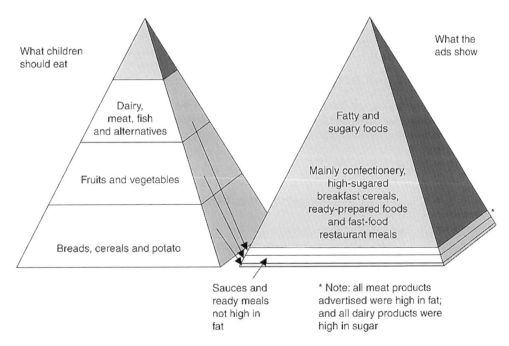

Fig. 12.2. The 'food pyramid' guide showing recommended proportions of food groups for a healthy diet and actual advertising content. (Adapted from Dalmeny *et al.*, 2003.)

advertising portrays a distorted picture of what children should be eating in only small amounts and infrequently. The fact that such messages are repeated day after day helps contribute to the impression that this is the norm, particularly when there are so few advertisements painting a picture of healthy eating.

The industry views are best summarized by Young (2003a) who, in a report that reviews the international research literature assessing the role of advertising in children's food choices, says that food advertising:

> does not dictate children's dietary patterns but it does have a role to play in food choice at the level of the brand. In addition, television programming offers a generous range of images about food and can shape food choices. Healthy and unhealthy eating with different kinds of foods are represented in all media in a host of different ways.

> (p. 1)

But, as we saw above, a range of foods and healthy and unhealthy eating practices are not represented in the advertising of food to children.

Incorporated Society of British Advertisers (2002), in speaking for the advertising industry in the UK, warned of the move to restrict advertising to children across Europe. They saw the danger of any restrictions as the first step in achieving widespread bans. They rest their case against restrictions on the following three principles:

1. The contention that, from an early age, children understand the role of advertising and that they have a right to access information and should not be artificially cut off from what is an important part of modern life.
2. Across the EU, advertisers respect children and existing laws and self-regulatory codes already afford protection for children.
3. Restrictions on television advertising to children would inevitably result in impoverishment of the quality and quantity of children's television programming.

Similar sentiments were expressed by Kerry Foods, a leading producer of dairy products in the UK and Irish markets, who said in their submission to the Broadcasting Commission of Ireland consultation on a children's advertising code that:

> As a brand leader in Childrens' [sic] cheese snacking we in Kerry Foods conduct childrens consumer research on a regular basis. The children can be as young as 6. In our experience advertising plays a key communication role in this category for both parties once respected and codes adhered to. Children have a general appreciation for advertising and its usage. They have the ability and necessary language to make their own judgement while understanding the objective of each 'manufacturer'; to deliver awareness, and provide product information. It is a relevant tool for both groups manufacturers and children.

> (Quoted in Quinn, 2004, p. 13)

Such views have become largely untenable as the formal evidence points to the fact that young children do find it difficult to distinguish between advertising and programme content (American Academy of Pediatrics, 1995; Jarlbro, 2001). Young (2003b, p. 4) says that:

there is no evidence that children under 5 years of age *see* advertising as anything but entertainment. Generally, an adequate understanding of advertising among children emerges by the age of 8 but some children do not apply this understanding until they are 12 years of age.

However, he sees this lack of differentiation as a positive aspect and from this argues that children's advertising does not need regulation as they do not understand its function.

The Swedish legislation does not deal with the debates over good/bad foods or appropriate/inappropriate toys; it sets a standard of no television advertising for children as a matter of fair play and based on the rights of the child. The 1994 Swedish report *Children and Television Advertising* by Bjurström (1994) was updated by Jarlbro in 2001, and both noted the widespread support among the Swedish public and the government for the policy on television advertising. In Sweden the findings from surveys are used as evidence that the Swedish public supports the current ban on advertising. This is an example of the needs/wants of the public being used to justify the continuation of an existing policy. It is also a clear demonstration of the importance of social context, with both Norway and Sweden operating controls on advertising aimed at children based on their welfare state provision (Cochrane and Clark, 1997).

Governments often adopt a formal approach to policy development based on the demonstration of malevolence or harm. This is in contrast to a more preventive approach using the precautionary principle, which is based on the principle of avoiding future harm to public health by careful forward planning (Raffensperger and Tickner, 1999). The Chief Medical Officer for England, Sir Liam Donaldson, in his annual report for 2002 argued for the application of the precautionary principle to the advertising of foods to children (Department of Health, 2003). He said:

> There is a case for adopting the precautionary principle for the marketing of foods to children. Industry should be asked to take a more responsible approach to the promotion (especially to children) of foods high in fat, salt and added sugars and balance this with the promotion of healthier options, including fruit and vegetables.
>
> (Department of Health, 2003)

The adoption of the precautionary principle could shift the balance for the development of policy from one of having to demonstrate harm beyond reasonable doubt to one based on probable threats from a foodstuff or the promotion of a message about a foodstuff.

The weighting of evidence is still based on the demonstration of harm. Currently there appears to be little drive from national governments or within the EU to seek changes in the regulation of advertising aimed at children. Within the European legislative frameworks, there also exists the potential to use and link the Television Without Frontiers Directive (European Commission Directorate-General Education and Culture, 1997) with Article 152 of the Amsterdam Treaty (European Commission, 1999), which calls for the EU to examine the possible impact of all major policies on public health.

The evidence that the heavy marketing of energy-dense foods and beverages to young children causes obesity is not unequivocal but is strong enough for the WHO/FAO (2003) report to say that the existing evidence is sufficient to warrant advertising targeted at children 'being placed in the "probable" category and thus becoming a potential target for interventions'. Young children are a prime target group for the advertising of these products because they have a significant influence on the foods bought by parents and are also increasingly consumers in their own right (Office for National Statistics, 1997; Borzekowski and Robinson, 2001). In the UK there is ample evidence that young people are increasingly spending more of their own money on food outside the home and thus outside the direct influence of parents. Both Lindstrom with Seybold (2003) and Quart (2003) report the increased direct spending power of young children and state that the threshold age is lowering for young people with disposable incomes. National Statistics in 2002 reported that children aged 7–15 years in the UK spent, on average, £12.30 per week. The single largest expenditure was on food and non-alcoholic drinks, 35% for boys and 30% for girls, accounting for over £4 of spending on food per week.

In a report commissioned by the UK Food Standards Authority, Hastings et al. (2003) systematically reviewed 122 studies that examined the effects of food promotion (i.e. food marketing) on children's food knowledge, preferences and behaviour. It concluded that: 'food promotion is having an effect, particularly on children's food preferences, purchase behaviour and consumption. This effect is independent of other factors and operates at both a brand and category level.' A summary of the findings of this review can be seen in Box 12.1.

Another argument used by the food and advertising industries is that the impact of pester power on food choice is exaggerated. A study often quoted by those promoting the view that advertising is a benign process comes from research on attitudes in Spain and Sweden by NOP Solutions for the Children's Programme (1999): both Spanish and Swedish (7% versus 9%) adults ranked pestering as the least problematic, despite children's television advertising being banned in Sweden. Restricting any measure of the impact of advertising to whether or not parents are aware of pester power ignores the wider implications of food advertising. The very term 'pester power' brings to mind images of direct action, with children pestering parents at the checkout, whereas Lindstrom with Seybold (2003) note the power that children possess is to influence, often exercised indirectly and in unspoken terms. Lindstrom's portrayal shows that teenagers globally have a wide range of influences on household purchases and the term 'pester power' is too narrow to adequately describe this process (Lindstrom with Seybold, 2003). Dixon and Banwell (2004) note that this debate needs to be informed by the changing role and place of the modern child in the family structure, whom they claim is metaphorically taking over the role of head-of-table position previously occupied by the 'father figure' based on a patriarchal system of control over food choice (see Beardsworth and Keil, 1997, pp. 77–83; Coveney, 1999; Atkins and Bowler, 2001). This is not to say that advertising has no role or is not important, but that there is a complex interplay of issues and that in the modern family influence and decisions about food are a result of a complex interplay of taste, preferences, convenience and the demands of modern

---

Box 12.1. Key findings from Hastings *et al.* (2003).

Advertising influences preferences
Reasonably strong evidence that food promotion influences children's food preferences, including evidence from three good quality experimental studies that children were significantly more likely to prefer high fat, salt or sugar foods over lower fat, salt or sugar alternatives following exposure to advertisements.

Advertising influences purchases
Strong evidence that food promotion influences children's food purchase-related behaviour, including increased requests for foods high in fat, sugar or salt. One study showed a significant association between children's exposure to television advertising and greater household purchase of advertised cereals. Two studies showed that exposure to television advertising increased pestering generally and in relation to advertised products.

Advertising influences consumption
Modest evidence of an effect of food promotion on children's consumption behaviour. Television viewing affects diet.

Advertising increases category sales
Some evidence that food promotion impacts on brand and category preferences (i.e. the effects of food promotion are not limited to brand switching and, therefore, potentially affect total category sales).

---

life, of which advertising is one. Another important dimension that is often lost is the secondary influence of advertising via peers and siblings. The advertising industry often quotes opinion polls which show advertising is less influential on children than on parents and older siblings, knowing that these groups see the advertising and influence younger children's behaviour too.

Discussion and Conclusion

The WHO/FAO (2003) report identifies the fast-food industry and the role of advertising as key components in the rise of obesity and sees the parameters for a dialogue with the food industries as: less saturated fat; more fruits and vegetables; effective food labelling; and incentives for the marketing and production of healthier products. The response from certain sections of the food industry to the WHO/FAO report was to respond with threats; for example, the sugar lobby in the USA threatened to 'scupper WHO' by lobbying for an end to US government funding (Boseley, 2003) and internationally by claiming that the report 'is scientifically deficient and therefore cannot be a basis for a global strategy on diet and physical health' (International Sugar Organization, 2004, p. 1). The power of the food industry and associated marketing industry is of crucial importance for public health nutrition and food policy and the role of advertising (Nestle, 1993, 2002; Hirschhorn, 2002). Yet, the industry is worried about the various issues and has responded in a number of ways. Some examples include:

- Cadbury Schweppes claims to have stopped advertising directly to children (later amended to no advertising to children below 8 years of age).
- McDonalds has set up a Global Advisory Council on Healthy Lifestyles (McDonalds Corporation, 2003; also see www.csr.com) and has developed a new range of healthy eating options.
- Coca Cola claims a policy of not advertising to under-12s. They have also established the Beverage Institute for Health and Wellness (http://www.beverageinstitute.org/).

Such developments show the food industry can adapt to demands from both the consumer and public health lobbying. Allied to this is a realization that, in working with public health bodies to deliver food which is healthier, they are also reducing the likelihood of lawsuits and consequent threat to shareholder value. The food industry has not yet fully exploited the promotion of healthy foods through mass advertising. The reality is that advertising is a crude but powerful tool for those wishing to influence branded food choice; it depends on having the goods to market and being able to make them available at prices and places where the consumer can access them. In modern society the psychological processes underpinning advertising are based on creating needs and wants, as opposed to logical/information-based direct approaches. In the developed world where food is no longer, for the majority, an issue for day-to-day survival, we have moved from a situation where food satisfies the physiological appetite to one where it demonstrates more about our social appetite and our cultural identity. This is an aspect of advertising that many health professionals and agencies fail to grasp. The promise of healthy eating and the role that food choice plays in this is not clearly understood, this is even more so with children.

There is currently a danger that the role and impact of advertising will be reduced to a concern about the possible impact on obesity; important as this is, it misses the point and runs the danger of not tackling the main determinants of health and what Egger and Swinburn (1997) have called the obesogenic environment (see Fig. 12.3). Advertising is but one part of the marketing mix. The others include price and availability. The problem with attempts to advertise healthy foods, such as fruit and vegetables, is that the value added to the food is minimal once it leaves the farm gate, and thus there is not a large margin for advertising and marketing budgets. Processed food, on the other hand, attracts added value after it leaves the farm gate, thus leaving more for the advertising and marketing of that foodstuff. This is the economics of advertising; advertising budgets are in effect part of the cost of the food. One solution that has been suggested to remedy this is to tax advertising of unhealthy or processed foods (Brownell and Horgen, 2004; House of Commons Health Committee, 2004). From an industry perspective this would be an unpopular approach and would be subject to objections, lobbying and the shifting of budgets from direct advertising as on television to less visible and less controllable media.

In addition, in any move to restrict current advertising of unhealthy practices and food there is a need to balance images used in advertising so as not to create a situation which sets up a dichotomy between thinness and obesity. Stearns (2002) in his cross-cultural analysis of fat shows how the issue of fat and media

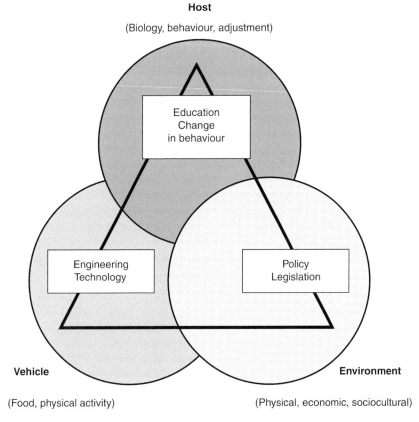

Fig. 12.3. The obesogenic environment. (Adapted from Egger and Swinburn, 1997.)

portrayals of obesity and slimness are culturally bound. Campaigns using advertising to promote health should not use 'thinness' as an ideal as this can be defined culturally and has an interpretative aspect – thinner than what or who?

Any proposed control and regulation of advertising aimed only at individual behaviour and responsibility, which are certainly key factors in the decision-making process, must also tackle the other parts of the obesogenic environment. This could include regulating the shopping environment, taxes on unhealthy foods and the development of new technologies to deliver health benefits.

The Strathclyde systematic review (Hastings *et al.*, 2003), for the first time, provides evidence for action limiting the impact of advertising directed to children on health grounds. Many health advocates wish for the power of advertising to be turned to the purpose of promoting healthy food without realizing the underlying processes informing advertising, such as the use of peripheral persuasion techniques, the absence of a clear product and the psychological process of asking for behavioural costs often without an immediate benefit. The Hastings report sets out the evidence for the impact on children's food choices; what it does not do and was not charged with doing was to set out the policy options from this evidence. Generally, regulation or statutory controls can take the following forms:

- A total ban on food advertising to children.
- A total ban on all advertising to children.
- More regulation based on some combination of the following quota systems: the times advertising is allowed; the amount of advertising to children by types/categories of food advertised; restrictions on the use of personalities to promote foodstuffs; and restrictions on the messages communicated.

A total ban would make operation and monitoring of the situation easy; restrictions or a partial ban would need to be clearly defined and standards for operation unambiguously set out. In most countries the first two approaches are likely to run into huge opposition; the latter approach, based on regulation, is more likely to be acceptable, although not without a battle. In respect of an outright ban, in the UK the Advertising Association warned that any attempt to ban food advertising on the basis that it could be harmful to children would be subject to appeal under the Human Rights Act as follows:

> Commercial freedom of speech is recognised and enshrined in the Human Rights Act (Article 10). Whilst there are derogations allowed for the protection of public health, for example, the panel is unable to offer any evidence that brand advertising of particular products impacts on dietary choice and thus on health, nor does any evidence exist that such advertising has long-term health implications for children or adults. Thus any proposal to ban or further restrict advertising of particular categories of food would be a de facto infringement of commercial freedom of speech and would face immediate challenge.
>
> (Advertising Association, 2000)

An approach based on regulation of advertising (whether enforced through legislation or voluntary agreements) is likely to be hard to monitor. For example, what is to stop fast-food restaurants advertising its healthy options such as fruit-and-vegetable bags and organic milk? They could still promote their brand and image to attract customers and then influence choice on the premises by comparative pricing. The way in which restrictions are applied across Europe differs, as does the age range for defining a child: below 12 years of age in Sweden to up to 18 years of age in Ireland.

The advertising industry uses the example of Sweden to demonstrate that an outright ban on food advertising is ineffective in terms of halting an increase in obesity, while health advocates point to it as an example of good policy making. There are two responses to this. First, as noted earlier, the original ban was not premised on stemming obesity or even on healthy eating but on a human rights standpoint, the rights of the child and the role of the state in protecting them from undue influences. Second, satellite television broadcasts in Swedish from the UK to Sweden, subject to UK regulations, bring commercial television with advertisements to children, so more and more Swedish children are subject to direct food advertising. The Swedish example shows that children are and have always been subject to the wider influences of marketing and the global economy, and regulatory frameworks make it harder for national governments to legislate just for their populations (Catford, 1995). The regulation of television advertising may force marketers to find other ways of getting their message across and some of these new media will be harder to regulate than television.

In recent years the Swedish ban of advertising on television to children has lost some of its strength. The Swedish Consumer Ombudsman has lost several cases in the Swedish Market Court dealing with marketing on television to children below 12 years of age. In two of the cases the advertisements were for foods (ice cream and breakfast cereal with high sugar content). The Market Court argued that if the product in question can be eaten by adults as well or if the programme the advertisements are shown in connection with can be regarded as targeting the whole family, then the advertisement cannot be considered aimed at children. The practice in the court decisions has shifted from previously focusing on the format of the advertisement (for example cartoons) to now focusing on the product itself (Filippa von Haartman, personal communication, Sweden, 2004).

Advertising is part of the bigger picture of marketing; it is a crude tool. In advertising there is an adage that only half of advertising spend is used efficiently but you cannot tell which half. For targeted campaigns television and other forms of advertising may not be the most appropriate means; using text messages on mobile phones or email marketing approaches means that you can target specifically and even personalize the message. The majority of current food advertising promises immediate returns; in the case of fast foods or energy-dense foods, the immediate pay-offs can be psychological, social or olfactory. Eating in a fast-food restaurant with your friends meets an immediate demand for sociability – the food may not be of gourmet quality standard but you get consistency (a Big Mac is a Big Mac), value for money, a strong tasting food and a feeling of satiation (Ritzer, 2000). In promoting fast-food restaurants, the message in advertisements is not focused on the food but on the peripheral aspects of eating there such as convenience, conviviality and value for money. Health messages in advertising promising a healthy future are not using the psychological impacts of advertising to best advantage. In Summer 2004 McDonalds promoted a healthier option menu and a £1 million healthy eating television advertising campaign aimed at children using cartoon characters called the Yum Chums to get the message across that it's fun when you eat right and be active. They call this 'edutainment'. Whether this remains a long-term viable strategy remains to be seen, but shows the conflation of advertising and education.

Debates over what is the prime influence on children's eating habits miss the policy implementation point: that of making policy that can have maximum impact. So while arguing that there is a case for the regulation of food advertising and particularly that directed at children, those who advocate such an approach are not saying that advertising is the most important determinant of food choice and behaviour, but that from a policy perspective this it is the one most easily regulated and likely to deliver results. Regulation of advertising may not be the most effective way to promote healthy eating but it may be the most efficient policy direction at a population level. Those who argue for the importance of structural factors, such as restrictions on advertising, are not saying that they are more or less important than other issues such as personal responsibility, but that they are more efficient in terms of their impact than policy initiatives to promote family responsibility. How do you support or encourage the adoption of positive behaviours in the domestic sphere? The answer is: not very easily; and from a policy perspective it is not the most efficient approach.

To our minds there is a case for the regulation of advertising directed at children. This is based on the following:

- The role of the state in promoting and protecting public health.
- The demonstrated impact of advertising on food choice.
- Psychologically that advertising has been shown to play an important part in determining the food choice and preferences of young children and adolescents.

Future debates will inevitably have to take account of the new media, their impact on food choice and their regulation. The debates will continue to rage over the magnitude of the impact of advertising on food choice, with the food and advertising industries continuing to defend a largely untenable position as the evidence points to the impact of advertising on food choice and which in common-sense terms is demonstrated every time a massive new advertising campaign is mounted to launch a new product range, e.g. cereal bars as breakfast alternatives. There is a need in the future to use econometric data and surveys to track the impact on food advertising on food behaviour.

References

Advertising Association (2000) *Position of the Advertising Association as contained in 'A submission to the Food Chain and Crops for Industry panel's consultation paper: Food's Contribution to Health in the Future' – The Foresight Programme.* Advertising Association, London.

Advertising Association (2001) *Student Briefing No. 6.* Advertising Association, London.

American Academy of Pediatrics (1995) Committee on Communications. Policy statement: children, adolescents, and advertising. *Pediatrics* 95, 295–297.

Atkins, P. and Bowler, I. (2001) *Food in Society: Economy, Culture, Geography.* Arnold, London.

Beardsworth, A. and Keil, T. (1997) *Sociology on the Menu.* Routledge, London.

Bjurström, E. (1994) *Children and Television Advertising, A Critical Study of International Research Concerning the Effects of TV Commercials on Children.* Report 1994/95:8. Swedish Consumer Agency, Stockholm.

Borzekowski, D.L. and Robinson, T.N. (2001) The 30-second effect: an experiment revealing the impact of television commercials on food preferences of preschoolers. *Journal of the American Dietetic Association* 101, 42–46.

Boseley, S. (2003) Sugar industry threatens to scupper WHO. *Guardian,* Monday 21 April, pp. 1–2.

Brownell, K.D. and Horgen, K.B. (2004) *Food Fight: The Inside Story of the Food Industry, America's Obesity Crisis, and What We Can Do About It.* McGraw-Hill, New York.

Caraher, M. and Baker, H. (2001) Designing an information leaflet: using consumer-oriented research to inform the development of a drug resource for children. *Drugs: Education, Prevention and Policy* 8, 243–260.

Caraher, M., Cowburn, G. and Currie, E. (2003) *Food in School: The Evidence: A Report to the Food in Schools Initiative, Department of Health*. Department of Health Management and Food Policy, City University, London.

Catford, J. (1995) The mass media is dead: long live the multimedia. *Health Promotion International* 10, 247–251.

Chapman, G. and MacLean, H. (1993) 'Junk food' and 'healthy food': meanings of food in adolescent women's culture. *Journal of Nutrition Education* 25, 108–113.

Coalition on Food Advertising to Children (2003) *Children's Health or Children's Wealth: The Case for Banning Food Advertising to Children*. Coalition on Food Advertising to Children, Flinders University, Adelaide, South Australia, Australia.

Cochrane, A. and Clarke, J. (1997) *Comparing Welfare States*. Open University and Sage, Milton Keynes, UK.

Conner, M. and Armitage, C.J. (2002) *The Social Psychology of Food*. Open University Press, Buckingham, UK.

Consumers International (1996) *Safe Food for All, The Consumer Agenda*. Consumers International, London.

Coveney, J. (1999) The government of the table: nutrition expertise and the social organisation of family habits. In: Germov, J. and Williams, L. (eds) *A Sociology of Food and Nutrition: The Social Appetite*. Oxford University Press, Melbourne, Victoria, Australia, pp. 259–276.

Dalmeny, K., Hanna, E. and Lobstein, T. (2003) *Broadcasting Bad Health: Why Food Marketing to Children Needs to be Controlled*. A Report by the International Association of Consumer Food Organizations for the World Health Organization Consultation on a Global Strategy for Diet and Health. The International Association of Consumer Food Organizations, London.

De Mooij, M. (1998) *Global Marketing and Advertising: Understanding Cultural Paradoxes*. Sage, London.

Department of Health (2003) *Health Check on the State of the Public Health*. Annual Report of the Chief Medical Officer 2002. Department of Health, London.

Dixon, J. and Banwell, C. (2004) Heading the table: parenting and the junior consumer. *British Food Journal* 106, 181–193.

Egger, G. and Swinburn, B. (1997) An 'ecological' approach to the obesity pandemic. *British Medical Journal* 315, 477–480.

Egger, G., Spark, R., Lawson, J. and Donovan, R. (1999) *Health Promotion Strategies and Methods*. McGraw-Hill, Sydney, New South Wales, Australia.

European Commission (1999) *Fourth Report on the Integration of Health Protection Requirements in Community Policies* (V/1999/408-EN). European Commission, Brussels.

European Commission Directorate-General Education and Culture (1997) *Television Without Frontiers Directive* (89/552/EEC, amended 1997 97/36/EC). European Commission, Brussels.

Fine, B., Heasman, M. and Wright, J. (1996) *Consumption in the Age of Affluence*. Routledge, London.

Garfield, S. (1994) *The End of Innocence: Britain in the Time of AIDS*. Faber and Faber, London, pp. 106–133.

Hastings, G., Stead, M., McDermott, L., Forsyth, A., MacKintosh, A., Rayner, M., Godfrey, C., Caraher, M. and Angus, K. (2003) *Review of the Research on the Effects of Food Promotion to Children, 2003*. Centre for Social Marketing, Glasgow, UK.

Hirschhorn, M.D. (2002) *How the Tobacco and Food Industries and Their Allies Tried to Exert Undue Influence over FAO/WHO Food and Nutrition Policies*. World Health Organization, Geneva, Switzerland.

Horne, P.J., Lowe, C.F., Bowdrey, M. and Egerton, C. (1998) The way to healthy eating for children. *British Food Journal* 100, 133–140.

House of Commons Health Committee (2004) *Obesity: Third Report of Session 2003–04*. The Stationery Office, London.

Ind, N. (1993) *Great Advertising Campaigns. How They Achieve Both Creative and Business Objectives*. Kogan Page, London.

International Sugar Organization (2004) *Memo (04)05 17 February Joint WHO/FAO Technical Report 916 on: 'Diet Nutrition and the Prevention of Chronic Diseases'*. International Sugar Organization, London.

ISBA (2002) *Briefing Paper Issue: Advertising and Children*. ISBA, London.

Jarlbro, G. (2001) *Children and Television Advertising. The Players, the Arguments and the Research during the Period 1994–2000*. Swedish Consumer Agency, Stockholm.

Jones, J.P. (1998) *How Advertising Works: The Role of Research*. Sage, London.

JP Morgan (2003) *Food Manufacturing: Obesity the Big Issue*. JP Morgan European Equity Research, London.

JP Morgan (2006) *Re-shaping the Food Industry*. JP Morgan European Equity Research, London.

Kotler, P., Roberto, N. and Lee, N. (2002) *Social Marketing: Improving the Quality of Life*, 2nd edn. Sage, Thousand Oaks, California.

Lewis, M.K. and Hill, A.J. (1998) Food advertising on British children's television: a content analysis and experimental study with nine-year olds. *International Journal of Obesity and Related Metabolic Disorders* 22, 206–214.

Lindstrom, M. with Seybold, P. (2003) *BRANDchild*. Kogan Page, London.

McDonalds Corporation (2003) *McDonald's Announces Members of Global Advisory Council on Healthy Lifestyles*. Press release, www.csr.wire.com (accessed 16 June 2003).

National Statistics (2002) *Special Focus: Children*. National Statistics, London.

Nestle, M. (1993) Food lobbies, the food pyramid and US nutrition policy. *International Journal of Health Services* 23, 483–496.

Nestle, M. (2002) *Food Politics: How the Food Industry Influences Nutrition and Health*. California State University Press, Berkeley, California.

NOP Solutions for the Children's Programme (1999) *Pester Power: A Report on Attitudes in Spain and Sweden*. NOP Solutions, London.

Office for National Statistics (1997) *Children's Spending 1995–96*. Office for National Statistics, London.

Ollila, E. (2003) *Global Health-Related Public Private Partnerships and the United Nations*. Globalism and Social Policy Programme website, www.gasp.org (accessed 11 June 2004).

Quart, A. (2003) *Branded*. Arrow, London.

Quinn, R.-B.M. (2004) *Children's Advertising Code: Phase Two Consultation Document Review of Adult Submissions Received*. Broadcasting Commission of Ireland, Dublin.

Raffensperger, C. and Tickner, J. (1999) *Protecting Public Health and the Environment: Implementing the Precautionary Principle*. Island Press, Washington, DC.

Ritzer, G. (2000) *The McDonaldization of Society*, new century edn. Pine Forge Press, Thousand Oaks, California.

Robinson, T.N. (1998) Does television cause childhood obesity? *Journal of the American Medical Association* 279, 959–960.

Stearns, P.N. (2002) *Fat History: Bodies and Beauty in the Modern World*. New York University Press, New York.

Taras, H.L. and Gage, M. (1995) Advertised foods on children's television. *Archives of Pediatrics and Adolescent Medicine* 149, 649–652.

UBS Warburg (2002) *Global Equity Research: Absolute Risk of Obesity*. UBS Warburg, London.

Vaughan, R. (1980) How advertising works: a planning model. *Journal of Advertising Research* 20, 27–33.

World Health Organization (2004) *Marketing Food to Children: The Global Regulatory Environment*. World Health Organization, Geneva, Switzerland.

World Health Organization/Food and Agriculture Organization (2003) *Diet, Nutrition and The Prevention of Chronic Diseases*. Technical Report Series No. 916. World Health Organization, Geneva, Switzerland.

Young, B. (2003a) *Advertising and Food Choice in Children: A Review of the Literature*. School of Psychology, The University of Exeter, Exeter, UK.

Young, B. (2003b) *Advertising and Food Choice in Children: A Review of the Literature. Summary*. School of Psychology, The University of Exeter, Exeter, UK.

This page intentionally left blank

13 Adolescents, Food Choice and Vegetarianism

KAREN TREW,[1] CHRISTINA CLARK,[2]
GLENDA MCCARTNEY,[1] JULIE BARNETT[2] AND
ORLA MULDOON[1]

[1]School of Psychology, Queen's University of Belfast, Belfast BT7 1NN, UK;
[2]School of Psychology, University of Surrey, Guildford GU2 7XH, UK

Introduction

Adolescence (ages 11 to 21 years) is one of the greatest periods of growth throughout the lifespan. It is characterized by dramatic hormonal and physical changes (Spear and Kulbok, 2001), as well as major changes in cognitive processes (Byrnes, 2003) and social roles and relationships. For most young people, early adolescence is marked by an accelerated rate of increase in height and weight associated with puberty (Coleman and Hendry, 2000).

Multiple individual, social, physical, environmental and macrosystem factors have been identified as important for the food choices of adolescents. Some of these influences, such as hunger and taste, impact on food choice throughout the lifespan. Other influences, such as rapid physical growth, are developmental factors uniquely associated with being an adolescent (Neumark-Sztainer et al., 1999; Story et al., 2002; Livingstone and Helsper, 2004). However, as Cusatis and Shannon (1996, p. 27) noted, 'while much has been written about aberrant adolescent nutrition practices (such as eating disorders), relatively little study has been devoted to factors that influence more typical eating behaviour across the general adolescent population'. Traditionally, the few studies that have been carried out in this area were limited in the set of predictor variables assessed (such as demographic variables; Anderson et al., 1994) or in the set of outcome measures (e.g. calcium intake; Harel et al., 1998).

The quality of the adolescent diet in the Western world has become of increasing concern to researchers and health professionals. Obesity in adolescents has reached epidemic proportions (e.g. Irving and Neumark-Sztainer, 2002; British Medical Association, 2003). Obesity rates have doubled in the UK and the USA over the last 20 years (British Medical Association, 2003) and obesity is considered to be the most common childhood disorder in Europe (International Obesity Task Force and European Association for Obesity, 2002).

The increase in the prevalence of obesity in adolescence has been linked with both the increased consumption of obesogenic foods and a decrease in physical activity amongst young people, especially girls, in the period of adolescence (e.g. Gregory *et al.*, 2000; British Medical Association, 2003). Obesity in adolescence has been found to persist into adulthood with consequences for long-term health (Story *et al.*, 2002; Mulvihill *et al.*, 2004).

It is generally accepted that dietary habits established during childhood and adolescence tend to be carried into adulthood and are difficult to alter (Coulson *et al.*, 1998; Hill *et al.*, 1998). For instance, early exposure to fruit and vegetables or to foods high in energy, sugar and fat has been related to adolescents' liking for, and consumption of, these foods (Hill *et al.*, 1998), a dietary practice that may continue into adulthood (Lien *et al.*, 2001). As Vereecken *et al.* (2004) noted, the World Health Organization recognizes that 'young people who develop healthy eating habits early in life are more likely to maintain them in maturity and to have reduced risk of chronic diseases, cancer, non-insulin dependent diabetes mellitus and osteoporosis' (p. 110).

An increase in energy intake is required to sustain the rapid physical changes in adolescents. However, recent studies show that the dietary intakes of adolescents are often inadequate when compared to national guidelines (Story *et al.*, 2002). The World Health Organization's 2001/2002 survey of Heath Behaviour in School-aged Children (HBSC) in 35 countries and regions found that fruit and vegetable consumption was relatively low with only about 30% of the young people eating fruit every day while a similar proportion drink sugared soft drinks every day in many countries and regions (Vereecken *et al.*, 2004). There is also evidence that adolescents' diets are low in dietary fibre, iron, calcium and other micronutrients (e.g. Gallagher, 2000; British Medical Association, 2003).

Theoretical Frameworks for Understanding Adolescents' Food Choices

The growing evidence of the importance of young people's dietary choices for the short- and long-term health and well-being of the population has been recognized by a range of international and national initiatives designed to promote healthy eating (British Medical Association, 2003). Many of these interventions have had limited impact. For example, Vereecken *et al.* (2004) note that the HSBC surveys found relatively low levels of fruit and vegetable consumption despite the efforts in many countries to promote fruit and vegetable consumption among children over the last decade. Story *et al.* (2002) suggest that the development of effective strategies for improving the dietary behaviour of young people requires an understanding of the multiple factors that impact on these behaviours.

The theory of planned behaviour (Ajzen and Madden, 1986) has been used by psychologists to establish the individual determinants of dietary behaviour in adult and adolescent populations (e.g. Newell *et al.*, 1990; Shannon *et al.*, 1990). However, studies derived from this model have found that determinants such as attitudes, subjective norms and self-efficacy show a stronger association with what individuals think they eat than with what they actually eat (Lechner *et al.*, 1998; de Bourdeaudhuij and van Oost, 2000). Recently, reviews of the research literature (e.g. Story *et al.*, 2002; Livingstone and Helsper, 2004) have adopted more complex theoretical frameworks of eating behaviour that take account of multiple factors that operate on multiple levels of influence. Story *et al.* (2002) built on social cognitive theory (Bandura, 1986) and Bronfenbrenner's (1979) ecological perspective in proposing an integrated composite theoretical model of factors that influence adolescents' eating behaviour. This framework has subsequently been endorsed by a range of researchers investigating diet in relation to the health of adolescents (e.g. British Medical Association, 2003; Vereecken *et al.*, 2004). In this model four general levels of influence are described:

- *Individual or intrapersonal influences* including biological factors (e.g. hunger), psychosocial influences (e.g. attitudes, beliefs, knowledge, self-efficacy, taste and food preferences), behavioural influences (e.g. meal and snack patterns and weight-control behaviours) and life-style factors (e.g. perceived barriers such as cost, time demands, convenience).
- *Social environmental or intrapersonal influences* from family, friends and peers, which may impact on food choice and dietary behaviours through modelling, reinforcement, social support and perceived norms.
- *Physical environmental influences*, which determine accessibility and availability of foods such as the range of school meals or the location of fast-food outlets that can impact on adolescents' food choices.
- *Macrosystem or societal influences*, which play a more distal and indirect role in determining eating behaviours, and include mass media and advertising, social and cultural norms of eating, food production and distribution systems, and policies and laws that regulate food-related issues, such as pricing.

Following a detailed review of the research on the impact of food advertising on children and young people's food choice which extended the work of Story *et al.* (2002), Livingstone and Helsper (2004) concluded that 'it is too simple to posit that the multiple factors each, separately, play a role in accounting for variation in food choice. Rather, we need to consider the possibility that these factors *interact* with each other, thereby *indirectly* affecting children's food choices' (p. 31). In their own work they explore the impact of advertising and television viewing and find that the weight of evidence suggests that television advertising has a modest direct effect on dietary choices, but they note that this finding must be viewed within the larger nexus of causality underlying children's food choice, health and obesity effects. For example, the young person's exposure to advertising is related to factors such as the sedentary nature of television viewing and its association with frequent snacking as well as the wide range of background and family factors included in Story *et al.*'s (2002) multifactorial model.

This chapter aims to complement the previous reviews in its focus on the determinants of adolescents' food choices. It builds on the work of Story *et al.* (2002) and selectively reviews psychological studies that have explored individual and social influences on food choices. In reviewing the literature, gender and the importance of weight control for adolescent girls emerged as pivotal factors in food choices (Wardle *et al.*, 2004). Gender differences are also notable in the account of teenage vegetarianism, which is included in this chapter to illustrate the further complexities involved in determining the influences on food choice.

Individual Determinants of Adolescents' Food Choices

Surveys find that adolescents have good knowledge about healthy eating practices. A meta-analysis of the literature on children, adolescents and adults found that nutrition knowledge and dietary behaviour were only weakly associated ($r = 0.10$; Axelson *et al.*, 1985). A similar lack of association has also been observed in recent studies (e.g. Brown *et al.*, 2000). For example, the majority of adolescents in a British Nutrition Foundation (Goldberg, 2003) survey claimed to like fruit and vegetables and to eat them often (52% of 11- to 13-year-olds and 55% of 13- to 16-year-olds). However, although fruit and vegetable consumption amongst these groups could be higher, both age groups showed a high awareness that they should be eating at least five portions of fruit and vegetables a day: of the 11–13-year-olds, 97% of girls and 84% of boys knew that they should eat this, whilst 97% of girls and 93% of boys in the 13–16 year age group were aware of this.

Research indicates that beliefs about food and weight may be more important than knowledge in altering food-related behaviours. For example, Nowak and Buettner (2003) found that the food intake of Australian adolescents was more related to their food beliefs and concerns than to their knowledge of nutritious food. Similarly, Story and Resnick (1986) found that despite being aware of the health consequences of eating food high in fat, sugar and salt, adolescents ate these foods because of their taste and convenience.

Self-reported food preferences or liking have been found to be one of the strongest predictors of adolescents' food choices, both in the UK (e.g. Shepherd and Dennison, 1996) and elsewhere (e.g. Woodward *et al.*, 1996). According to Birch (1999), food preferences are formed as a result of early childhood experiences with food, positive and negative conditioning, food exposure, and genetic predispositions (e.g. sensitivity to sour tastes). In turn, taste has emerged as the motivational factor with the greatest influence on food preference (e.g. Norton *et al.*, 2000). Focus groups of American adolescents have shown that adolescents rated taste and the appearance of food as primary factors that influenced their food selection (Neumark-Sztainer *et al.*, 1999). Adolescents also said that following a healthy diet was difficult because taste was very important to them, with 'junk' food tasting better than more healthy foods, such as vegetables. Similarly, American adolescents reported that taste, followed by hunger and price, were the most important factors in their choice of snacks from vending machines (French *et al.*, 1999).

In contrast, health and nutrition do not rank as important influences on food choice in adolescents (Story *et al.*, 2002). For example, Horacek and Betts (1998) found that only a quarter of American college students were motivated by health or weight when making dietary decisions. Research that compared the students motivated by health concerns with the majority of college students who were motivated by other factors (e.g. hunger) found those motivated by health concerns ate less fat and had higher nutrient intakes than their peers (Neumark-Sztainer et al., 1999). It seems that eating behaviours are related to other health-related behaviours amongst adolescents (Cusatis and Shannon, 1996). For example, Neumark-Sztainer et al. (1997) found that boys and girls who engaged in health-promoting behaviours, such as tooth-brushing, exercise and seat-belt use, were less likely to have unhealthy eating behaviours than those engaging in risk-taking activities, smoking and problematic school behaviours. In general, although adolescents are concerned about school, family and friends, they do not tend to worry about healthy eating. According to Neumark-Sztainer et al. (1999) and Story and Resnick (1986), adolescents tend to display a lack of urgency in responding to health-related dietary consequences. Indeed, other studies indicate that nutrition becomes more important with age (e.g. Glanz et al., 1998).

There has been little consistent evidence of associations between personality factors and dietary behaviour, but research on food choices in young children, and on attitudes in children and adults, has demonstrated the existence of individual differences in food neophobia (MacNicol et al., 2003). In a study of Scottish adolescents, MacNicol et al. (2003) found that a tendency to fussy/picky attitudes and high food neophobia, defined as an individual's unwillingness to try new food, was more common in girls than boys and associated with a lack of dietary knowledge, neuroticism, lower socioeconomic status and the consumption of unhealthy foods. However, it is unclear, from this cross-sectional study, whether food neophobia and pickiness should be regarded as causes or consequences of dietary behaviour. Further longitudinal research is required to establish the contribution of personal characteristics to individual differences in adolescents' food choices.

Social Determinants of Adolescents' Food Choices

Adolescence is associated with the need for peer acceptance, the search for identity and a growing independence and autonomy (Adams and Berzonsky, 2003). Although an increase in parent–adolescent conflict around puberty is so widely observed in Western cultures that it is assumed to be developmentally functional (Granic et al., 2003), most adolescents remain connected to their families and experience few long-term problems. Nevertheless, the major transitions of adolescence are thought to be vulnerable times that can contribute to the development of problems such as eating disorders for some young people (Polivy et al., 2003). One of the ways in which adolescents may express independence or rebellion is through eating less healthy foods or not eating as an act of parental defiance. According to Hill et al. (1992), some adolescents strive for nutritional autonomy and eat less healthy foods not because of their taste but as an act of parental defiance and peer solidarity.

Social independence, when linked with the greater purchasing power available to many young people for meals, snacks and drinks, has been associated with changes in dietary behaviour. Instead of relying solely on family foods, the adolescent's sources of food may also include food outlets, vending machines and school canteens. For example, the international HBSC study found that, in general, the percentage of young people who ate breakfast every morning dropped sharply with age, with average breakfast consumption dropping from 73% among 11-year-olds to 64% among 15-year-olds (Vereecken *et al.*, 2004). Barker *et al.* (2000) found that British adolescents who were socially independent (defined as going out in the evenings with friends, smoking and eating a meal with family infrequently) ate more crisps, snacks and chocolate, and drank more soft drinks, than their socially more dependent peers. They also ate fewer vegetables, less brown bread and breakfast cereals.

Peer influences through increased social activity also affect the food choices of adolescents (Cusatis and Shannon, 1996). It has been suggested that adolescents may be reluctant to eat healthily because of a fear of appearing weird or different from their friends (Brown *et al.*, 2000). However, Jas (1998) found that peer pressure did not seem to be an issue in 16-year-olds' choice of soft drinks. Although there is some disagreement over the influence of peer groups on adolescents' food choices (Dennison and Shepherd, 1995; Feunekes *et al.*, 1998), there is general agreement that family influence tends to have a positive effect on food choices in adolescence. Conformity to parents is positively predictive of dietary diversity and family meals are positively predictive of good fruit, vegetable and dairy intakes (de Bourdeaudhuij and van Oost, 2000; Videon and Manning, 2003). In a comparison of family and peer influences on adolescents' food choices, Woodward *et al.* (1996) found that family usage was a better predictor of food choice than friends' usage.

Parental use of food rules (both restrictions and obligations) in childhood appears to lead to less unhealthy food choices later in life, although not to more healthy choices. According to de Bourdeaudhuij (1997), there appears to be a distinction between positive healthy eating and negative healthy eating rules. The former are characterized by what one should eat (and eat more of) and the latter by what one should eat less of. These two concepts are not always presented together; unhealthy foods are used as rewards or withheld as punishments, creating confusion over the conceptualization of 'good' and 'bad' foods (Hill *et al.*, 1998).

Research indicates that adolescents' food preferences change depending on the environment in which they find themselves. In their study of adolescents in Northern Ireland, Brown *et al.* (2000) reported that the food preferences at home were different from those expressed in the school or social environments. Whilst adolescents' food preferences at home were for home-made meals, fast-food meals were the most popular preference for school meals and meals consumed in a social situation. Further, Croll *et al.* (2001) found that fast foods tend to be viewed as adolescent foods consumed away from home, while healthy foods were adult foods consumed at home. Equally, healthy foods were often characterized by adolescents as those they have to eat at home and unhealthy foods as those they were told they could not eat by their parents. Despite the school being reported as the main source of nutritional and food risk education, cafeteria food tended to be associated with high-fat and high-sugar foods (e.g. Cusatis and Shannon, 1996).

Research has shown significant differences in dietary behaviour according to socioeconomic status. For example, Wrieden (1996) found that children from higher socioeconomic backgrounds ate vegetables and potatoes (not chips) more frequently than children from less affluent backgrounds. Similarly, Warwick *et al.* (1999) and Inchley *et al.* (2001) found that children from lower socioeconomic backgrounds consumed more chips and less fruit/vegetables than children from more affluent groups. Overall, lower socioeconomic status is associated with both an increased tendency to skip breakfast more frequently and consume less healthy foods and a decreased tendency to consume more healthy foods (Sweeting *et al.*, 1994; Vereecken and Maes, 2000; MacNicol *et al.*, 2003).

Gender and Adolescents' Food Choices

Gender differences in food choice are widely reported (Wardle *et al.*, 2004). Haste (2004) noted that 'the goals of fitness and desirable weight are salient for both sexes but expressed in different ways. Girls and boys monitor their bodies differently, and they perceive themselves differently in relation to people the same age and sex as themselves' (p. 7). Wrieden (1996) found that boys consumed more chips, nuts, baked beans and orange juice than girls, whilst girls ate more apples and green vegetables than boys. Similarly, Vereecken *et al.* (2004) report that in nearly all of the 35 countries and regions included in the World Health Organization survey of eating habits, more girls than boys reported eating fruit and vegetables every day and more boys reported that they drink sugared soft drinks every day. In most countries and increasingly with age, more girls than boys reported missing breakfast. Although gender differences in sweet or chocolate consumption were negligible, Vereecken *et al.* (2004) suggest that the observed gender differences in eating patterns relate to girls' increased concerns about weight and shape rather than health.

Studies show that adolescents, especially females, are concerned about their body image (Wardle and Beales, 1986; Worsley and Skrzypiec, 1997). The unrealistic thin beauty ideal promoted in the media is one of the primary influences associated with the cultural pressure for adolescent girls to be thinner than is required for good health (Morris and Katzman, 2003; Livingstone and Helsper, 2004). The emotional stress of the perceived pressure to enhance their body image is often associated with inappropriate dietary restrictions and poor nutritional choices. Preoccupation with body weight and diet is so common in adolescent girls that it is considered by some to be part of normal development (e.g. Cooper and Goodyer, 1997). Prevalence figures indicate that between 25% and 77% of adolescent girls report to be 'on a diet' (Hill *et al.*, 1992; Button *et al.*, 1996; Roberts *et al.*, 1999). In almost all studies of dieting in developing and developed countries, across age groups and economic groups, women and girls report more concerns about body weight and make more attempts at weight control than men and boys (Wardle *et al.*, 2004). Indeed, few boys report actual dieting (Vereecken and Maes, 2000).

Some studies suggest that 'dieting' is interpreted in different ways. Neumark-Sztainer and Story (1998) found that American adolescents viewed 'being on a diet' in a much broader way than health professionals. For example, in addition to 'eating less/cutting down', British adolescent girls (Roberts *et al.*, 2001) viewed dieting as being 'good for their health'. Similarly, adolescents sampled in a range of other studies associated dieting with eating healthy food (e.g. Lytle *et al.*, 1997; Neumark-Sztainer and Story, 1998; Nichter, 2003). Roberts *et al.* (2001) found that the most popular definition of healthy eating was 'increased fruit/vegetables/salads', a definition that was similar to how many girls perceived dieting. In this respect it is interesting to note that a number of surveys report that dieting adolescents have an increased consumption of food/vegetables and a lower consumption of less nutritious food items (e.g. Nowak, 1998; Vereecken and Maes, 2000; Lattimore and Halford, 2003).

In a recent review of dieting in adolescence, the Adolescent Health Committee of the Canadian Paediatric Society (2004) noted that 'the spectrum of behaviours captured by dieting represents a range from healthy to unhealthy. . . However, a significant percentage of teenagers, girls in particular, engage in unhealthy behaviours to control weight' (p. 487). Wardle *et al.* (2004) examined food choices in a large-scale study of university students in 23 countries to establish the contribution of dieting, as compared with a belief in healthy eating, to gender differences in food choices. In almost all of the countries, women were more likely than men to be dieting and to attach greater importance to healthy food choices. They were also more likely than men to avoid high-fat foods, to eat fruit and fibre, and limit intake of salt. Analysis indicated that for this well-educated group of young people, health beliefs and dieting status accounted for almost half of the gender differences in dietary behaviours. Wardle *et al.* (2004) concluded that their results were consistent with the view that part of the reason women generally make more healthy food choices than men is that health is a more important motivation to them, whereas men are less enthusiastic about the benefits of healthy eating.

Adolescents and Vegetarianism

Traditionally health, together with taste and ethics, were assumed to be the major reasons why young people choose to adopt a vegetarian diet (Haste, 2004). However, the growing body of research, which is reviewed below, reveals a far more complex picture.

According to the British Nutrition Foundation Survey (Goldberg, 2003) more girls (16.8% of 11–13-year-olds and 15% of 14–16-year-olds) than boys (11.5% of 11–13-year-olds and 10.5% of 14–16-year-olds) claimed to be vegetarian. However, there appear to be problems with how individuals defined vegetarianism. For example, studies indicate that teenage vegetarians do not eat red meat but eat chicken (e.g. Worsley and Skrzypiec, 1997), even to a greater degree than non-vegetarians. Haste (2004) in a recent survey of 687 British children and young people aged 11–21 years found that 9.5% of the sample could be categorized as vegetarian in the conventional definition of the term, as they were flesh-avoiders who excluded red meat in combination with fish and/or white meat from their diet. However, when flesh-avoiders were defined more generally to include those who excluded just red meat or fish, 39% of boys and half the girls were classified as flesh-avoiders.

Little is known about the reasons why adolescents adopt vegetarian diets. Using an ethnographic approach, Kenyon and Barker (1998) interviewed 30 teenage girls between the ages of 13 and 19 years (15 vegetarians and 15 non-vegetarians). They found that dissatisfaction with the killing of animals and similar ethical concerns were the predominant issues to arise from the interviews. Overall, they found that meat was a negative symbol for adolescent vegetarian girls. Similarly, dislike of meat and adverse effects of meat consumption were cited as reasons for avoiding animal products in studies of British (Santos and Booth, 1996; Haste, 2004), Australian (Worsley and Skrzypiec, 1998) and Swedish (Larsson *et al.*, 2003) adolescents.

Kenyon and Barker (1998) found that only a few adolescent interviewees (20%) made any references to meat being unhealthy or vegetarianism being a healthier diet. The finding that female vegetarian students did not evoke health reasons is also similar to that made by Santos and Booth (1996). In contrast, Haste (2004) noted that flesh-avoiders had a somewhat differing worldview than flesh-eaters, which reflected their awareness and sensitivity to health issues. Beardsworth and Bryman (2004) argue that motives behind meat avoidance are complex and suggest that there is 'an interweaving of ethical, health, gustatory and environmental factors' (p. 315).

There also seem to be more personal reasons for adopting a reduced meat diet. Meat avoidance in female adolescents has been linked to their perception of meat as a fattening food. For example, some of the girls favouring a meatless diet were concerned about being slim and tended to restrict their energy intake (Worsely and Skrzypiec, 1997). Indeed, some have attributed the popularity of vegetarianism amongst adolescent girls to their belief that it will help them to slim (Ryan, 1997). Research indicates that teenage vegetarians weigh less than non-vegetarian adolescents, which may reinforce this dietary pattern amongst young people (e.g. Hebbelnick *et al.*, 1999). Indeed, Perry *et al.* (2001) reported that teenage vegetarians were more weight- and body-conscious, dissatisfied with their bodies and involved in a variety of healthy and unhealthy weight-control behaviours than non-vegetarians. In particular, vegetarians more often reported having been told by their doctor that they had an eating disorder. Similarly, Klopp *et al.* (2003) reported that self-reported vegetarians were more likely to display disordered eating attitudes and behaviours than non-vegetarians. This finding, however, is not unequivocal. Exploring the link between vegetarianism and weight concerns in a sample of Swedish and Norwegian adolescents, Larsson *et al.* (2002) found no significant difference in weight preoccupation between vegetarians and non-vegetarians.

Research also indicates an urban/rural divide in the acceptance of adolescent vegetarianism. In a study of Norwegian adolescents and their attitudes towards meat, Kubberod *et al.* (2002) found that adolescents who were in regular contact with animals showed more relaxed attitudes towards animal production, showed no disgust reactions towards red meat or blood in meat, and justified the necessity of slaughtering animals for food.

Relatively little is known about the support or lack of support for vegetarian practices from close others. An American study of adolescents and their food choices showed that teenagers perceived parents to be one of the most influential factors on their food choices, and that they influenced it in a number of ways (Neumark-Sztainer et al., 1999). Indeed, Beardsworth and Keil (1992) reported that family and peers might facilitate or inhibit becoming a vegetarian. Regarding inhibitory influences, research indicates that parental opposition often suppressed inclinations towards vegetarianism and that vegetarian tendencies were dormant for a number of respondents until they reached a degree of independence from parental control. Similarly, Santos and Booth (1996) and Larsson et al. (2003) suggested that eating more vegetarian foods after moving away from home could possibly be the result of no longer being under the control of parents.

Regarding facilitating influences, in a study of Australian adolescents, Worsley and Skrzypiec (1997, 1998) found that support for vegetarian practices was high especially from mothers (50%) and classmates (30%). However, a third of teenage vegetarians reported that it was difficult to avoid eating meat at home, thus feeling pressured to eat meat despite their own wishes. Interestingly, male teenagers expected less support from their friends than from their female peers. Overall, vegetarian girls reported to know more people who were vegetarian but they did not have more vegetarian friends. Worsley and Skrzypiec (1997, 1998) also examined Australian adolescents' reasons for being or not being vegetarian. Weight loss, animal welfare, adverse effects of meat and pressure from others were offered as reasons for vegetarianism and liking meat too much, being pressured by others, such as peers or parents, to eat meat, believing vegetarianism to be unhealthy and not liking the alternatives were the most important reasons advanced for not being vegetarian.

The link between rebelliousness and vegetarianism has been explored only infrequently. It was argued earlier that adolescents adopt and maintain behaviours for a variety of reasons that are unique to their age group, such as to assert their independence, to rebel, or to establish an identity (Hill et al., 1992). Worsley and Skrzypiec (1997) argue that the label of 'vegetarian' represents a mixture of socially desirable goals about concerns for the environment and animal welfare and may symbolize an adolescent's differentiation from his/her family and mainstream society. Sims (1978) compared American vegetarians and non-vegetarians, and found that vegetarianism was linked to egalitarianism. Vegetarianism thus opposed social hierarchies and promotes equality between humans and between humans and animals. These antiestablishment leanings may appeal to adolescents who need to balance the need for self-expression with the needs of others and those of the wider community, which may be accompanied by rebellion against adult behavioural norms and social hierarchies. Similarly, rebelliousness was mentioned as one reason for avoiding animal food products in a British study of vegetarian students (Santos and Booth, 1996) and a Swedish study of vegan adolescents (Larsson et al., 2003).

Discussion and Conclusion

Adolescents' dietary behaviour has traditionally been viewed as a topic for social scientists studying problem behaviour and does not regularly feature in accounts of normal adolescent development (e.g. Coleman and Hendry, 2000). For example, a recent handbook of research on adolescence (Adams and Berzonsky, 2003) includes a chapter on eating disorders (Polivy *et al.*, 2003) but there is no reference to the growing body of research on normal dietary behaviour. This chapter suggests that the psychological literature on adolescent eating behaviour has practical as well as theoretical significance for those concerned with the health and development of children and young people. For example, the review of factors which have been found to influence adolescents' choice of a vegetarian diet should inform those concerned with the normal social changes that occur during adolescence as well as those specifically interested in the dietary behaviours of young people.

In terms of methodology, the evidence reviewed in this chapter shows that large-scale international quantitative surveys have been complemented by detailed qualitative studies but the cross-sectional nature of almost all of the work has limited the analysis of causality and directionality. Furthermore, most research is correlational, as would be expected for an emergent topic, but additional insight into cause-and-effect relationships requires experimental investigations that involve random allocation of participants and changes in dependent behaviour. For example, Freeman and Bunting (2003) provide an account of a randomized trial which tested the effectiveness of a child-to-child approach to promote healthier snacking in children using the innovative 'rubbish bag' method to record what the children actually ate during the school break, as well as the traditional attitude and knowledge scales.

The growing concern of governments and policy makers with the 'obesity epidemic' should help to provide funding to carry out the research that is required to empirically test models of adolescent eating behaviour and develop effective, empirically based programmes and strategies for the promotion of healthy eating and prevention of obesity. For example, in view of findings of the international HBSC survey on eating habits, Vereecken *et al.* (2004) commend the model proposed by Story *et al.* (2002) as an appropriate framework for developing interventions that would enable young people to 'receive consistent messages on healthy eating in multiple settings and from a variety of sources, including home, schools, health care settings, community organizations, the mass media and government agencies' (p. 118).

References

Adams, G.R. and Berzonsky, M.D. (2003) *Blackwell Handbook of Adolescence.* Blackwell, Oxford, UK.

Adolescent Health Committee, Canadian Paediatric Society (2004) Dieting in adolescence. *Paediatrics and Child Health* 9, 487–491.

Ajzen, I. and Madden, T.J. (1986) Prediction of goal-directed behaviour: attitudes, intentions and perceived behavioural control. *Journal of Experimental Social Psychology* 22, 453–474.

Anderson, A., MacIntyre, S. and West, P. (1994) Dietary patterns among adolescents in the west of Scotland. *British Journal of Nutrition* 71, 111–122.

Axelson, M.L., Federline, T. and Brinberg, D.A. (1985) A meta-analysis of food and nutrition-related research. *Journal of Nutrition Education* 17, 51–54.

Bandura, A. (1986) *Social Foundations of Thought and Action: A Social Cognitive Theory*. Prentice Hall, Englewood Cliffs, New Jersey.

Barker, M.E., Wilman, C. and Barker, D.J P. (2000) Behaviour, body composition and diet in adolescent girls. *Appetite* 35, 161–170.

Beardsworth, A.D. and Bryman, A.E. (2004) Meat consumption and meat avoidance among young people: an 11-year longitudinal study. *British Food Journal* 106, 313–327.

Beardsworth, A.D. and Keil, E.T. (1992) The vegetarian option: varieties, conversions, motives and careers. *Sociological Review* 40, 253–293.

Birch, L. (1999) Development of food preferences. *Annual Review of Nutrition* 19, 41–62.

British Medical Association (2003) *Adolescent Health*. British Medical Association, London.

Bronfenbrenner, U. (1979) *The Ecology of Human Development: Experiments by Nature and Design*. Harvard University Press, Cambridge, Massachusetts.

Brown, K., McIlveen, H. and Strugnell, C. (2000) Nutritional awareness and food preferences of young consumers. *Nutrition and Food Science* 30, 230–235.

Button, E.J., Sonuga-Barke, E.J.S., Davies, J. and Thompson, M. (1996) A prospective study of self-esteem in the prediction of eating problems in adolescent schoolgirls: questionnaire findings. *British Journal of Clinical Psychology* 35, 193–203.

Byrnes, J.P. (2003) Cognitive development during adolescence. In: Adams, G.R. and Berzonsky, M.D. (eds) *Blackwell Handbook of Adolescence*. Blackwell, Oxford, UK, pp. 227–246.

Coleman, J.C. and Hendry, L.B. (2000) *The Nature of Adolescence*. Routledge, London.

Cooper, P.J. and Goodyer, I. (1997) Prevalence and significance of weight and shape concerns in girls aged 11–16 years. *British Journal of Psychiatry* 171, 542–544.

Coulson, N.S., Eiser, C. and Eiser, J.R. (1998) Nutrition education in the National Curriculum. *Health Education Journal* 57, 81–88.

Croll, J.K., Neumark-Sztainer, D. and Story, M. (2001) Healthy eating: what does it mean to adolescents? *Journal of Nutrition Education* 33, 193–198.

Cusatis, D.C. and Shannon, B.M. (1996) Influences on adolescent eating behaviour. *Journal of Adolescent Health* 18, 27–34.

De Bourdeaudhuij, I. (1997) Family food rules and healthy eating in adolescents. *Journal of Health Psychology* 2, 45–56.

De Bourdeaudhuij, I. and van Oost, P. (2000) Personal and family determinants of dietary behaviour in adolescents and their parents. *Psychology and Health* 15, 751–770.

Dennison, C.M. and Shepherd, R. (1995) Adolescent food choice: an application of the theory of planned behaviour. *Journal of Human Nutrition and Dietetics* 8, 9–23.

Feunekes, G.I.J., de Graaf, C., Meyboom, S. and van Staveren, W.A. (1998) Food choice and fat intake of adolescents and adults: associations of intakes within social networks. *Preventive Medicine* 27, 645–656.

Freeman, R. and Bunting, G. (2003) A child-to-child approach to promoting healthier snacking in primary school children: a randomised trial in Northern Ireland. *Health Education* 103, 17–27.

French, S.A., Story, M., Hannan, P., Breitlow, K.K., Jeffery, R.W., Baxter, J.S. and Snyder, M.P. (1999) Cognitive and demographic correlates of low-fat vending snack choices among adolescents and adults. *Journal of the American Dietetic Association* 99, 471–475.

Gallagher, K. (2000) Dietary practices and nutrition knowledge of adolescents from contrasting social backgrounds. *Journal of Consumer Studies and Home Economics* 22, 207–211.

Glanz, K., Basil, M., Maibach, E., Goldberg, J. and Snyder, D. (1998) Why Americans eat what they do: taste, nutrition, cost, convenience and weight control concerns as influences on food consumption. *Journal of the American Dietetic Association* 98, 1118–1126.

Goldberg, G.R. (2003) *Plants: Diet and Health. The Report of a British Nutrition Foundation Task Force*. Blackwell Publishing, Oxford, UK.

Granic, I., Dishion, T.J. and Hollenstein, T. (2003) The family ecology of adolescence: a dynamic perspective on normative development. In: Adams, G.R and Berzonsky, M.D. (eds) *Blackwell Handbook of Adolescence*. Blackwell, Oxford, UK, pp. 60–91.

Gregory, J., Lowe, S., Bates, C.J., Prentice, A., Jackson, L.V., Smithers, G., Wenlock, R. and Farron, M. (2000) *National Diet and Nutrition Survey: Young People aged 4 to 18 years*. Vol. 1. *Report of The Diet and Nutrition Survey*. The Stationery Office, London.

Harel, Z., Riggs, S., Vaz, R., White, L. and Menzies, G. (1998) Adolescents and calcium: what they do and do not know and how much they consume. *Journal of Adolescent Health* 22, 225–228.

Haste, H. (2004) *My Body, My Self. Young People's Values and Motives about Healthy Living*. Nestle Social Research Programme, London.

Hebbelnick, M., Clarys, P. and de Malsche, A. (1999) Growth, development, and physical fitness of Flemish vegetarian children, adolescents, and young adults. *American Journal of Clinical Nutrition* 70, 579S–585S.

Hill, A.J., Oliver, S. and Rogers, P.J. (1992) Eating in the adult world: the rise of dieting in childhood and adolescence. *British Journal of Clinical Psychology* 31, 95–105.

Hill, L., Casswell, S., Maskill, C., Jones, S. and Wyllie, A. (1998) Fruit and vegetables as adolescent food choices in New Zealand. *Health Promotion International* 13, 55–65.

Horacek, T.M. and Betts, N.M. (1998) Students cluster into four groups according to the factors influencing their dietary intake. *Journal of the American Dietetic Association* 98, 1464–1467.

Inchley, J., Todd, J., Bryce, C. and Currie, C. (2001) Dietary trends among Scottish schoolchildren in the 1990s. *Journal of Human Nutrition and Dietetics* 14, 207–216.

International Obesity Task Force and European Association for Obesity (2002) *Obesity in Europe: The Case for Action*. International Obesity Task Force, London.

Irving, L.M. and Neumark-Sztainer, D. (2002) Integrating the prevention of eating disorders and obesity: feasible or futile? *Preventative Medicine* 34, 299–309.

Jas, P. (1998) Aspects of food choice behaviour in adolescents. *Nutrition and Food Science* 3, 163–165.

Kenyon, P.M. and Barker, M.E. (1998) Attitudes towards meat-eating in vegetarian and non-vegetarian teenage girls in England – an ethnographic approach. *Appetite* 30, 185–198.

Klopp, S.A., Heiss, C. and Smith, H.S. (2003) Self-reported vegetarianism may be a marker for college women at risk for disordered eating. *Journal of the American Dietetic Association* 103, 745–747.

Kubberod, E., Ueland, O., Tronstad, A. and Risvik, E. (2002) Attitudes towards meat and meat-eating among adolescents in Norway: a qualitative study. *Appetite* 38, 53–62.

Larsson, C.L., Klock, K.S., Nordrehaug Astrom, A., Haugejorden, O. and Johansson, G. (2002) Lifestyle-related characteristics of young low-meat consumers and omnivores in Sweden and Norway. *Journal of Adolescent Health* 31, 190–198.

Larsson, C.L., Ronnlund, U., Johansson, G. and Dahlgren, L. (2003) Veganism as status passage: the process of becoming a vegan among youths in Sweden. *Appetite* 41, 61–67.

Lattimore, P.J. and Halford, C.G. (2003) Adolescence and the diet–dieting disparity: healthy food choice or risky health behaviour. *British Journal of Health Psychology* 8, 451–463.

Lechner, L., Brug, J., de Vries, H., van Assema, P. and Mudde, A. (1998) Stages of change for fruit, vegetable and fat intake: consequences of misconception. *Health Education Research* 13, 1–13.

Lien, N., Lytle, L.A. and Klepp, K.I. (2001) Stability in consumption of fruit, vegetables, and sugary foods in a cohort from age 14 to age 21. *Preventive Medicine* 33, 217–226.

Livingstone, S. and Helsper, E. (2004) *Advertising Foods to Children: Understanding Promotion in the Context of Children's Daily Lives: A Review of the Literature Prepared for the Research Department of the Office of Communications.* Office of Communications, London.

Lytle, L.A., Eldridge, A.L., Kotz, K., Piper, J., Williams, S. and Kalina, B. (1997) Children's interpretation of nutrition messages. *Journal of Nutrition Education* 29, 128–136.

MacNicol, S.A.M., Murray, S.M. and Austin, E.J. (2003) Relationship between personality, attitudes and dietary behaviour in a group of Scottish adolescents. *Personality and Individual Differences* 34, 1–12.

Morris, A.M. and Katzman, D.K. (2003) The impact of the media on eating disorders in children and adolescents. *Paediatric Child Health* 8, 287–289.

Mulvihill, C., Nemeth, A. and Vereecken, C. (2004) Body image, weight control and body weight. In: Currie, C., Roberts, C., Morgan, A., Smith, R., Setterobulte, W., Samdel, O. and Rasmussen, V.B. (eds) *Young People's Health in Context: Health Behaviour in School-aged Children (HSBC) Study: International Report from the 2001/2002 Survey.* Health Policy for Children and Adolescents No. 4. WHO Regional Office for Europe, Copenhagen, pp. 120–130. Available at: http://www.who.dk/document/e82923.pdf (accessed 20 December 2004).

Neumark-Sztainer, D. and Story, M. (1998) Dieting and binge eating among adolescents: what do they really mean? *Journal of the American Dietetic Association* 98, 446–450.

Neumark-Sztainer, D., Story, M., Toporoff, E., Himes, J.H., Resnick, M.D. and Blum, W.M. (1997) Covariations of eating behaviour with other health-related behaviour among adolescents. *Journal of Adolescent Health* 20, 450–458.

Neumark-Sztainer, D., Story, M., Perry, C. and Casey, M.A. (1999) Factors influencing food choices of adolescents: findings from focus-group discussions with adolescents. *Journal of the American Dietetic Association* 99, 929–937.

Newell, G.K., Hammig, C.L., Jurich, A.P. and Johnson, D.E. (1990) Self-concept as a factor in the quality of diets of adolescent girls. *Adolescence* 25, 117–130.

Nichter, M. (2003) *Fat Talk: What Girls and Their Parents Say about Dieting.* Harvard University Press, London.

Norton, P.A., Falciglia, G.A. and Ricketts, C. (2000) Motivational determinants of food preferences in adolescents and pre-adolescents. *Ecology of Food and Nutrition* 39, 169–182.

Nowak, M. (1998) The weight-conscious adolescent: body image, food intake and weight-related behaviour. *Journal of Adolescent Health* 23, 389–398.

Nowak, M. and Buettner, P. (2003) Relationship between adolescents' food-related beliefs and food intake behaviour. *Nutrition Research* 23, 45–55.

Perry, C.L., McGuire, M.T., Neumark-Sztainer, D. and Story, M. (2001) Characteristics of vegetarian adolescents in a multiethnic urban population. *Journal of Adolescent Health* 29, 406–416.

Polivy, J., Herman, P.C., Mills, J.S. and Wheeler, H.B. (2003) Eating disorders in adolescence. In: Adams, G.R. and Berzonsky, M.D. (eds) *Blackwell Handbook of Adolescence.* Blackwell, Oxford, UK, pp. 521–549.

Roberts, S.J., McGuiness, P.J., Bilton, R. and Maxwell, S.M. (1999) Dieting behaviour among 11–15 year-old girls in Merseyside and the northwest of England. *Journal of Adolescent Health* 25, 62–67.

Roberts, S.J., Maxwell, S.M., Bagnall, G. and Bilton, R. (2001) The incidence of dieting amongst adolescent girls: a question of interpretation? *Journal of Human Nutrition and Dietetics* 14, 103–109.

Ryan, Y.M. (1997) Meat avoidance and body weight concerns: nutritional implications for teenage girls. *Proceedings of the Nutrition Society* 56, 519–524.

Santos, M.L.S. and Booth, D.A. (1996) Influences on meat avoidance among British students. *Appetite* 27, 197–205.

Shannon, B., Bagby, R., Wang, M.O. and Trenkner, L.L. (1990) Self-efficacy: a contributor to the explanation of eating behavior. *Health Education Research* 5, 395–407.

Shepherd, R. and Dennison, C.M. (1996) Influences on adolescent food choice. *Proceedings of the Nutrition Society* 55, 345–357.

Sims, L.S. (1978) Food-related value-orientations, attitudes and beliefs of vegetarians and non-vegetarians. *Ecology of Food Nutrition* 7, 23–35.

Spear, H.J. and Kulbok, P.A. (2001) Adolescent health behaviour and related factors: a review. *Public Health Nursing* 18, 82–93.

Story, M. and Resnick, M.D. (1986) Adolescents' views on food and nutrition. *Journal of Nutrition Education* 18, 188–192.

Story, M., Neumark-Sztainer, D. and French, S. (2002) Individual and environmental influences on adolescent eating behaviours. *Journal of the American Dietetic Association* 102, S40–S51.

Sweeting, H., Anderson, A. and West, P. (1994) Socio-demographic correlates of dietary habits in mid to late adolescence. *European Journal of Clinical Nutrition* 48, 736–748.

Vereecken, C. and Maes, L. (2000) Eating habits, dental care and dieting. In: Currie, C., Hurrelman, K., Settertobulte, W., Smith, R. and Todd, J. (eds) *Health and Health Behaviour among Young People.* Health Policy for Children and Adolescents No. 1. WHO Regional Office for Europe, Copenhagen, pp. 83–89. Available at: http://www.who.dk/document/e67880.pdf (accessed 22 November 2004).

Vereecken, C., Ojala, K. and Delgrande, J. (2004) Eating habits. In: Currie, C., Roberts, C., Morgan, A., Smith, R., Setterobulte, W., Samdel, O. and Rasmussen, V.B. (eds) *Young People's Health in Context: Health Behaviour in School-aged Children (HSBC) Study: International Report From the 2001/2002 Survey.* Health Policy for Children and Adolescents No. 4. WHO Regional Office for Europe, Copenhagen, pp. 110–119. Available at: http://www.who.dk/document/e82923.pdf (accessed 20 December 2004).

Videon, T.M. and Manning, C.K. (2003) Influences on adolescent eating patterns: the importance of family meals. *Journal of Adolescent Health* 32, 365–373.

Wardle, J. and Beales, S. (1986) Restraint, body image and food attitudes in children from 12 to 18 years. *Appetite* 7, 209–217.

Wardle, J., Haase, A.M., Steptoe, A., Nillapun, M., Jonwutiwes, K. and Bellisle, F. (2004) Gender differences in food choice: the contribution of health beliefs and dieting. *Annals of Behavioural Medicine* 27, 107–116.

Warwick, J., McIlveen, H. and Strugnell, C. (1999) Food choices of 9–17 year olds in Northern Ireland – influences and challenges. *Nutrition and Food Science* 14, 229–236.

Woodward, D.R., Boon, J.A., Cumming, F.J., Ball, P.J., Williams, H.M. and Hornsby, H. (1996) Adolescents' reported usage of selected foods in relation to their perceptions and social norms for those foods. *Appetite* 27, 109–117.

Worsley, A. and Skrzypiec, G. (1997) Teenage vegetarianism: beauty or the beast? *Nutrition Research* 17, 391–404.

Worsley, A. and Skrzypiec, G. (1998) Teenage vegetarianism: prevalence, social and cognitive contexts. *Appetite* 30, 151–170.

Wrieden, W. (1996) Fruit and vegetable consumption of 10–11 year old children in a region of Scotland. *Health Education Journal* 14, 185–193.

14 Intra-family Influences on Food Choice at Mid-life

Department of Food Science, Penn State University, 205 A Borland, University Park, PA 16802, USA

Introduction

Many economic, cognitive, psychological, physiological and social factors influence food choices of individuals at mid-life (Nestle *et al.*, 1998; Gedrich, 2003). For instance, both social norms and social class influence the foods preferred by men versus women (Mooney and Lorenz, 1997; Fagerli and Wandel, 1999; Jensen and Holm, 1999; Hupkens *et al.*, 2000; Roos *et al.*, 2001). At mid-life, most individuals live in families, another important social influence on food choice. In 2000, 97% of Americans lived in households, of which single individuals maintained only 26% (US Bureau of the Census, 2000). Most of the remaining 74% were families, i.e. two or more persons who share a common residence and are related by blood, adoption or marriage.

A family is a system in which members participate in establishing an equilibrium state of interaction called homeostasis (Noller and Fitzpatrick, 1993). When families share meals, patterns of food choice (rules) are established through overt or covert negotiation (Charles and Kerr, 1988; Kemmer *et al.*, 1998), another characteristic of a family system (Broderick, 1993). Studies indicate some similarity in spousal food consumption, especially if couples eat meals together and have young children (Laitinen *et al.*, 1997; Macario and Sorenson, 1998; Hannon *et al.*, 2003). Positive family food interactions (discussion, decision making, eating together) have some positive effects on partners' diet quality, especially the husband's (Schafer *et al.*, 1999), while negative interactions have been correlated with poor diet quality for both partners (Kintner *et al.*, 1981). Families influence children's food preferences (Borah-Giddens and Falciglia, 1993; Young *et al.*, 2004), especially when young (Skinner *et al.*, 1998; Cullen *et al.*, 2002), although other factors soften the effect as children mature (Rozin, 1996). By eating meals together (Neumark-Sztainer *et al.*, 2003), modelling behaviours (Tibbs *et al.*, 2001; Young *et al.*, 2004) and setting rules

©The Authors 2006. *The Psychology of Food Choice*
(eds R. Shepherd and M. Raats)   263

(Fisher *et al.*, 2002), parents influence food and nutrient intake (Tibbs *et al.*, 2001; Fisher *et al.*, 2002; Gonzales *et al.*, 2002; Young *et al.*, 2004).

While families are recognized to influence members' food choices, little is known of the processes used within the family to influence those of adult members. In this chapter I review:

1. The dynamics of setting food choices in families at mid-life.
2. Gender, gender roles and their influence on household tasks and food chores.
3. Marital power and its expression in household tasks, food chores and food choices.

Using data from family social science and psychology, I argue that both gender and power influence family food choices and our efforts to alter food choice in families will be ineffectual until we have greater understanding of how these affect family decision making. Most studies reviewed were done with Caucasians, although a few were done exclusively with blacks. Some panel studies involved a small proportion of blacks and Hispanics. Thus the conclusions would not apply to all ethnic groups.

Dynamics of Family Food Choice at Mid-life

Adjustment and its effects

Family formation and maturation involves food choice adjustments. During engagement, cohabitation and the initial years of marriage, food choices and domestic roles are negotiated around the evening meal, where couples strongly desire to eat the same foods (Craig and Truswell, 1988; Kemmer *et al.*, 1998; Brown and Miller, 2002a,b; Marshall and Anderson, 2002; Bove *et al.*, 2003). The convergence process can occur with minimal interaction (similar preferences), active negotiation or moulding efforts, or even conflict (Kemmer *et al.*, 1998; Brown and Miller, 2002b; Bove *et al.*, 2003). Changes focus on meat, milk fat level and vegetables and the proper meal of meat and potatoes is retained, adopted or modified (Craig and Truswell, 1988; Brown and Miller, 2002a,b; Marshall and Anderson, 2002; Bove *et al.*, 2003). Outcomes might not be satisfactory for both partners, especially if a sense of obligation or a desire to please leads to one partner's preferences dominating meals (Brown and Miller, 2002b), so use of side dishes, ingredients omission, eating out, choices at other meals or meals with in-laws serve as ways to satisfy individual preferences (Brown and Miller, 2002b; Marshall and Anderson, 2002; Bove *et al.*, 2003). In a small longitudinal study, 6 months into marriage more wives had made cooperative changes in food choices but by 2.5 years, more husbands had (Craig and Truswell, 1988). Whether this reflected the greater initial influence of the husband or the greater initial desire of the wife to please the husband is not clear, but the outcome of these initial decisions lays the framework for future changes in food choices.

Entry of children into the family can spark re-examination and readjustment of food choices (Schafer and Keith, 1981; Devine *et al.*, 1998; Lupton, 2000;

Brown and Miller, 2002b). New parents may increase serving and eating fruits and vegetables for the child's sake (Devine *et al.*, 1998). Often young children's mothers show the most concern about children's food intake (Schafer and Keith, 1981; Gillespie and Achterberg, 1989), are more likely to make dietary changes for their children's sake than older women (Devine and Olson, 1991) but also may satisfy children's preferences over their own needs and better judgement (Kirk and Gillespie, 1990; Devine and Olson, 1991). Re-entry of an older child into the family can also influence food choices (Devine *et al.*, 1998).

Middle-aged adults are more likely to consider altering food choice for health reasons as the first signs of chronic disease can appear in the fourth decade (Jensen and Holm, 1999). Although a woman may have more success changing food choices once children leave home (Devine and Olson, 1991), dietary changes needed to address a husband's disease risk or disease are more often accepted by the family or couple than those needed to address the wife's risk or disease (Sexton *et al.*, 1987; Cigoli *et al.*, 1994; Bovbjerg *et al.*, 1995; Aish, 1996; Devine *et al.*, 1998; Hepworth, 1999; Savoca and Miller, 2001; Kristofferzon *et al.*, 2003). However, the willingness of the unaffected partner, regardless of sex, to accept the food choice alterations is critical to long-term maintenance of a new dietary pattern (Zimmerman *et al.*, 1988; White *et al.*, 1991; Shattuck *et al.*, 1992; Russell *et al.*, 1994; Bovbjerg *et al.*, 1995).

Families influence health because primary attitudes and behaviours about food as well as other life-style patterns are learned within them (Campbell, 1994). While some data suggest a protective effect of marriage on men's rather than women's health (Sobal *et al.*, 1992; Schofield *et al.*, 2000), others have found increasing similarity in some cardiovascular disease risk factors among spouses over years married (Knuiman *et al.*, 1996) and some effect of a shared family environment on such risk factors (Harrap *et al.*, 2000). Only a few studies have examined how family roles and interactions might affect members' health. Fisher *et al.* (1993) examined the link between four domains of family life (world view, emotion management, structure/organization and problem solving) and the health of husband and wife in 225 families with at least one adolescent child. The health indicators included anxiety, depression, weight problems, general well-being, preventive behaviours, drinking, smoking and work productiveness measured by self-report questionnaires. Examination of family structure/organization (Fisher *et al.*, 1992) revealed that the general well-being (plus less depression, drinking, anxiety and smoking) of both partners was positively correlated with clear organization of household tasks (i.e. roles) and rules and greater interpersonal closeness (called cohesion). However, husband's health was also positively associated with traditional gender roles and adaptability that facilitated job productiveness while wife's health was associated with a balance of personal time versus time in traditional family roles. Wickrama *et al.* (2001) examined risk of hypertension in 367 husbands and wives followed for 5 years and found that, in addition to personal health risks (diet, exercise and weight), wives', but not husbands' risk, was increased by work–family role conflict and parental role stress. De Bourdeaudhuij and van Oost (1998a) found that adolescent healthful behaviours (not smoking or drinking, better food choices, regular sleep pattern and physical activity) were more likely in families ($n = 522$) that had greater family cohesion and regularity in roles and rules, two components of family system theory. Although the variance explained varies, these studies suggest the effects of family roles and interactions on health outcomes including diet warrant further examination.

Family roles and food choice

Food choice decisions in families are embedded in the job (or role) of household food provision (shopping and preparation). Recent US household survey data indicate that, in most families, women occupy this role that some consider a powerful gatekeeper (Lewin, 1943; Harnack et al., 1998). However, many studies in European and American households reveal that the food provider role, when occupied by a woman, includes explicit expectations of how and what foods are served in the family, especially for the main meal eaten together (Murcott, 1983; Kerr and Charles, 1986; Pill and Parry, 1989; DeVault, 1991; Jensen and Holm, 1999; Brown and Miller, 2002b; Marshall and Anderson, 2002), a desired social organizer of family life (DeVault, 1987; Kemmer, 1999). The woman's role responsibilities include taking the needs and preferences of other family members into account and granting 'privilege' to particular food choices (DeVault, 1987; Mennell et al., 1992). Because women face multiple and often contradictory demands for food choices as they fulfil their obligation to satisfy their spouse and train, feed and please children, they often take on additional sub-roles (family diplomat, peacekeeper, etc.) that allow them to make compromises with their own preferences (Kirk and Gillespie, 1990; Mennell et al., 1992; Gregory, 1999; Blake and Bisogni, 2003). In contrast, men taking this role assumed their preferences were acceptable (DeVault, 1991). Because the provision role is gendered, the expectations do not empower the female gatekeeper to easily implement her own preferences or those she might want to instil. The interplay of gender and power around food choices has been documented qualitatively for families where work and family roles must be balanced (DeVault, 1990; Bradbard et al., 1997; de Bourdeaudhuij, 1997; Brown and Miller, 2002b; Krummel et al., 2002; Blake and Bisogni, 2003).

Despite this evidence, little quantitative research has examined how gendered role expectations and power differentials affect family food choices. Partly this reflects the use of theoretical models like social learning theory or the theory of planned behaviour, which focus on the individual rather than the family unit and assume individual independence rather than interdependence. Even the food choice model (Furst et al., 1996) has been criticized for focusing on the individual instead of making the family with its interactive processes the focal point (Stratton and Bromley, 1999). When the individual is the focus, outcomes are more often measured rather than the process leading to them. Baranowski and Hearn (1997) note that little is known of how families facilitate change (or conversely how they inhibit change) in food choices and suggest examining family functioning and internal relationships in more detail. Functioning involves patterns of interaction and interdependence and is a reflection of adaptability, cohesion and communication (Gorall and Olson, 1995). Adaptability, a characteristic needed in families to institute changes in food choice, reflects the ability of the family to alter its power structure, role relationships and rules in response to demands for change. Gender influences internal relationships through ascribed roles. Thus, understanding the construction of gender and power in families could help us understand how family food choices might be more successfully altered.

Gender, Gender Roles and Division of Household Tasks

Gender and sex are two distinct constructs. Sex is the distinction between male and female based on biological factors (Schofield *et al.*, 2000). Gender is used to signify differential power, based on social stratification, in social relationships between the sexes both within the family and without (Scott, 1986; Losh-Hesselbart, 1987). Gender is demonstrated through social roles that are taught and enacted until attitudes and behaviours describing the role become 'natural'. Since it is linked to the distribution of merit, privilege, power and resources through overt and covert processes, gender must be constantly constructed, i.e. one must 'do gender'. Thus gender is the product of social processes that provide the cultural meaning of masculinity and femininity (Fox and Murry, 2000).

Gender roles emerged out of structure functionalism wherein males and females had specific roles in the family unit. Men's focus was outside the family with the role of family wage earner while women's focus was inside the family with the role of childcare and housework (Parson and Bales, 1955). Exchange theory posited that marital partners trade services provided by their roles (i.e. cooked meals for wages) based on their relative value in order to gain personal rewards (Szinovacz, 1984), that exchanges are regulated by norms of reciprocity and fairness, and that marital satisfaction would be greater when rewards outweigh costs (Pina and Bengston, 1993). Blood and Wolfe (1960) noted that wages represent economic power and postulated that women's entry into the workforce would shift power so that family roles might be renegotiated. Over the last 30 years, as researchers followed women's entry into the workforce, gender roles in family sociology have come to represent the marital and family roles partners assume when balancing work and family (Greenstein, 2000).

Gender role attitudes are the overall attitudes and beliefs individuals have about the appropriate roles for men and women in work and family relationships (Scott *et al.*, 1996). These beliefs are the elements that make up a gender ideology (Greenstein, 1996a). Measurement assumes a scale where scores at one end identify those favouring traditional gender roles and differential power relationships while scores at the other end identify those favouring shared roles or egalitarianism (Amato and Booth, 1995). Scores in the middle are often called transitional. However, depending on item content, scales can focus on roles in the public sphere, feminism and equal rights as well as marital and parental roles (Beere, 1990). Comparisons among studies must be done carefully because scales differ in the roles and activity domains addressed (McHugh and Frieze, 1997).

For the specific arena of family decision making, Scanzoni and Fox (1980) proposed the term 'gender role preference' as an estimate of an individual's preference for the gendered roles of wife, mother, father and husband. Preferences are attained through day-to-day decisions that balance costs with rewards and so seem particularly applicable to food choice decisions.

Changes in gender role attitudes

Since the 1960s, women have increasingly entered the workforce. In the 1960s, 90% of husbands and 30% of wives worked. In 1994, the numbers were 74% and 60%, respectively (Rogers and Amato, 2000). During this same period, gender role attitudes have become less traditional. In both the USA and Europe, analysis of annual national social surveys from 1977 to 1996 indicated increasing egalitarian views among working women about combining work and family responsibilities while men's views changed more slowly (Scott et al., 1996; Harris and Firestone, 1998; Brewster and Padavic, 2000). However, more conservative views emerging in the last decade have slowed changes in attitudes (Brewster and Padavic, 2000). Examination of longitudinal data from national samples of US married couples support the differential rise in egalitarian views and revealed that while married men are more willing to share the provider role, they still felt that women should fulfil their traditional roles in the home (Amato and Booth, 1995; Zuo, 1997; Smith and Beaujot, 1999). Marital discord increases with the rise in wife's egalitarianism (Amato and Booth, 1995; Rogers and Amato, 2000) and a major contributor is work–family demands and perceptions of unfair distribution of household labour. Thus although attitudes about women's role in the workforce have become more liberal, attitudes about women's role as wife and mother, particularly among men, have changed less.

Gender role expression through household task performance

From 1980 onwards, numerous studies have indicated that household labour remains highly segregated with men doing mainly masculine tasks (car maintenance, yard work) and women doing mainly feminine (shopping, preparing meals, washing dishes, cleaning the house, washing and ironing) (Coverman and Sheley, 1986; Gershuny and Robinson, 1988; Hochschild, 1989a; Blair and Lichter, 1991; Broman, 1991; Manke et al., 1994; Sullivan, 1997; Coltrane, 2000; Haynes, 2000; Cunningham, 2001). Blair and Lichter (1991) found this segregated pattern was dampened somewhat by education, higher female earnings, fewer years of marriage and household egalitarian views about employment. But husbands would still have had to reallocate 50% of their time from male tasks to female tasks to reach equity. Although women's housework contributions declined somewhat and men's increased somewhat between 1988 and 1993, the average married woman still did three times as much routine housework as the average married man (32 versus 10 h per week; Coltrane, 2000), even in dual-earner couples (Biernat and Wortman, 1991; Manke et al., 1994).

Using national US survey data, Greenstein (1996a) demonstrated that the gender role ideology of each partner interacts to affect the husband's relative contribution (rather than absolute contribution) to domestic housework overall and the traditional feminine tasks in particular. Gender ideology was determined by six statements, five assessing views of women working outside the home and one about sharing housework if both partners work outside the home. Husbands were more likely to participate in feminine household tasks only if both the wife and husband had egalitarian gender role ideologies and least likely if both had traditional ideologies or if the wife was traditional, regardless of the male ideology. A traditional man married to an egalitarian woman or an egalitarian man married to a traditional woman was not likely to do any more domestic labour or feminine chores than a husband in a couple sharing traditional views. One interpretation is that the wife's gender ideology is the key factor but congruence of attitudes is critical for change. Many other studies from the 1990s verified that, in addition to partner's employment hours and earnings, the spouse's gender role ideology and congruence were consistent predictors of how domestic tasks, including food chores, were shared in the household (Coltrane, 2000).

Using a representative sample of two-earner households ($n = 382$), Twiggs *et al.* (1999) found evidence that gender role attitudes were associated with a hierarchy of acceptable feminine tasks for men. Sharing washing dishes (made less onerous by dishwashers) and grocery shopping were more likely than helping to clean house, do laundry or prepare meals. Thresholds for sharing meal preparation were highest and, if a man was sharing this, he was more likely to be sharing all other feminine tasks. Unfortunately, no distinctions were reported about types of meals prepared (i.e. breakfast versus dinner) where thresholds might also exist. This pattern has been noticed by others (Biernat and Wortman, 1991; Sullivan, 1997) and suggests the gendered meanings attached to various tasks differ and allow husbands to shift contribution without altering their beliefs about appropriate gender roles.

Gender roles, perceived fairness, gratitude and division of household tasks

Division of household labour influences women's perceptions of fairness and marital satisfaction. Studies in the 1990s indicated the most important predictor of a wife's perceptions of fairness in household labour was the proportion of routine housework (particularly feminine tasks) her husband does (Sanchez and Kane, 1996; Coltrane, 2000). However, women found division fair if they were doing two-thirds of the housework and men one-third, an arrangement that men also found fair (Lennon and Rosenfield, 1994). This suggested that either trade-offs (house repairs for meals) or the potential meaning (loving, caring, support, etc.) of the work done by men was more important than the actual amount (Hochschild, 1989a; Thompson and Walker, 1989; Pina and Bengston, 1993; Sanchez and Kane, 1996).

Gender role ideology influences the wife's evaluation of a husband's contribution to household labour. While traditional women may be dissatisfied with their husband's contribution, they reduce or eliminate personal feelings of unfairness, especially if the husband is also traditional, and are less likely to feel this impacts marital quality (Pina and Bengston, 1993; Greenstein, 1996b; Lavee and Katz, 2002). Women with more egalitarian views who experience traditional family work roles more often report unfairness and lower marital quality (McHale and Crouter, 1992; Pina and Bengston, 1993) and disagreements increase (Lye and Biblarz, 1993). Even if discontent with division of housework, traditional wives and wives with traditional husbands are more likely to avoid overt conflict than egalitarian wives or wives with egalitarian husbands (Kluwer et al., 1997).

Hochschild (1989a,b) described an 'economy of gratitude' wherein the interaction of partners' gender role ideologies define what is a gift (something extra) and what is an entitlement (expected). A traditional partner would view the wife's housework as an entitlement but the husband's as a gift while an egalitarian partner might see the husband's help as an entitlement and a greater share from the wife as a gift (Greenstein, 1996a). Emotional interdependence also affects perceptions of unfairness differently for men and women. Less emotionally involved men are unlikely to view the skewed division of household labour as unfair while less emotionally involved women are (Sanchez and Kane, 1996). Both traditional gender role ideology and greater emotional attachment could affect a wife's degree of gratitude for a husband's lesser contribution to housework. Interestingly, in second marriages the strongest predictor of husband's involvement in household chores was his gender role ideology, despite the wife's feelings of entitlements, but if second husbands do even somewhat more housework than the wife's first, this tempers the wife's feelings of entitlements and inflates her gratitude (Pyke and Coltrane, 1996).

Thus, gender role ideology affects partners' relative contribution to household chores, the feminine chores most likely shared, the meanings and degree of fairness associated with household tasks performed by partners, and expressions of gratitude. Except for partners with shared egalitarian views, task allocation and the interaction of gratitude, love and trade-offs likely favours men's interests and preferences.

Gender role construction within families

Because the unequal division of household labour persists despite changes in women's work patterns, time available and resources, scholars argue that gendered roles are actively constructed through day-to-day activities and decision making (Scanzoni and Fox, 1980; DeVault, 1987; Thompson and Walker, 1989; Zvonkovic et al., 1996). Couples can establish a 'myth of equality' based on communication patterns that rationalize gendered patterns, hide the issues and avoid explicit negotiation (Zvonkovic et al., 1996; Knudson-Martin and Mahoney, 1998). Partners can use many evasive strategies to avoid housework that perpetuate the gendered adult role pattern (Thompson and Walker, 1989) or women can actively defend their gatekeeper role by assuming manager–helper relationships, setting standards and criticizing their partner's efforts (Thompson and Walker, 1989; Allen and Hawkins, 1999).

Children receive gender role training in families and, by adolescence, have learned the roles used in their household (Losh-Hesselbart, 1987; Benin and Edwards, 1990; Blair, 1992; Cunningham, 2001). Parents reinforce the roles through housework assignments that involve girls more in feminine tasks than boys (Blair, 1992). Based on time diary data from children aged 12–17 years, girls in dual- or single-earner families perform four times the amount of traditional feminine chores compared with boys (Benin and Edwards, 1990), a pattern confirmed for children aged 9–12 years (McHale *et al.*, 1990), regardless of time of week tasks were performed (Manke *et al.*, 1994). Both cross-sectional survey and longitudinal panel data indicate that the parents' gender role attitudes influence the type of tasks assigned the same-sex child (Blair, 1992) and the child's gender role attitudes at age 18 years (Cunningham, 2001). The mother's attitudes and the father's actual participation had the strongest effect on expectations (Thorn and Gilbert, 1998; Cunningham, 2001).

Influence of gender and gender roles on family food chores

This review indicates that, while attitudes towards women's role in the workforce have become more liberal, men's and women's attitudes about women's and girls' family roles have changed less. Gendered roles are reflected in family food chores, which remain women's work (Losh-Hesselbart, 1987; DeVault, 1990; Warde and Hetherington, 1994; Jensen and Holm, 1999; Kemmer, 1999) and are labelled 'feminine' (Coltrane, 2000; Kroska, 2003). They are further differentiated from other chores by when and how often they are done and the degree of visible and invisible work involved (Thompson and Walker, 1989; DeVault, 1991; Milkie and Peltola, 1999; Coltrane, 2000). This gendered division may depend on family life stage (Warde and Hetherington, 1994; Coltrane, 2000) but is likely in place at mid-life.

Schafer and Schafer (1989) examined how gender affects roles in food chores in a representative sample of Iowa families that varied in family life cycle stage. Regardless of employment status, partners shared the perception that the wife should and actually did most of the food chores across mid-life. Although younger employed wives felt husbands should do more and perceived more participation by husbands, wives were still doing 80% or more of these chores. Despite the inequities, both partners perceived each other's share to be fair. Using a representative, national sample of US dual-earner, two-child families, Miller and Ackerman (1990) found that wages, employment hours, parental education and age of older children were poor predictors of why wives were doing most of the food chores and suggested examining other factors, like sex role preferences. In 1994, over 90% of US married or cohabiting women were involved in food planning and preparation and 88% in shopping (Harnack *et al.*, 1998). Men were more likely to be involved in shopping (36%) than planning (23%) or preparation (27%), especially if younger, lacking children or if their wife was employed full-time.

Qualitative studies illuminate the process of establishing and adhering to food chore roles. Brown and Miller (2002a) grouped Caucasian couples with young children ($n = 20$) based on spouses' gender role preference scores, and interviewed both spouses to learn how food chore responsibilities were established and handled. Scores were transitional or egalitarian, not traditional. Couples in which both were transitional or the husband was transitional reported that, although the husband was more involved in food chores when first married, arrival of the first child resulted in the transfer of food chore responsibility to the wife, based on traditional role expectations, even if the wife continued to work, something seen by others (Gupta, 1999). Although many transitional wives (and their husbands) were satisfied with these roles, wives who wanted more help with cooking and clean-up did not request this, deferring to the husband's breadwinner role. Egalitarian women married to transitional men were more likely to ask for their husband's help with clean-up and expected their roles to change in the future. In contrast, egalitarian couples used three strategies to share food chores that were established early in their relationship and sustained even with the arrival of children. This suggests that both partners must hold strong egalitarian beliefs to sustain a non-traditional role pattern after children arrive. In a more ethnically diverse sample, parents reported they might trade-off food chores by necessity but most women indicated they were the primary household food managers and felt responsible for what their family ate (Devine et al., 2003). Traditional (and transitional) gendered food chore roles are likely most prevalent as suggested by Harnack et al. (1998), Brown and Miller (2002a) and numerous studies from Europe (e.g. Kemmer, 1999).

Studies using mealtime observations and interviews have documented that food chore gender roles are demonstrated, assigned and transmitted to children. Mothers are the primary organizers of family meals (preparing, serving and doing most of the clean-up) (Feiring and Lewis, 1987; Grieshaber, 1997; Gill, 1998). They are the social directors of mealtime conversation (Feiring and Lewis, 1987) and often serve as diplomats or peacekeepers (Kirk and Gillespie, 1990; Blake and Bisogni, 2003). Vuchinich (1987) found that mothers act as peacemakers when conflict arises at meals and teach their daughters how to do this. Daughters more often are expected to help with meals and the daily food preparation routine produces boys and girls socialized to gendered roles that are well established before entering school (Grieshaber, 1997; Gill, 1998).

In sum, household food chores are accomplished through gendered roles that are sustained through practice and passed on to children. The couple's gender role preferences may interact in a manner similar to that found by Greenstein (1996a) to affect the degree to which husbands participate in food chores and shape perceptions of fairness. Within a gendered family food system, marital power may influence food choice decision making.

Power in Families: Expression in Decision Making about Household Chores

Power has been defined as actor's ability to produce an intended outcome through effects on others (Rogers, 1974; Szinovacz, 1987). When actors are part of a family system, the distribution of resources (income, education, occupational status) and the values, norms and roles of the players affect how power is accrued and used (Rogers, 1974; Scanzoni and Polonko, 1980; Szinovacz, 1987). The exercise of power is a multidimensional, dynamic process that involves power bases, power processes and power outcomes (Cromwell and Olson, 1975; Blumberg and Coleman, 1989) and is often expressed through decision making (Blood and Wolfe, 1960; Szinovacz, 1987). Within the family each individual has potential power that is defined by a power basis, the tangible and intangible resources that person can employ to affect others, and power means, the strategies used by the person to achieve intended effects on others. The outcome of applying power is also determined by the scope, extent, amount, temporal reach and costs (Szinovacz, 1987). Thus, when examining power in families, the players, their relationships and resources, the type of decision, its relative importance and its frequency must be clearly defined. This review focuses on marital power or that shared between the couple or parental dyad.

In quantitative studies of power, the usual independent variables include economic power (contributions to household income), structural power (education, occupational status, gender) (Cast, 2003) and relationship power (emotional dependence), all thought to influence the dependent variables of decision-making outcomes and/or a measure of general overall power. How the independent variables interact to produce marital power is a key research question. The finding of overt, latent and invisible marital power adds complications. Both overt and latent power could be detected in decision making using an appropriate framework but invisible power is more likely connected to relationship and economic power, and detected only through discourse or qualitative analysis. There is no well-defined way to measure and study these various types of power. In this section, I present a brief review of relevant types of power and their influence on division of family household labour, followed by an outline of a decision-making framework that may be useful in examining the role of power in food choices.

Overt, latent and invisible power and household chores

According to Lukes (1974), power in political systems is demonstrated overtly by having the final say over the most important decisions, is exercised covertly when one person prevents grievances from being discussed (so conflict is hidden) and latently when conflicts of interest are prevented from even occurring through ideology that precludes alternatives and influences people to accept the status quo as natural and inevitable. In a key study of household decision making about domestic labour, childcare and sexuality, using Lukes' ideas, Komter (1989) found that marital power includes the exercise of overt power in observable negotiation or conflict as decision making (i.e. manifest power); of latent power that results in the less powerful partner anticipating the other partner's negative response and consciously deciding not to negotiate, resulting in latent grievances; and of invisible power where an inequitable situation is unconsciously accepted by the less powerful with gender role-based reasoning. In her sample, all of the women, regardless of employment, were doing most of the domestic work and more women than men wanted this changed. Cautiousness, sanctioning, waiting, ignoring and appeals to reason (i.e. power processes) were used to affect change and men used the last three more successfully than their wives. Invisible power was detected by men's greater self-esteem, slanted estimation of contributions to household chores and both partners' rationalization of inequities in face of the wife's discontent. Invisible power appeared to contribute to egalitarian women's inability to achieve equity in household tasks by promoting the status quo of gendered roles.

Structural, relational and economic power and household chores

Power patterns and perceptions are established early in relationships. In a 4-year longitudinal study of dating couples ($n = 101$), less than 20% reported power was shared and more often men were viewed as more powerful (Sprecher and Felmlee, 1997). Men were more likely to report having greater general power, greater decision-making power and less emotional involvement while women were more likely to report equal general and decision-making power and more emotional involvement. These patterns did not change over the length of the study and were not related to likelihood of break-up, suggesting that power bases are influenced by gender and emotional involvement (relational power) and are established early in a relationship.

Within the first 2 years of marriage, decisions about responsibilities for feminine household chores are made and patterns established. In a 2-year longitudinal study of newly-wed couples ($n = 207$), Cast (2003) found that women were doing more of these chores than men and that partners having more structural power (occupational status and education) and relationship power (less love for spouse), who feel it is their partner's role to do the feminine chores, are more able to use their own expectations to influence their partner to do this and also to successfully fend off arguments to the contrary.

The transition to parenthood most often creates a traditional gendered division of labour by reshaping the wife's responsibilities but not the husband's. Using two waves of US national survey data, Sanchez and Thomson (1997) found that the wife's responsibility for feminine household chores increased by 10% with birth of two or more children while her contribution to total household employment hours dropped by 18%. The effect on wife's employment hours was greatest if both partners had traditional gender ideologies and the husband was full-time employed. While the husband might do more feminine tasks right after childbirth, by 6 months postpartum the husband's role has shifted to being breadwinner and parent, while the wife's focus has shifted to being caretaker of house and child rather than worker (Cowan and Cowan, 1988). There is some evidence that love or relational power can affect this role transition. Over the first 2.5 years of marriage, Johnson and Huston (1998) found that the more the wife loved the husband, the more her preferences for division of childcare chores changed towards those of her husband after birth of the first child, irrespective of the wife's income. In contrast, the wife's preferences had no effect on husband's postnatal preferences, regardless of his love or her income. The influence of relational power on preferences may help to explain why many wives consider the gendered division of household labour fair and suggests that husband's invisible power can be magnified by their partner's love. Thagaard (1997) found that close emotional ties between spouses and a rich economy of gratitude resulting from mutually satisfactory work and family roles create the perception that power is shared.

At mid-life, economic and structural power also affect the balance of marital power. Several British studies examined how family income management affects power measured as 'degree of financial deprivation when money was tight' and as 'access to personal spending money' (Vogler and Pahl, 1994; Pahl, 1995). Of three patterns of management (joint, 20%; male-managed, 40%; female-managed, 40%) found, only 'joint pooling with equal access and decision-making' resulted in little gender discrimination in financial deprivation or personal spending money. In both other systems, men were better off by both measures and female deprivation was higher in female-managed systems than male at all income levels. Women's 'control' of money was more responsibility than power, especially if she received an allotment rather than access to total income. Power seemed to reside in decision making, which most men either controlled or only nominally shared. Pahl (1995) suggested gendered role expectations influenced the greater deprivation in female-managed systems, i.e. husband as breadwinner and wife as family caretaker, also noted by Kerr and Charles (1986). Vogler (1998) argued that husband's gender ideology influenced household income distribution and marital power (overt, covert and latent as per Lukes). If allocation is gendered and male breadwinner and female caretaker roles are assumed to define responsibilities, covert power eliminated discussion. If discourse (latent power) is patriarchal and the wife is viewed as non-earner or secondary earner, then egalitarian roles with shared income and truly shared decision making are unlikely to emerge. In an Australian study of 831 married or cohabiting employed men and women, men's economic power, defined as men's percentage contribution to family income, and gender role attitudes were the most significant predictors of men's involvement in feminine housework and household tasks overall (Baxter, 1992). As men earn more of the household income relative to their partners, their involvement declines. However, only actual hours of employment affect time women spend on housework, implying they have little economic power. These studies suggest that a husband's economic power must decline relative to his wife's and his gender role attitudes must become more liberal before egalitarian household labour arrangements emerge.

Several US qualitative studies indicate this power and gender role shift will be rare and difficult. Studying 15 couples with equitable division of household work, Risman and Johnson-Sumerford (1998) observed that sharing power (*n* = 9) depended upon equal or greater status of wife's employment, elimination of the male breadwinner belief, emotional closeness and shared egalitarian beliefs about household roles. Among the other six, the wife appeared more powerful and the husbands acquiescent. Finding truly equitable division of labour among volunteer couples (*n* = 75) was difficult and, among these 15, only one couple had renegotiated their roles after a decade of traditional gender roles.

This took 4 years and required the continuing investment of the wife's energy to maintain.

In a study of 30 dual-earner couples in which 22 were status-reversed (wife had higher educational attainment, higher status job and earned at least 50% more than her husband), Tichenor (1999) found that, without a mutual commitment to egalitarianism, status reversal did not lead to greater power or less housework for the wife. Compared with conventional couples, status-reversed women avoided actions that might be construed as powerful by not exercising control over decisions, emphasizing the co-ownership of assets, minimizing the income differences through manipulation of checking accounts and by redefining the provider role (jointly with their husbands) so husbands could still fulfil this. Their husbands rarely performed more than a third of the domestic labour and the wives felt guilty about not doing more. These status-reversed couples restructured the meanings of terms and behaviours to make their relationship appear more conventional. Dabbs (1994) found that traditional working-class wives who earned more than their husbands also discounted their power.

The breadwinner status quo is also maintained by attitudes towards the wife's income. A wife's earnings are seen as marginal, extra or non-essential, low priority and 'discounted' so that the wife is not seen as a co-provider (Hood, 1986; Blumberg and Coleman, 1989; Thompson and Walker, 1989; Pahl, 1995; Potuchek, 1997; Zuo, 1997; Tichenor, 1999), allowing the husband's job higher priority (Zvonkovic *et al.*, 1996). Although the wife's contribution might be significant, gratitude is less when this does not match gender norms in and outside the family. Indeed, a recent survey indicates that the pattern of gratitude for men and women's earnings still differs (Deutsch *et al.*, 2003). Gratitude for men's income was based on its relative proportion, rather than actual contribution to household income, reflecting appreciation of the breadwinner role. Men were grateful for the wife's actual earnings unless her relative share threatened to turn her into the provider. Thus gendered breadwinning remains the norm for men and a critical part of 'doing gender' which is reinforced by the level of gratitude expressed.

Examining marital power through decision making

Scanzoni and Polonko (1980) proposed a model for study of explicit family decision making that linked the social context, power processes used and outcomes. Scanzoni argued that it is the pursuit of gender role preferences through implicit or explicit decision making that creates the gendered household labour structure (Scanzoni and Fox, 1980). In couples with shared traditional values, familial roles and possible outcomes are prescribed, so implicit rather than explicit decision making occurs. Shared egalitarian views might force active negotiation and decision making as roles and outcomes are not well-defined (Scanzoni and Fox, 1980; Sillars and Kalbflesch, 1989). Lack of change in gendered behaviour, despite change in attitudes, reflects lack of explicit decision-making processes needed to alter reality.

Studies using the Scanzoni model indicated that process and outcomes were distinct for any given issue area, and that the importance of the issue to each partner as well as past cooperativeness influences the power processes used

(Godwin and Scanzoni, 1989a,b). Additionally, in dual-earner couples, only if the wife was much more egalitarian than her husband (disparity scores of 10+) did she have more process power than her husband (Kingsbury and Scanzoni, 1989). Minimal disparity (equally egalitarian) resulted in the husband having more ability to institute or resist change (process power).

While this model offers insight into explicit decision making, many food choice decisions are routine and likely affected by the latent and invisible power in the relationship. A qualitative study of marital problem-solving situations (74% about managing domestic chores or work–family conflicts) in multi-ethnic, middle-class couples ($n = 27$) revealed three phases: mobilizing the discussion, problem definition and planning the solution (Ball *et al.*, 1995). Wives usually mobilize the discussion by finding a favourable 'time or situation' but husbands could veto it altogether. When defining the problem, men tended to control the content and women the form (reciprocity of exchanges). Men defined the outcomes 78% of the time, often by ignoring the wife's recommendations. Thus the husband's latent power influenced the timing of discussions, while his overt power affected discussion content and outcomes.

Szinovacz (1987) outlined a more detailed dynamic model of family power relations that can be used to examine a particular decision-making (or controlling) event involving power exertion. This model includes the independent variables of: (i) structural context, (ii) member characteristics and (iii) situational contingencies, the multidimensional process variable of (iv) power exertion strategies, and the dependent variables of (v) control outcomes and (vi) outcome evaluations, all of which must be clearly defined and measured to produce comparable findings (Mizan, 1994).

The model offers a rich framework from which to draw research questions, variables of interest and ideas for the antecedents of phenomenon. For the purposes of this chapter, it allows the consideration of societal norms and obligation within the structural context, emotional commitment (relational power), gratitude versus expectation, personal locus of control, gender role ideologies or preferences and perceived fairness within member characteristics, comparison of distributive versus integrative conflict as situational contingencies and the effect of reciprocity of resources exchanged in outcome evaluations. Although the model focuses more on overt power, latent and invisible power could be revealed through outcome evaluations of practices and of discontent or dissatisfaction or unquestioned inexplicable inequities. Szinovacz suggested focusing on specific situations and examining the controlling events through direct observation as well as self-reports from all family members involved. For instance, understanding the power processes involved in family food choice would require examining the decision-making points from shopping to meal consumption (Brown and Miller, 2002a).

Involvement of Power in Family Food Choices

Many empirical studies have reported the father's influence on the foods served at family meals in both the USA (Bryan and Lowenberg, 1958; Cosper and

Wakefield, 1975; Burt and Hertzler, 1978; Weidner *et al.*, 1985; DeVault, 1987; Kirk and Gillespie, 1990; Bradbard *et al.*, 1997; Brown and Miller, 2002b; Krummel *et al.*, 2002) and in parts of Europe (Murcott, 1983; Kerr and Charles, 1986; Pill and Parry, 1989; Mennell *et al.*, 1992; de Bourdeaudhuij, 1997; Stratton and Bromley, 1999). The influence of children's preferences was also noted (Kirk and Gillespie, 1990; Bradbard *et al.*, 1997; Krummel *et al.*, 2002). Because of his influence, some advised that fathers be involved in interventions to influence dietary change (Burt and Hertzler, 1978; Weidner *et al.*, 1985; de Bourdeaudhuij, 1997) or suggested that changes will require intra-family interaction (Yetley and Roderuck, 1980; Baranowski and Hearn, 1997). In 80% of these studies, only women were participants. Power was not measured in any. Instead, a form of latent power emerged in which women knew husbands' reactions from experience and so no longer considered 'new foods'. In the most direct identification of the husband's power, DeVault (1990) described women's work to feed their family as 'invisible'. Conflict was avoided by deference to and accommodation of the desire of husbands, reflecting a power imbalance.

Observational studies of family meals reveal both husband's and male children's power. When dinner table conflicts arise, children verbally attacked mothers twice as often as fathers, who were the least likely target among family members. Mothers were more likely than fathers to be peacemakers, ending conflicts with compromise or a 'draw', while fathers appeared generally more powerful (Vuchinich, 1987). In a small longitudinal study of families with young children, most fathers influenced family meal food choices. Boys challenged their mother's food rules, sometimes with the father's silent blessing, while girls accepted rules with little protest enabling continuance of patriarchal family relationships (Grieshaber, 1997).

Only a few studies have examined influences on food choice decision making in families using multiple perspectives. Using a random sample of families (*n* = 336), Schafer and Keith (1981) found that among five factors, family members, especially the husband, had the most influence on wife's food choices at mid-life. Examining member influence on altering food choices in families with adolescents (*n* = 92), de Bourdeaudhuij and van Oost (1998b) found mothers could only alter fat content of meal food choices if they were acceptable to the father and, to a lesser extent, the children. The power to resist or disapprove choices lay with fathers as well as adolescents who used direct communication strategies to squash presentation of disliked foods. Brown and Miller (2002b) found that the wife only had overt power to alter food choices if she and her husband shared egalitarian values where a pattern of negotiation, established early in the marriage, continued. If both partners shared or the husband had more traditional gender role values, the husband's power to veto or resist changes was established early in the marriage and wives found altering food choices later difficult.

When traditional gender role norms hold sway, what power processes might gain husband's compliance? Such techniques include rewarding, punishing, claiming expertise (punishment or reward due to higher authority), appeal to legitimacy (through internal norms) and appeal to referents (external norms) (French and Raven, 1960; Marwell and Schmitt, 1967). In couples where the wife had greater economic power but respected traditional gender norms, wives used logic and persuasion, avoiding ultimatums and vetoes, so that men retained 'face' (Tichenor, 1999). Disputes may also be settled by indirect means such as ingratiation, aversion stimulation, hinting, instilling guilt or deceit (Rudd and Burant, 1995). However, in a study of power processes used by miners' wives ($n = 45$) to alter men's use of leisure time, bargaining and 'giving orders' only worked if the husband held non-traditional views (Collis, 1999). Bargaining declined, reflecting husband's latent power as wives anticipated losing arguments. Manipulation, supplication, sanctioning (having set mealtimes) or disengagement had limited success. When influence strategies failed, wives turned to limited coping and adjustment strategies to deal with the status quo. This illustrates the difficulty women might face in non-egalitarian relationships, where husbands hold overt, latent and invisible power, when attempting to change food choices.

Few studies have examined strategies used to alter husband's food choices. Early in marriage, efforts to actively change food choices involved 'tricking', requesting specific recipes and monitoring choices (nagging) (Bove *et al.*, 2003). Later, hidden substitutions, not purchasing foods and sometimes enforcing choices are used (Gregory, 1999; Krummel *et al.*, 2002; Blake and Bisogni, 2003). Sometimes, wives formed coalitions with children to overrule a husband's preferences or establish a domain of influence within the husband's preferences where latitude allows changes, but only in couples with shared egalitarian views did overt discussion/negotiation occur (Brown and Miller, 2002b). Altering established food choices is difficult unless the husband had few dislikes or is not 'picky'.

Conclusions

Because food chores are part of gendered feminine household chores wherein gender role ideology influences who does these and how, food choice decisions for family meals are likely influenced by gender role expectations. More equitable sharing of household chores including food chores only emerges if both partners share egalitarian values and only with this sharing does shared decision making about food choices emerge. The connection between the ideal male provider (breadwinner) and masculinity has been evident for over a century (Hood, 1986; Deutsch *et al.*, 2003). This ideal is expressed as a deep-seated gender ideology that is continuously reinforced by couple interaction (Zvonkovic *et al.*, 1996; Tichenor, 1999). Male marital power is embedded in this traditional breadwinner role and only if this is diminished so that wives are co-providers and partners share egalitarian values do wives share power including decision-making power. Power and gender role expectations shape the economy of gratitude so that traditional husbands, viewed as the primary breadwinner, can claim more love and gratitude for that role. It is likely that this 'gratitude' shapes women's deference to their husband's food preferences and thus food choices in traditional households (e.g. Kerr and Charles, 1986). This deference to male preferences and power means that food choices at family meals are restricted to those that both husband and wife like at best (Jansson, 1995; Brown and Miller,

2002b) and is likely to limit possible food choices overall. Since US survey data indicate that women still do the majority of food chores and couples with truly egalitarian behaviour are hard to find, it is likely that most US households operate in a traditional gender role setting. The deference to male preferences and power means that just targeting the female gatekeeper as change agent does not guarantee the infiltration of family meals with healthful food choices.

Murcott (1995) warns that 'we should not separate food choice from social influences' and that we will only understand food choice behaviour when we understand the social relationships in which it is embedded. We actually know little about how the interaction of gender, gender roles, power and partner trade-offs affect food decision making and food choice although we can measure the outcome as individual food intake. Understanding these interactions is critical. Contrasting the traditional ideology of English mid-life families with the more egalitarian pattern of Sweden, Jansson (1995) proposed that predominant gender role patterns could affect the implementation of national dietary guidelines. Further research should examine intra-family decision making in more detail and rectify the predominantly female (and mother) perspective of the published literature. Only when we understand the interaction patterns among family members around food will we be able to understand key determinants of food choices in mid-life families.

References

Aish, A. (1996) A comparison of female and male cardiac patients' responses to nursing care promoting nutritional self-care. *Canadian Journal of Cardiovascular Nursing* 7, 4–13.

Allen, S.M. and Hawkins, A.J. (1999) Maternal gatekeeping: mothers' beliefs and behaviors that inhibit greater father involvement in family work. *Journal of Marriage and the Family* 61, 199–212.

Amato, P.R. and Booth, A. (1995) Changes in gender role attitudes and marital quality. *American Sociological Review* 60, 58–66.

Ball, F.L.J., Cowan, P. and Cowan, C.P. (1995) Who's got the power? Gender differences in partners' perceptions of influence during marital problem-solving discussions. *Family Process* 34, 303–321.

Baranowski, T. and Hearn, M.D. (1997) Health behavior interventions within families. In: Gochman, D.S. (ed.) *Handbook of Health Behavior Research IV: Relevance for the Professionals and Issues for the Future.* Plenum Press, New York, pp. 303–323.

Baxter, J. (1992) Power attitudes and time: the domestic division of labor. *Journal of Comparative Family Studies* 23, 165–182.

Beere, C.A. (1990) *Gender Roles: A Handbook of Tests and Measures.* Greenwood Press, New York.

Benin, M.H. and Edwards, D.A. (1990) Adolescents' chores: the difference between dual- and single-earner families. *Journal of Marriage and the Family* 52, 361–373.

Biernat, M. and Wortman, C.B. (1991) Sharing of home responsibilities between professionally employed women and their husbands. *Journal of Personality and Social Psychology* 60, 844–860.

Blair, S.L. (1992) The sex typing of children's household labor: parental influence of daughters' and sons' housework. *Youth and Society* 24, 178–203.

Blair, S.L. and Lichter, D.T. (1991) Measuring the division of household labor: gender segregation of housework among American couples. *Journal of Family Issues* 12, 91–113.

Blake, C. and Bisogni, C.A. (2003) Personal and family food choice schemas of rural women in upstate New York. *Journal of Nutrition Education and Behavior* 35, 282–293.

Blood, R.O. and Wolfe, D.M. (1960) *Husbands and Wives: The Dynamics of Married Living.* Free Press, New York.

Blumberg, R.L. and Coleman, M.T. (1989) A theoretical look at the gender balance of power in the American couple. *Journal of Family Issues* 10, 225–250.

Borah-Gidens, J. and Falciglia, G.A. (1993) A meta-analysis of the relationship in food preferences between parents and children. *Journal of Nutrition Education* 25, 102–107.

Bovbjerg, V.E., McCann, B.S., Brief, D.J., Follette, W.C., Retzlaff, B.M., Dowdy, A.A., Walden, C.E. and Knopp, R.H. (1995) Spouse support and long-term adherence to lipid-lowering diets. *American Journal of Epidemiology* 141, 451–460.

Bove, C.F., Sobal, J. and Rauschenbach, B.S. (2003) Food choices among newly married couples: convergence, conflict, individualism and projects. *Appetite* 40, 25–41.

Bradbard, S., Michaels, E.F., Fleming, K. and Campbell, M. (1997) *Understanding the Food Choices of Low-income Families: Summary of Findings.* US Department of Agriculture, Alexandria, Virginia.

Brewster, K.L. and Padavic, I. (2000) Changes in gender ideology, 1977–1996: the contributions of intra-cohort change and population turnover. *Journal of Marriage and the Family* 62, 477–487.

Broderick, C.B. (1993) *Understanding Family Process.* Sage Publications, Newbury Park, California.

Broman, C.L. (1991) Gender, work–family roles, and psychological well-being of blacks. *Journal of Marriage and the Family* 53, 509–520.

Brown, J.L. and Miller, D. (2002a) Gender role preference and family food chores. *Journal of Nutrition Education and Behavior* 34, 100–108.

Brown, J.L. and Miller, D. (2002b) Couples' gender role preferences and management of family food preferences. *Journal of Nutrition Education and Behavior* 34, 215–223.

Bryan, M.S. and Lowenberg, M.E. (1958) The father's influence on young children's food preferences. *Journal of the American Dietetic Association* 34, 30–35.

Burt, J.V. and Hertzler, A.A. (1978) Parental influence on the child's food preference. *Journal of Nutrition Education* 10, 127–128.

Campbell, T. (1994) Families influence health. *The Futurist* 28, 59.

Cast, A.D. (2003) Power and the ability to define the situation. *Social Psychology Quarterly* 66, 185–201.

Charles, N. and Kerr, M. (1988) *Women, Food and Families.* Manchester University Press, Manchester, UK.

Cigoli, V., Binda, W. and Marta, E. (1994) Marital relationships and type II diabetes. *Family Systems Medicine* 12, 295–314.

Collis, M. (1999) Marital conflict and men's leisure: how women negotiate male power in a small mining community. *Journal of Sociology* 35, 60–76.

Coltrane, S. (2000) Research on household labor: modeling and measuring the social embeddedness of routine family work. *Journal of Marriage and the Family* 62, 1208–1233.

Cosper, B.A. and Wakefield, L.M. (1975) Food choices of women. *Journal of the American Dietetic Association* 66, 152–155.

Coverman, S. and Sheley, J.F. (1986) Change in men's housework and child-care time, 1965–1975. *Journal of Marriage and the Family* 48, 413–422.

Cowan, C.P. and Cowan, P.A. (1988) Who does what when partners become parents: implications for men, women and marriage. *Marriage and Family Review* 13, 105–132.

Craig, P.L. and Truswell, A.S. (1988) Changes in food habits when people get married: analysis of food frequencies. In: Truswell, A.S. and Wahlqvist, M.L. (eds) *Food Habits in Australia*. Rene Gordon, Melbourne, Victoria, Australia, pp. 94–111.

Cromwell, R.E. and Olson, D.H. (1975) *Power in Families*. John Wiley, New York.

Cullen, K.W., Lara, K.M. and de Moor, C. (2002) Familial concordance of dietary fat practices and intakes. *Family and Community Health* 25, 65–75.

Cunningham, M. (2001) The influence of parental attitudes and behaviors on children's attitudes toward gender and household labor in early adulthood. *Journal of Marriage and the Family* 63, 111–122.

Dabbs, J.M. (1994) Women and men in central Appalachia: a qualitative study of marital power. Dissertation, University of North Texas, Denton, Texas.

De Bourdeaudhuij, I. (1997) Perceived family members' influence on introducing healthy food into the family. *Health Education Research* 12, 77–90.

De Bourdeaudhuij, I. and van Oost, P. (1998a) Family characteristics and health behaviors of adolescents and families. *Psychology and Health* 13, 785–803.

De Bourdeaudhuij, I. and van Oost, P. (1998b) Family members' influences on decision making about food: differences in perception and relationship with healthy eating. *American Journal of Health Promotion* 13, 73–81.

Deutsch, F.M., Roksa, J. and Messke, C. (2003) How gender counts when couples count their money. *Sex Roles* 48, 291–304.

DeVault, M.L. (1987) Doing housework: feeding and family life. In: Gerstel, N. and Gross, H.E. (eds) *Families and Work*. Temple University Press, Philadelphia, Pennsylvania, pp. 178–191.

DeVault, M.L. (1990) Conflict over housework: a problem that (still) has no name. In: Kriesberg, L. (ed.) *Research in Social Movements, Conflict and Change*. JAI Press, Greenwich, Connecticut, pp. 189–202.

DeVault, M.L. (1991) *Feeding the Family: The Social Organization of Caring as Gendered Work*. Chicago University Press, Chicago, Illinois.

Devine, C.M. and Olson, C. (1991) Women's dietary prevention motives: life stage influences. *Journal of Nutrition Education* 23, 269–274.

Devine, C.M., Connors, M., Bisogni, C.A. and Sobal, J. (1998) Life-course influences on fruit and vegetable trajectories: qualitative analysis of food choices. *Journal of Nutrition Education* 30, 361–370.

Devine, C.M., Connors, M.M., Sobal, J. and Bisogni, C.A. (2003) Sandwiching it in: spillover of work onto food choices and family roles in low- and moderate income urban households. *Social Science & Medicine* 56, 617–630.

Fagerli, R.A. and Wandel, M. (1999) Gender differences in opinions and practices with regard to a healthy diet. *Appetite* 32, 171–190.

Feiring, C. and Lewis, M. (1987) The ecology of some middle class families at dinner. *International Journal of Behavioral Development* 10, 377–390.

Fisher, J.O., Mitchell, D.C., Smiciklas-Wright, H. and Birch, L.L. (2002) Parental influences on young girls' fruit and vegetable, micronutrient and fat intakes. *Journal of the American Dietetic Association* 102, 58–64.

Fisher, L., Ransom, D.C., Terry, H.E. and Burge, S. (1992) The California Family Health Project: IV. Family structure/organization and adult health. *Family Process* 31, 399–419.

Fisher, L., Ransom, D.C. and Terry, H.E. (1993) The California Family Health Project: VII. Summary and integration of findings. *Family Process* 32, 69–86.

Fox, G.L. and Murry, V.M. (2000) Gender and families: feminist perspectives and family research. *Journal of Marriage and the Family* 62, 1160–1172.

French, J.R.P. and Raven, B. (1960) The bases of social power. In: Cartwright, D. and Zander, A. (eds) *Group Dynamics*, 2nd edn. Harper and Row, New York, pp. 607–623.

Furst, T., Connors, M., Bisogni, C.A., Sobal, J. and Falk, L.W. (1996) Food choice: a conceptual model of the process. *Appetite* 26, 247–266.

Gedrich, K. (2003) Determinants of nutritional behavior: a multitude of levers for successful interventions? *Appetite* 41, 231–238.

Gershuny, J. and Robinson, J.P. (1988) Historical changes in the household division of labor. *Demography* 25, 537–552.

Gill, G.K. (1998) The strategic involvement of children in housework: an Australian case of two-income families. *International Journal of Comparative Sociology* 39, 301–314.

Gillespie, A. and Achterberg, C. (1989) Comparison of family interaction patterns related to food and nutrition. *Journal of the American Dietetic Association* 89, 509–512.

Godwin, D.D. and Scanzoni, J. (1989a) Couple decision-making: commonalities and differences across issues and spouses. *Journal of Family Issues* 10, 291–310.

Godwin, D.D. and Scanzoni, J. (1989b) Couple consensus during marital joint decision-making: a context, process, outcome model. *Journal of Marriage and the Family* 51, 943–956.

Gonzales, E.N., Marshall, J.A., Heimendinger, J., Crane, L.A. and Neal, W.A. (2002) Home and eating environments are associated with saturated fat intake in children in rural West Virginia. *Journal of the American Dietetic Association* 102, 657–663.

Gorall, D.M. and Olson, D.H. (1995) Circumplex model of family systems: integrating ethnic diversity and other social systems. In: Mikesell, R.H., Lusterman, D.D. and McDaniel, S.H. (eds) *Integrating Family Therapy: Handbook of Family Psychology and Systems Theory*. American Psychological Association, Washington, DC, pp. 217–233.

Greenstein, T.N. (1996a) Husbands' participation in domestic labor: interactive effects of wives' and husbands' gender ideologies. *Journal of Marriage and the Family* 58, 585–595.

Greenstein, T.N. (1996b) Gender ideology and perceptions of the fairness of the division of household labor: effects on marital quality. *Social Forces* 74, 1029–1042.

Greenstein, T.N. (2000) Economic dependence, gender and the division of labor in the home: a replication and extension. *Journal of Marriage and the Family* 62, 322–335.

Gregory, S. (1999) Gender roles and food in families. In: McKie, L., Bowlby, S. and Gregory, S. (eds) *Gender, Power and the Household*. St Martin's Press, Inc., New York, pp. 60–75.

Grieshaber, S. (1997) Mealtime rituals: power and resistance in the construction of mealtime rules. *British Journal of Sociology* 48, 649–666.

Gupta, S. (1999) The effect of transitions in marital status on men's performance of housework. *Journal of Marriage and the Family* 61, 700–711.

Hannon, P.A., Bowen, D.J., Moinpour, C.M. and McLerran, D.F. (2003) Correlations in perceived food use between the family food preparer and their spouses and children. *Appetite* 40, 77–83.

Harnack, L., Story, M., Martinson, B., Neumark-Sztainer, D. and Stang, J. (1998) Guess who's cooking? The role of men in meal planning, shopping and preparation in US families. *Journal of the American Dietetic Association* 98, 995–1000.

Harrap, S.B., Stebbing, M., Hopper, J.L., Hoang, H.N. and Giles, G.G. (2000) Familial patterns of co-variation for cardiovascular risk factors in adults: The Victorian Family Heart Study. *American Journal of Epidemiology* 152, 704–715.

Harris, R.J. and Firestone, J.M. (1998) Changes in predictors of gender role ideologies among women: a multivariate analysis. *Sex Roles* 38, 239–252.

Haynes, F.E. (2000) Gender and family ideas: an exploratory study of black middle-class Americans. *Journal of Family Issues* 21, 811–837.

Hepworth, J. (1999) Gender and the capacity of women with NIDDM to implement medical advice. *Scandinavian Journal of Public Health* 27, 260–266.

Hochschild, A.R. (1989a) *The Second Shift*. Viking, New York.

Hochschild, A.R. (1989b) The economy of gratitude. In: Franks, D.D. and McCarthy, E.D. (eds) *The Sociology of Emotions: Original Essays and Research Papers*. JAI Press, Greenwich, Connecticut, pp. 95–113.

Hood, J.C. (1986) The provider role: its meaning and measurement. *Journal of Marriage and the Family* 48, 349–359.

Hupkens, C.L.H., Knibbe, R.B. and Drop, M.J. (2000) Social class differences in food consumption: the explanatory value of permissiveness and health and cost considerations. *European Journal of Public Health* 10, 108–113.

Jansson, S. (1995) Food practices and division of domestic labor: a comparison between British and Swedish households. *The Sociological Review* 43, 462–477.

Jensen, K.O. and Holm, L. (1999) Preferences, quantities, and concerns: socio-cultural perspectives on the gendered consumption of foods. *European Journal of Clinical Nutrition* 53, 351–359.

Johnson, E.M. and Huston, T.L. (1998) The perils of love or why wives adapt to husbands during transition to parenthood. *Journal of Marriage and the Family* 60, 195–204.

Kemmer, D. (1999) Food preparation and the division of domestic labor among newly married and cohabiting couples. *British Food Journal* 101, 570–579.

Kemmer, D., Anderson, A. and Marshall, D. (1998) Living together and eating together: changes in food choice and eating habits during the transition from single to married/cohabiting. *The Sociological Review* 46, 48–72.

Kerr, M. and Charles, N. (1986) Servers and providers: the distribution of food within the family. *Sociology Review* 34, 115–157.

Kingsbury, N.M. and Scanzoni, J. (1989) Process power and decision outcomes among dual-career couples. *Journal of Comparative Family Studies* 20, 231–246.

Kintner, M., Boss, P.G. and Johnson, N. (1981) The relationship between dysfunctional family environments and family member food intake. *Journal of Marriage and the Family* 43, 633–641.

Kirk, M.C. and Gillespie, A.H. (1990) Factors affecting food choices of working mothers with young families. *Journal of Nutrition Education* 22, 161–168.

Kluwer, E.S., Heesink, J.A.M. and van de Vliert, E. (1997) The marital dynamics of conflict over the division of labor. *Journal of Marriage and the Family* 59, 635–653.

Knudson-Martin, C. and Mahoney, A.R. (1998) Language and processes in the construction of equality in new marriages. *Family Relations* 47, 81–91.

Knuiman, M.W., Divitini, M.L., Bartholomew, H.C. and Welborn, T.A. (1996) Spouse correlations in cardiovascular risk factors and the effect of marriage duration. *American Journal of Epidemiology* 143, 48–53.

Komter, A. (1989) Hidden power in marriage. *Gender and Society* 3, 187–216.

Kristofferzon, M., Lofmark, R. and Carlsson, M. (2003) Myocardial infarction: gender differences in coping and social support. *Journal of Advanced Nursing* 44, 360–374.

Kroska, A. (2003) Investigating gender differences in the meaning of household chores and child care. *Journal of Marriage and the Family* 65, 456–473.

Krummel, D.A., Humphries, D. and Tessaro, I. (2002) Focus groups on cardiovascular health in rural women: implications for health. *Journal of Nutrition Education and Behavior* 34, 38–46.

Laitinen, S., Hogstrom, P. and Rasanen, L. (1997) Similarity of food choices among young Finnish couples. *Journal of Human Nutrition and Dietetics* 10, 353–360.

Lavee, Y. and Katz, R. (2002) Division of labor, perceived fairness and marital quality: the effect of gender ideology. *Journal of Marriage and the Family* 64, 27–39.

Lennon, M.C. and Rosenfield, S. (1994) Relative fairness and the division of household work: the importance of options. *American Journal of Sociology* 100, 506–531.

Lewin, K. (1943) Forces behind food habits and methods of change. In: *The Problem of Changing Food Habits*. Bulletin No. 108. National Academy of Science, National Research Council, Washington, DC, pp. 35–65.

Losh-Hesselbart, S. (1987) Development of gender roles. In: Sussman, B.M. and Steinmetz, K.S. (eds) *Handbook of Marriage and the Family*. Plenum Press, New York, pp. 535–563.

Lukes, S. (1974) *Power: A Radical View*. Macmillan, London.

Lupton, D. (2000) The heart of the meal: food preferences and habits among rural Australian couples. *Sociology of Health and Illness* 22, 94–109.

Lye, D.E. and Biblarz, T.J. (1993) The effects of attitudes toward family life and gender roles on marital satisfaction. *Journal of Family Issues* 14, 157–188.

Macario, E. and Sorensen, G. (1998) Spousal similarities in fruit and vegetable consumption. *American Journal of Health Promotion* 12, 369–377.

McHale, S.M. and Crouter, A.C. (1992) You can't always get what you want: incongruence between sex-role attitudes and family work roles and its implications for marriage. *Journal of Marriage and the Family* 54, 537–547.

McHale, S.M., Bartko, W.T., Crouter, A.C. and Perry-Jenkins, M. (1990) Children's housework and psychosocial functioning: the mediating effects of parents' sex role behaviors and attitudes. *Child Development* 61, 1413–1426.

McHugh, M.C. and Frieze, I.H. (1997) The measurement of gender-role attitudes: a review and commentary. *Psychology of Women Quarterly* 21, 1–16.

Manke, B., Seery, B.L., Crouter, A.C. and McHale, S.M. (1994) The three corners of domestic labor: mothers', fathers' and children's weekday and weekend housework. *Journal of Marriage and the Family* 56, 657–668.

Marshall, D.W. and Anderson, A.S. (2002) Proper meals in transition: young married couples on the nature of eating together. *Appetite* 39, 193–206.

Marwell, G. and Schmitt, D.R. (1967) Dimensions of compliance-gaining behavior: an empirical analysis. *Sociometry* 30, 350–364.

Mennell, S., Murcott, A. and van Otterloo, A.H. (1992) *The Sociology of Food: Eating, Diet and Culture*. Sage Publications, Newbury Park, California, pp. 95–146.

Milkie, M.A. and Peltola, P. (1999) Playing all the roles: gender and the work–family balancing act. *Journal of Marriage and the Family* 61, 476–490.

Miller, J.S. and Ackerman, N.M. (1990) Predictors of time allocation of food tasks in dual-earner families. *Home Economics Research Journal* 18, 286–302.

Mizan, A.N. (1994) Family power studies: some major methodological issues. *International Journal of Sociology of the Family* 24, 85–91.

Mooney, K.M. and Lorenz, E. (1997) The effects of food and gender on interpersonal perceptions. *Sex Roles* 36, 639–653.

Murcott, A. (1983) It's a pleasure to cook for him: food, mealtimes and gender in some South Wales households. In: Garmarnikow, E., Morgan, D.H.J., Purvis, J. and Taylorso, D. (eds) *The Public and the Private*. Heinemann, London, pp. 78–90.

Murcott, A. (1995) Social influences on food choice and dietary change: a sociological attitude. *Proceedings of the Nutrition Society* 54, 729–735.

Nestle, M., Wing, R., Birch, L., DiSogra, L., Drewnowski, A., Middleton, S., Sigman-Grant, M., Sobal, J., Winston, M. and Economos, C. (1998) Behavioral and social influences on food choice. *Nutrition Reviews* 56, S50–S74.

Neumark-Sztainer, D., Hannan, P.J., Story, M., Croll, J. and Perry, C. (2003) Family meal patterns: associations with socio-demographic characteristics and improved dietary intake among adolescents. *Journal of the American Dietetic Association* 103, 317–322.

Noller, P. and Fitzpatrick, M. (1993) *Communication in Family Relationships*. Prentice-Hall, Englewood Cliffs, New Jersey.

Pahl, J. (1995) His money, her money: recent research on financial organization in marriage. *Journal of Economic Psychology* 16, 361–376.

Parson, T. and Bales, R.F. (1955) *Family, Socialization and Interaction Process*. Free Press, Glencoe, Illinois.

Pill, R. and Parry, O. (1989) Making changes – women, food and families. *Health Education Journal* 48, 51–54.

Pina, D.L. and Bengston, V.L. (1993) The division of household labor and wives' happiness: ideology, employment and perceptions of support. *Journal of Marriage and the Family* 55, 901–912.

Potuchek, J.L. (1997) *Who Supports the Family? Gender and Breadwinning in Dual Earner Marriages*. Stanford University Press, Stanford, California.

Pyke, K. and Coltrane, S. (1996) Entitlement, obligation and gratitude in family work. *Journal of Family Issues* 17, 60–82.

Risman, B.J. and Johnson-Sumerford, D. (1998) Doing it fairly: a study of postgender marriages. *Journal of Marriage and the Family* 60, 23–40.

Rogers, M.F. (1974) Instrumental and infra-resources: the bases of power. *American Journal of Sociology* 79, 1418–1433.

Rogers, S.J. and Amato, P.R. (2000) Have changes in gender relations affected marital quality? *Social Forces* 79, 731–753.

Roos, G., Prattala, R. and Koshi, K. (2001) Men, masculinity and food: interviews with Finnish carpenters and engineers. *Appetite* 37, 47–56.

Rozin, P. (1996) The socio-cultural context of eating and food choice. In: Meiselman, H.L. and MacFie, H.J.H. (eds) *Food Choice, Acceptance and Consumption*. Chapman and Hall, London, pp. 83–104.

Rudd, J.E. and Burant, P.A. (1995) A study of women's compliance-gaining behaviors in violent and non-violent relationships. *Communication Research Reports* 12, 134–144.

Russell, B.S., Harris, B.V., Huster, G.A. and Sprecher, D.L. (1994) Effect of premature myocardial infarction in men on the eating habits of spouses and offspring. *Journal of the American Dietetic Association* 94, 859–864.

Sanchez, L. and Kane, E.W. (1996) Women and men's construction of perceptions of housework fairness. *Journal of Family Issues* 17, 358–387.

Sanchez, L. and Thomson, E. (1997) Becoming mothers and fathers: parenthood, gender and the division of labor. *Gender and Society* 11, 747–772.

Savoca, M. and Miller, C. (2001) Food selection and eating patterns: themes found among people with type 2 diabetes mellitus. *Journal of Nutrition Education and Behavior* 33, 224–233.

Scanzoni, J. and Fox, G.L. (1980) Sex roles, family and society: the seventies and beyond. *Journal of Marriage and the Family* 42, 743–756.

Scanzoni, J. and Polonko, K. (1980) A conceptual approach to explicit marital negotiation. *Journal of Marriage and the Family* 42, 31–44.

Schafer, R.B. and Keith, P.M. (1981) Influences on food decisions across the family life cycle. *Journal of the American Dietetic Association* 78, 460–466.

Schafer, R.B. and Schafer, E. (1989) Relationship between gender and food roles in families. *Journal of Nutrition Education* 21, 119–126.

Schafer, R.B., Schafer, E., Dunbar, M. and Keith, P.M. (1999) Marital food interaction and dietary behavior. *Social Science & Medicine* 38, 787–796.

Schofield, T., Connell, R.W., Walker, L., Wood, J.F. and Butland, D.L. (2000) Understanding men's health and illness: a gender-relations approach to policy, research and practice. *Journal of the American College of Health* 48, 247–255.

Scott, J.W. (1986) Gender: a useful category of historical analysis. *American Historical Review* 91, 1053–1075.

Scott, J., Alwin, D.F. and Braun, M. (1996) Generational change in gender-role attitudes: Britain in a cross-national perspective. *Sociology* 30, 471–492.

Sexton, M., Bross, D., Hebel, J.R., Schumann, B.C., Gerace, T.A., Lasser, N. and Wright, N. (1987) Risk-factor changes in wives with husbands at high-risk of coronary heart disease (CHD): the spin-off effect. *Journal of Behavioral Medicine* 10, 251–261.

Shattuck, A.L., White, E. and Kristal, A. (1992) How women's adopted low fat diets affect their husbands. *American Journal of Public Health* 82, 1244–1250.

Sillars, A.L. and Kalbflesch, P.J. (1989) Implicit and explicit decision-making styles in couples. In: Brinberg, D. and Jaccard, J. (eds) *Dyadic Decision-Making*. Springer Verleg, New York, pp. 179–215.

Skinner, J., Carruth, B.R., Moran, J. III, Houck, K., Schmidhamme, J., Reed, A., Coletta, F., Cotter, R. and Ott, C. (1998) Toddler's food preferences: concordance with family members' preferences. *Journal of Nutrition Education* 30, 17–22.

Smith, P.J. and Beaujot, R. (1999) Men's orientation toward marriage and family roles. *Journal of Comparative Family Studies* 30, 471–487.

Sobal, J., Rauschenbach, B.S. and Frongillo, E.A. (1992) Marital status, fatness and obesity. *Social Science & Medicine* 35, 915–923.

Sprecher, S. and Felmlee, D. (1997) The balance of power in romantic heterosexual couples over time from his and her perspectives. *Sex Roles* 37, 361–379.

Stratton, P. and Bromley, K. (1999) Families' accounts of the causal processes in food choice. *Appetite* 33, 89–108.

Sullivan, O. (1997) Time waits for no (wo)man: an investigation of the gendered experience of domestic time. *Sociology* 31, 221–239.

Szinovacz, M.E. (1984) Changing family roles and interactions. *Marriage and Family Review* 7, 163–201.

Szinovacz, M.E. (1987) Family power. In: Sussman, B.M. and Steinmetz, K.S. (eds) *Handbook of Marriage and the Family*. Plenum Press, New York, pp. 651–693.

Thagaard, T. (1997) Gender, power and love: a study of the interaction between spouses. *Acta Sociologica* 40, 359–376.

Thompson, L. and Walker, A.J. (1989) Gender in families: women and men in marriage, work and parenthood. *Journal of Marriage and the Family* 51, 845–871.

Thorn, B.L. and Gilbert, L.A. (1998) Antecedents of work and family role expectations of college men. *Journal of Family Psychology* 12, 259–267.

Tibbs, T., Haire-Joshu, D., Schechtman, K.B., Brownson, R.C., Nanney, M.S., Houston, C. and Auslander, W. (2001) The relationship of parental modeling, eating patterns and dietary intake among African–American parents. *Journal of the American Dietetic Association* 101, 535–541.

Tichenor, V.J. (1999) Status and income as gendered resources: the case of marital power. *Journal of Marriage and the Family* 61, 638–650.

Twiggs, J.E., McQuillan, J. and Ferree, M.M. (1999) Meaning and measurement: reconceptualizing measures of the division of household labor. *Journal of Marriage and the Family* 61, 712–724.

US Bureau of the Census (2000) *Households and Families: 2000*. Census 2000 Brief. US Government Printing Office, Washington, DC.

Vogler, C. (1998) Money in the household: some underlying issues of power. *The Sociological Review* 46, 687–713.

Vogler, C. and Pahl, J. (1994) Money, power and inequality within marriage. *The Sociological Review* 42, 263–288.

Vuchinich, S. (1987) Starting and stopping spontaneous family conflicts. *Journal of Marriage and the Family* 49, 591–601.

Warde, A. and Hetherington, K. (1994) English households and routine food practices: a research note. *The Sociological Review* 42, 758–778.

Weidner, G., Archer, B.H. and Matarazzo, J.D. (1985) Family consumption of low fat foods: stated preference versus actual consumption. *Journal of Applied Social Psychology* 15, 773–779.

White, E., Hurlich, M., Thompson, R.S., Woods, M.N., Henderson, M.M., Urban, N. and Kristal, A. (1991) Dietary change among husbands of participants in a low-fat dietary intervention. *American Journal of Preventive Medicine* 7, 319–325.

Wickrama, K.A.S., Lorenz, F.O., Wallace, L.E., Peiris, L., Conger, R.D. and Elder, G.H. (2001) Family influence on physical health during the middle years: the case for hypertension. *Journal of Marriage and the Family* 63, 527–539.

Yetley, E.A. and Roderuck, C. (1980) Nutrition knowledge and health goals of young spouses. *Journal of the American Dietetic Association* 17, 31–40.

Young, E.M., Fors, S.W., Fasha, E.D. and Hayes, D.M. (2004) Associations between perceived parent behaviors and middle school student fruit and vegetable consumption. *Journal of Nutrition Education and Behavior* 36, 2–12.

Zimmerman, R.S., Gerace, T.A., Smith, J.C. and Benezra, J. (1988) The effects of a worksite health promotion program on the wives of fire fighters. *Social Science & Medicine* 26, 537–543.

Zuo, J. (1997) The effect of men's breadwinner status on their changing gender beliefs. *Sex Roles* 37, 799–816.

Zvonkovic, A.M., Greaves, K.M., Schmiege, C.J. and Hall, L.D. (1996) The marital construction of gender through work and family decisions: a qualitative analysis. *Journal of Marriage and the Family* 58, 91–100.

15 Food Choices in Later Life

MARGARET LUMBERS[1] AND MONIQUE RAATS[2]

[1]Food, Consumer Behaviour and Health Research Centre, School of Management, University of Surrey, Guildford GU2 7XH, UK; [2]Food, Consumer Behaviour and Health Research Centre, Department of Psychology, University of Surrey, Guildford GU2 7XH, UK

Maintaining Health, Independence and Quality of Life

Almost all countries are experiencing increases in the proportion of older people in their populations (Kinsella and Velkoff, 2001). In Western countries, 20% of today's population is aged 60 years or over and it is predicted that by 2050 the proportion will be 32% (Population Division of the Department of Economic and Social Affairs of the United Nations Secretariat, 2005). The fastest growing age group in the world is those aged 80 years or older (United Nations Department of Economic and Social Affairs Population Division, 2002). Public health policies need to focus on maximizing the quality of life as well as the number of years of healthy life (Drewnowski et al., 2003).

Progressive and irreversible biological changes are part of the ageing process and result in a growing risk of chronic disease, cognitive and functional impairment, and an increased likelihood of dying (e.g. Verbrugge and Jette, 1994; Khaw, 1997; Bowling and Ebrahim, 2001). Ageing is associated with a decline in many of the body's physiological functions, resulting in structural changes, loss of lean mass and a relative increase in fat mass over time (Prinsley and Sandstead, 1990). Morley and Silver (1988) defined the loss of appetite associated with ageing, sometimes called the anorexia of ageing, as the physiological decrease in food intake occurring to counterbalance reduced physical activity and a lower metabolic rate not compensated for in the long term. Ageing is associated with a functional decline of taste and smell that could potentially lead to decreases in food palatability and a potential failure to develop sensory-specific satiety (Rolls, 1999).

The three key elements of successful ageing as described by Rowe and Kahn (1998) are decreasing the risk of diseases and disease-related disability; maintaining physical and mental functioning; and being actively engaged with life. The term 'active' not only refers to being physically or economically active, but also to continued societal participation. Social, physical and psychological well-being are all part of successful ageing (Khaw, 1997). Concepts such as productive ageing (i.e. the ability to contribute directly and indirectly in older age) and healthy ageing (i.e. the ability to remain physically and mentally fit) have been identified and brought together in the World Health Organization's (2002) active ageing policy framework. Campion (1998) describes healthy ageing as an ideal situation where morbidity and disability are compressed into a relatively short period before death, preceded by a long period in which people age with their vigour and functional independence intact.

While definitions of health tend to focus on mental, physical and social aspects of well-being, Pörn (1993) defines health as a person's capacity to achieve their life goals. One of the most highly valued life goals among older people is maintaining independence. Interestingly, the role of food and diet in maintaining this goal is rarely studied (McKie, 1999), although Swedish women were found to value being active and continuing with familiar shopping and cooking routines in order to retain their ability to live independently (Sidenvall *et al.*, 2001).

Theories about social life and old age have developed from seeing old age as one of dependency. More recently the emphasis within theory development about social life and old age has been to move away from considering old age as a problem in itself, to focusing on the ability of old people to improve their own quality of their life (Fennell *et al.*, 1994). Studies of mealtimes on geriatric wards in Sweden showed that older patients were not even given the chance to feed themselves and therefore adopted the role of dependent patient (Sidenvall *et al.*, 1994). Hockey and James (1993) argue that dependence is socially constructed, and that loss of individual freedom is expected to become a problem for people growing older in developed countries leading to 'infantalization' of the Western world, where older people are in danger of being seen by society as not being capable of taking care of themselves or knowing what is best for them.

In a qualitative study of food-related work by older women with and without disease, Gustafsson *et al.* (2003) found that they adopted various strategies including public health support services (rehabilitation, medication, transportation service for disabled persons), improved self-management skills (better planning, learning new approaches to doing things) and adaptation (simplifying cooking and using partly prepared or even ready-cooked meals) to maintain independence. Similar strategies were observed in another study of free-living older people including the observation that maintaining independence was the most valued factor (Mack *et al.*, 1997). Becoming dependent can give way to feelings of personal humiliation and of being socially marginalized (Hockey and James, 1993). Gustafsson *et al.* (2003) found that women felt that over-reliance on their husbands could potentially lead to increased dependence, a finding cited by Pound and Gompertz (1998).

There is also evidence of stability in the face of life transitions. Using a life course framework in a qualitative study with women aged 44 to 75 years, Edstrom and Devine (2001) found that women described consistent orientations to food and nutrition at interviews 10 years apart. Even when they had dealt with expected and unexpected changes in health, social environment and roles, 14 of the 17 women perceived their food and nutrition-related thoughts, beliefs and strategies to have been consistent over the 10-year period. The relatively few women who felt they had changed attributed this to changes in work and family roles, a disabling health problem, and ageing and family demands. Many described having been consistent despite having undergone major life transitions during the study period (e.g. personal health changes, the death of family members, life stage changes in family roles).

Experiencing Food Insecurity

Food security is defined as having access at all times to enough nutritious food for an active and healthy life (Anderson, 1990). Carlson *et al.* (1999) defined food insecurity as the limited or uncertain availability of nutritionally adequate and safe foods, or having limited or uncertain ability to acquire food in socially acceptable ways. Food insecurity has been studied in relation to older people (e.g. Wolfe *et al.*, 1996, 1998, 2003; Quandt and Rao, 1999; Lee and Frongillo, 2001a,b; Sharkey and Schoenberg, 2005).

Wolfe *et al.* (2003) sought to broaden the conceptualization of older people's experience of food insecurity, showing it to have four components: quantitative, qualitative, psychological and social. The quantitative component relates to the actual amount of food and energy able to be accessed and consumed. The qualitative component relates to diet quality, i.e. not being able to access the right quality and type of food. The psychological component refers to older people's feelings resulting from their knowledge and perception of their food situation and includes two sub-components: (i) feelings of worry and anxiety that result from knowing and perceiving the uncertainty of their food situation and lack of the right foods for health; and (ii) feelings of deprivation, anger and embarrassment resulting from knowing and perceiving their lack of food choice and the need to make compromises. The social component also includes two sub-components: (i) accessing food in socially unacceptable ways (e.g. using a food pantry); and (ii) socially or culturally less normative patterns of eating such as having to skip meals or replace main meals with sandwiches rather than preparing a 'real' meal.

Common to these four components of food insecurity (Wolfe *et al.*, 2003) are the dimensions of severity, time and compromised food choice, the latter also found by Quandt *et al.* (2001a). Major causes of food insecurity among older people include financial difficulties, poor health, limited mobility and lack of social support (Cook and Brown, 1992; Cohen *et al.*, 1993; Frongillo *et al.*, 2003). The inability to obtain necessary foods can be due to not being able to get to shops as a result of lack of transport or functional limitations. The inability to prepare food can be due to health problems (e.g. Lee and Frongillo, 2001b) and/or a lack of cooking skills. Quandt *et al.* (2001a) found that some older people prioritized health-care costs, thus having less money to spend on food.

Social Aspects of Procuring Food

The social life of many older people is focused around food and eating (e.g. Walker and Beauchene, 1991). Indeed, the procurement of food is an activity of social significance in all societies, but can be of greater importance yet more difficult to achieve for the older community. Research with older women (Sidenvall *et al.*, 2001) found that they valued being active through continuing with familiar routines whereby they could live independently, and that they gained physical exercise and social contacts when they went shopping. Hare *et al.* (1999) and Wilson *et al.* (2004) also found that food shopping is seen as a 'social activity' and an 'opportunity to meet friends'. The inaccessibility of large out-of-town supermarkets and the nature of home delivery schemes mitigate against maintaining social networks of support in the community associated with the procurement of food for older consumers. Attempts have been made to address limited accessibility of foodstuffs in disadvantaged communities by implementing innovative community projects and charity retailing initiatives (Piacentini *et al.*, 2001). These developments may have eased the constraints on some consumers but there is little research that explores the precise nature of the grocery shopping needs of older disadvantaged consumers and how they take advantage of these interventions within the wider retail environment (Piacentini *et al.*, 2001).

The management of food in everyday life is an important area where individual freedom might become restricted and dependence enforced on individuals. This is exemplified in those who find it difficult to get to the shops as discussed above. Older people have been found to be among those more likely to be limited to shopping for groceries at retail locations closer to home and report they are dissatisfied with the food shopping facilities (Bromley and Thomas, 1995). The nature of retailing has been changing, in particular the growth of large 'out-of-town' hyper- or supermarkets and the closure of the traditional community-based local shops (Burt, 1989; Borghesani *et al.*, 1997). While the degree to which this development has advanced differs between countries, the direction of the development has been the same. According to Lang (1994), governments and supermarkets through their planning and location strategies are responsible for the decline of local communities, compromising older people's ability to shop for food. Respondents interviewed by Wilson *et al.* (2004) stated that they missed the social environment provided by local, independent stores that had since closed in their area (see also Baron *et al.*, 2001). In addition, local shops or convenience stores generally charge higher prices and have a limited choice of foods (Barrett, 1997).

Particularly, those older people on low incomes and in poor health have reported difficulty in either getting to the shops or shopping (e.g. Mason and Bearden, 1979; Stitt *et al.*, 1995; Wylie *et al.*, 1999). Research from the USA (Arcury *et al.*, 1998; Quandt and Rao, 1999; Locher *et al.*, 2005) highlights food procurement problems that older people living in rural communities experience resulting from inadequate public transportation. The interaction between mobility and social support is important. A study by Bromley and Thomas (1995) of small town shopping behaviour demonstrated that disadvantaged consumers are more likely to be limited to shopping for groceries at retail locations closer to home, while families with cars and higher incomes shop at supermarkets outside the immediate area. Piacentini *et al.* (2001) found that the level of disadvantage experienced by older consumers is reduced where families are able to offer social support by doing the main food shop for their older relative. However, local shops were used more when older people had to rely on neighbours and home-helps for shopping and consequently they did not get best value for money (Piacentini *et al.*, 2001). Poor mobility meant that individuals were less able to exercise control over food shopping and feelings of disadvantage were exacerbated, particularly where social networks were weak.

Research has been carried out to understand older people's needs with regard to retailing (e.g. Lambert, 1979; Mason and Bearden, 1979; Lumpkin *et al.*, 1985; Kerin *et al.*, 1992; Leighton and Seaman, 1997a,b; Goodwin and McElwee, 1999; Hare *et al.*, 2001). In a study of older consumers in the USA, Mason and Bearden (1979) found that more than 30% of their sample felt food shopping was a problem, reasons given included: difficulties seeing labels; package sizes too large; foods primarily marketed to older people; meat being packaged; feeling overcharged; supermarkets being too cold; trolleys difficult to manoeuvre; and buses difficult to use. Leighton and Seaman (1997a,b) found older consumers in the UK to report similar difficulties, finding the main problems to be reaching high and low shelves, carrying baskets and reading price displays. Investigating food shopping experiences of older consumers using the critical incident technique, Hare *et al.* (2001) identified positive and negative aspects of food shopping activity. The main factors that were found to contribute to the quality of the shopping experience were merchandise-related, retail practices and staff issues. The internal store environment, accessibility, external shopping environment and personal factors were also identified and featured both positive and negative incidents, with social aspects only having positive incidents.

Food Preparation in Later Life

Women have been found to view the meals they cook and serve as 'gifts' and value being able to eat with friends and relatives (Sidenvall *et al.*, 2001). Charles and Kerr (1988) found that cooking for others was regarded as an incentive for women to cook traditional, so-called 'proper' meals. Similarly, Sidenvall *et al.* (2000) found that newly widowed women reported a loss of motivation to cook on the death of their husband. When living alone, the meaning of cooking as an expression of their friendship is lost; hence people are less likely to enjoy meals and run the risk of becoming malnourished (Lyon and Colquhoun, 1999). Many women regard cooking as a source of joy (Warde, 1997), especially cooking for others (Charles and Kerr, 1988; Sidenvall *et al.*, 2000). Davidson (2001) found that, for older women, widowhood could lead to a new-found sense of freedom and autonomy, whereas widowers can feel less free because of their need to take on tasks previously carried out by their spouse. In a study comparing men's and women's experiences in bereavement, Bennett *et al.* (2003) found that men believed women are better equipped to deal with widowhood, explaining this in terms of women's domestic abilities and social skills, and men's inability to talk about their emotions. It was also found that women believed men received more support than they did; this was confirmed (Bennett *et al.*, 2003).

Effort in food preparation, the presence of physical disabilities, and lack of enjoyment and skills in cooking may have implications for food selection and meal preparation among older people. Due to functional limitations it can be difficult for older people to obtain acceptable food (Lee and Frongillo, 2001b). Also, physiological decline (e.g. sight, hearing, dental health) and other conditions may result in older people having related mobility problems; thus they may find it difficult not only to procure but also to prepare food, which further restricts access to adequate amounts and types of food and limits variety and satisfactory nutrient intake (e.g. Rovner and Ganguli, 1998; Keller *et al.*, 1999).

Little is known about how older people perceive convenience food products that can be eaten immediately or at least prepared with minimum effort (Swoboda and Morschett, 2001). Even if time may be more plentiful among older people, the effort in obtaining and preparing food may still be important. In younger people a high level of work necessary for preparation might affect food selection and reduce nutritional intake (Meiselman *et al.*, 1994). Similar effects might be expected among older people, especially in those who lack the skill to cook (Hughes *et al.*, 2004). However, it does not mean that convenience foods are preferred to the conventional products. For older people, the meaning of healthy eating has been shown to match that of a 'proper' meal consisting of meat or fish, potatoes and a vegetable (Winter Falk *et al.*, 1996; McKie, 1999). 'Proper food' meant fresh natural ingredients, whereas convenience foods were seen as rubbish or junk food. Older women in Sweden showed no positive attitudes towards ready-to-heat or ready-to-serve foods (Sidenvall *et al.*, 2000). In a survey of 1843 Europeans aged 65 years and over, de Almeida *et al.* (2001) found that the most important factors influencing older people's food choices were quality and freshness (54%). Older people defined healthy eating as 'less fat' (37%), 'more fresh vegetables and fruit' (34%) and 'natural foods' (11%).

Caraher *et al.* (1999) investigated whether differences in cooking skills might be a factor in health differences and whether these differences could be construed as inequality. Based on data from the 1993 Health and Lifestyles Survey of England, socioeconomic status and education were associated with people's knowledge about cooking. Although Caraher *et al.* (1999) found there to be variation between sexes, age groups, income and social class, the greatest variation was with gender. Acquisition of cooking skills was structurally determined, primarily along gender lines but also by social class and income. Mothers were the prime source of information on cooking skills in all social classes although many people were unsure of cooking techniques, with a large number of men claiming to have no cooking skills. Older men may particularly lack the motivation, knowledge and skills for meal preparation, resulting in less healthy food choices (Caraher *et al.*, 1999).

It is important to note that the relationship between cooking skills and food choice is complex. It is often assumed that better or more comprehensive skills lead to more frequent cooking and the use of raw/fresh ingredients (e.g. Fieldhouse, 1995). A qualitative study of the relationship between cooking and meal preparation skills and food choice led Short (2003) to suggest that campaigns and policies should focus more broadly on domestic food preparation and culture in terms of responsibilities for food provision and the sociocultural understanding of 'cooking', rather than just on distinct and separate aspects such as 'practical cooking skills'.

In a study of older men living alone, Hughes *et al.* (2004) found that men with good cooking skills reported better physical health and higher intake of vegetables. The study revealed that poor cooking skills and low motivation to change eating habits may constitute barriers to improving energy intake, healthy eating and appetite in older men. In an intervention in which older men were taught cooking skills, Keller *et al.* (2004) reported that participants gained confidence in cooking, increased their cooking activities at home, developed healthier cooking skills, and improved cooking variety through the programme. The men also identified social benefits, suggesting that community-based nutrition and cooking education for older men is a beneficial nutrition education activity to support. Participants reported wishing to improve cooking skills out of interest but also as a preventive measure, in case family roles changed due to their wives becoming ill or dying. Keller *et al.* (2004) suggest that this might be a form of behaviour change resulting from what Laditka and Pappas-Rogich (2001) termed 'anticipatory caregiving anxiety'.

Social Aspects of Meals

Despite the focus by many scientists and food providers on individual foods, most food is eaten as part of a meal. The factors controlling what and how much is eaten should take into account that foods are selected and consumed in combination (Meiselman, 2000). Meals are also complex and difficult to define. They are social events, as well as food events (Sobal, 2000). A 'proper' or 'ideal' meal is typically eaten with others, with eating alone not considered a 'real meal' for many people (Douglas, 1972; Murcott, 1982). Eating with the family has been found to be highly valued (Quandt *et al.*, 1997). In most societies, food and meals convey social meaning, as well as providing nutritional sustenance (Quandt *et al.*, 2001b). Apart from the material benefits, foods and meals are said to act as the social 'glue'. Across almost all societies, commensality, the process of eating together or giving and receiving food, reinforces social relations and group memberships (Counihan and van Esterik, 1997). Specific foods or significant eating occasions are usually embedded with core social values and culture.

The importance of ambience on food intake and food choice has been reviewed by Stroebele and de Castro (2004). As Meiselman (1992a,b) has stated, there is sufficient research relating to sensory and physiological intake and appetite, but the effect of other situational and social factors has been ignored. Stroebele and de Castro (2004) found in their review that changes in intake can be detected with different numbers of people being present, food accessibility, eating location, room ambience and food colour. In institutional food service settings, low quality ratings were reported for food presentation, food variety and physical setting (e.g. Meiselman *et al.*, 1989, 2000; Cardello *et al.*, 1996). These are usually equipped sparsely and the lack of table-cloths, silverware and attractive food presentation may be major contributors to perceptions and attitudes towards institutional foods. Gibbons and Henry (2005) compared older people's intakes of identical meals in two eating environments, showing increased intakes when eating in a restaurant environment as compared to a canteen-style environment.

McAlpine *et al.* (2003) found that when older adults ate in social groups, this enhanced food intake; a well-established phenomenon in younger adults (de Castro, 1994). In a comparison of data from different age groups, de Castro (2002) found that older people ate with fewer other people present and earlier in the day than younger people. They were, however, just as responsive as younger groups to social facilitation of intake, palatability, cognitive restraint, time of day, day of week and location, but showed blunted responses to self-reported hunger. De Castro (2002) suggests that inadequate intakes in older people might be improved through interventions involving non-physiological factors (e.g. such as the number of other people present at meals, palatability of meals, meal time of day and meal location).

Oldenburg (1999) uses the term 'third place' to describe accessible and happy gathering places for adults beyond family and work, which can include venues for eating out. As well as providing nourishment, eating out may offer non-obligatory social interaction for older people. Cheang (2002) studied older adults congregating in a fast-food restaurant to be with friends to 'play'. Although little social support was exchanged, they perceived the restaurant setting as an environment over which they had control and within which they had freedom. Cheang (2002) found that, contrary to the many studies that portray older people as needy and seeking support, these community-dwelling physically independent older people have found a place in which to have a good time in public. Such venues are thus important in the lives of older people and support healthy ageing. On the other hand, participants in Cheang's (2002) study regarded social centres for seniors negatively and described them as being overly structured and places for old folks.

Eating Alone

Structural and demographic changes in society have increased the probability of eating alone. Older people's living arrangements appear to be changing, with elderly people increasingly less likely to live with other family members or unrelated individuals and more likely to live alone (Sundström, 1994; Kinsella and Velkoff, 2001). The findings of community-based studies in which the relationship between diet quality, social support and living arrangements has been investigated have not been consistent (Payette and Shatenstein, 2005). Many studies have found that the presence of social networks has a positive effect on diet (e.g. McIntosh *et al.*, 1989; Davis *et al.*, 1990; Walker and Beauchene, 1991; Toner and Morris, 1992; Keller *et al.*, 1997; Prothro and Rosenbloom, 1999; Shatenstein *et al.*, 2004), whereas other studies (e.g. Rothenberg *et al.*,

1993) have found that diet quality was not affected by a poor social network. Using data from the nationally representative Third National Health and Examination Survey in the USA, Sahyoun and Zhang (2005) showed that people with fewer social contacts had significantly lower healthy eating scores, consumed fewer calories, ate less varied diets, and consumed fewer portions of fruit and vegetables.

Living and eating alone are prevalent amongst older people because of the relatively high proportion of widows and widowers (Arber and Evandrou, 1993). Many studies suggest that widowhood has the potential to have a negative impact on food intake (Maddison and Walker, 1967; Davis *et al.*, 1990; Murphy *et al.*, 1990; Walker and Beauchene, 1991; Rosenbloom and Whittington, 1993; Keller *et al.*, 1997; Donkin *et al.*, 1998; Charlton, 1999; Quandt *et al.*, 2000; Shahar *et al.*, 2001; Johnson, 2002). For example, in a case–control study Rosenbloom and Whittington (1993) found that, following widowhood, the widowed group lost significantly more weight and had poorer eating habits, including more meals eaten alone, less enjoyment from eating and lower appetite levels. Evidence from a bereavement project that focused on health and wellness issues, including nutritional self-care skills (Caserta *et al.*, 2004), suggests that there is scope to develop food-related interventions as well as those that simply address the issues of grief and loss issues alone.

Loneliness, rather than simply living alone, may be the real cause of reduced intakes (Murphy *et al.*, 1990; Walker and Beauchene, 1991). Although never-married older people have been found to be more isolated than married individuals, they are similar to them with respect to loneliness and life satisfaction (Gubrium, 1974). Dissatisfaction with available relationships may be a more powerful indicator of loneliness than the number of social contacts (Revenson and Johnson, 1984). The number of social contacts *per se* had no relationship to food choice and dietary adequacy (Walker and Beauchene, 1991). Social interaction at mealtimes has been found to improve dietary adequacy in a variety of settings including among those living independently and those in sheltered housing, hospitalized or other care centres (Hanson, 1978). Suda *et al.* (2001) showed that the presence of a Meals-on-Wheels delivery volunteer during meals could improve recipients' dietary intakes.

Gustafsson *et al.* (2003) found social withdrawal was a clear adaptation strategy of many women in their study. When women were unable to behave in a way they viewed as acceptable for their own social group, they withdrew. Other researchers (Nijhof, 1995; Sidenvall *et al.*, 1996; Jacobsson *et al.*, 2000) reported similar behaviour in people suffering from stroke and Parkinson's disease who were found to be ashamed of their eating disability.

Formal Support from Food-related Services

The projected growth in the number of older people in need of care will lead to a growing demand for formal systems of food provision. Given the significance of the meal, very little research has been undertaken to investigate user satisfaction with food-related services among older people including Meals-on-Wheels, luncheon clubs, delivery services and home-helps. As stated earlier, poor nutritional intakes can be attributed to difficulties in undertaking everyday activities such as shopping and cooking. However, work with older women suffering Parkinson's disease (Andersson and Sidenvall, 2001) suggests that complete dependence on external support can have negative consequences for nutritional status. For older people there is an increasing need for community-based services to postpone and minimize dependency and health problems in old age. However, the provision of formal systems of food provision requires evaluation using effective methods.

Although United States' Older Americans Act Nutrition Programs home-delivered meals provide an important source of food assistance through the traditional model of five nutritionally balanced meals per week (each meeting at least 33% of daily nutrient requirements), substantial proportions of homebound participants still report not having enough food to eat (Ponza et al., 1996; American Dietetic Association, 2002). As part of a cross-sectional field study evaluating whether the addition of breakfast as a second home-delivered meal can improve the well-being of at-risk older adults, Gollub and Weddle (2004) found that participants receiving the additional breakfasts had fewer depressive symptoms and greater energy/nutrient intakes and levels of food security. Kretser et al. (2003) tested the feasibility of an enhanced Meals-on-Wheels service in terms of number of meals provided, i.e. comparing the provision of five meals per week (consisting of hot meals made from scratch; meeting 33% of the Daily Reference Intake) with a programme of three meals and two snacks per day, 7 days a week (consisting of frozen meals, nutritional supplements, and shelf-stable and fresh food items; meeting 100% of the Daily Reference Intake). Participants receiving the enhanced meal programme improved more in terms of health outcomes.

Locher et al. (2005) examined the relationships that exist between social isolation, social support, social capital (e.g. the provision of support through community-based services) and nutritional risk in the south-eastern USA and found that social isolation and lower income contribute most to nutritional risk, particularly for black women, white women and white men. However, in the case of black men, social support and social capital were most important in predicting nutritional risk, i.e. lower levels of trust in community and regular religious participation. The authors suggest that targeted programmes need to be developed. For example, homebound older adults could be sent frozen meals, groceries and food commodities directly to their homes to overcome their lack of access to appropriate services.

When comparing the provision of meals to older people in three environments (restaurants, 'part-of-day' care and 'around-the-clock' care), Sydner and Fjellström (2005) found that care recipients were given different opportunities concerning what, how, when and with whom to eat, depending on where their meals were served. In restaurants, older people were able to choose from a variety of foods as well as determine when and with whom meals could be eaten. In the care settings, both 'part-of-day' care and 'around-the-clock' care, choices, in terms of foods, meal timing and companions, were limited. This was especially the case in the units providing 'around-the-clock' care, where the most vulnerable older people lived. These findings echo those of Sidenvall et al. (1994) who looked at the social and cultural aspects of meals in geriatric care, Spalding's (1999) study of older people on acute hospital wards and Pearson *et al.* (2003) who looked at the role of staff at mealtime in nursing homes. Sydner and Fjellström (2005) stress the importance of not only ensuring the client's nutritional needs are met, but also care needs to be taken to address the cultural and social meaning of food and meals in people's lives, especially in situations of dependence on others.

Dietary Change in Later Life

Dietary patterns and other modifiable life-style factors are associated with mortality from all causes, coronary heart disease, cardiovascular diseases and cancer (e.g. Trichopoulou *et al.*, 1995, 2000, 2003; Huijbregts *et al.*, 1997; Haveman-Nies *et al.*, 2002). Recent studies (Mozaffarian *et al.*, 2003; Knoops *et al.*, 2004; Song *et al.*, 2004; Trichopoulou and Critselis, 2004) have provided evidence that Mediterranean-style diets as well as limited red meat and high cereal-fibre consumption reduce cardiovascular disease and cancer in older adults. Data from the cross-cultural Food Habits in Later Life study, looking at the extent of health in Sweden, Greece, Australia and Japan, suggest that diet as compared with other social and life-style variables is an important predictor of survival (e.g. Wahlqvist *et al.*, 1997, 1999, 2005).

Successful intervention strategies are needed to achieve dietary change. A number of authors have reviewed the literature pertinent to understanding the efficacy of nutrition interventions for older people (Contento *et al.*, 1995, 2002; Fletcher and Rake, 1998; Sahyoun *et al.*, 2004; Higgins and Clarke Barkley, 2003a,b,c,d, 2004a,b,c). In their review of 23 interventions to promote healthy eating in free-living elderly individuals aged 65 years and over, Fletcher and Rake (1998) concluded that there was some evidence of effectiveness but that most were of poor quality.

Sahyoun *et al.* (2004) reviewed 25 nutrition interventions targeting adults aged over 55 years and concluded that the interventions were limited in their ability to induce behaviour change. The authors suggest that success was more likely if interventions limited educational messages to one or two; used reinforcing and personalized messages; provided hands-on activities, incentives, cues and access to health professionals; and used appropriate theories of behaviour change. Based on these findings Sahyoun *et al.* (2004) suggest that designing nutrition interventions for older adults be guided by the use of a theoretical framework based on the a social ecological model for planning public health interventions recommended by the Institute of Medicine (Smedley and Syme, 2000).

Contento *et al.* (2002) reviewed and analysed evaluation measures used in behavioural intervention studies carried out with older people over 65 years of age. Only two of the 15 studies measured intervening variables (Hackman and Wagner, 1990; Crockett *et al.*, 1992), i.e. measures that might give some indication as to why or why not an intervention is or is not working. Most studies focused on collecting measures of knowledge (e.g. Hermann *et al.*, 1990) or behavioural outcomes using 24 h recalls (e.g. Bedell and Shackleton, 1989) or food frequency questionnaires (e.g. Dennison et al., 1991) analysed for nutrients or foods. Contento et al. (2002) concluded that judgements regarding the effectiveness of nutrition education will be easier once more work is done to develop and test evaluation instruments with each new target audience, to ensure that they are appropriate and have adequate psychometric properties. This finding is echoed by Higgins and Clarke Barkley (2003d), who conclude that there continues to be a great need for research to develop behavioural and educational theoretical frameworks, as well as designs, intervention strategies and evaluation methods.

The barriers for health-care professionals to providing nutrition education include misconceptions and stereotypes about older people and about their nutritional concerns; lack of attention to and lack of funding for older adult education programmes; and difficulties recruiting older learners (Higgins and Clarke Barkley, 2004c). Barriers to older people's responding to nutrition education can be grouped as attitudinal, motivational, environmental, and those related to low literacy and poverty (Higgins and Clarke Barkley, 2004c).

Marketing to Older Consumers

In the past, older consumers were not viewed as an important market segment by the business community (Mason and Bearden, 1979). There is evidence that the advertising and marketing industries somewhat ignore the mature market (e.g. Goerlich and Stipp, 1995; Lee, 1997; Long, 1998; Carrigan and Szmigin, 1999). Long (1998) in the UK and Lee (1997) in USA have both found evidence of marketers viewing older people negatively. There is a concern amongst marketers that a product that is appealing to older consumers is less attractive to younger consumers (Mazis et al., 1992; Sawchuck, 1995; Thomas and Wolfe, 1995). Moschis (2003) distinguishes three distinct stages in terms of the development of the 'mature market': (i) prior to the 1980s, when older consumers were not considered to be a significant segment, and were ignored; (ii) the 1980s, in which the 'mature' market was defined both in terms of size and buying power (see Bartos, 1980); and (iii) the stage since the early 1990s, in which there has been a dual trend, one of companies with marketing programmes targeted at the mature market and a second of companies being hesitant to develop products or messages aimed at this market.

Marketers frequently conduct research to try to understand the purchasing behaviour of the so-called 'grey market'. In the past too little attention has been placed on the aspirations of older consumers, their shopping habits and store choice behaviour, or their response to alternative forms of food delivery (Tantiwong and Wilton, 1985). Older people are not homogeneous in their food preferences and the existence of different market segments within the older community makes it difficult to make generalizations (Szmigin and Carrigan, 2001). Reviewing the methods used to segment the mature market, Bone (1991) found across 33 studies that segmentation based on chronological age is the most common method. She then however goes on to argue that five other variables can better be used: discretionary income; health; activity level; discretionary time; and response to others. The Center for Mature Consumer Studies, as described in Moschis (1996) and Moschis *et al.* (1997), has developed what they call gerontographics: segmentation based factors associated with biological, social and experiential ageing. Their model consists of four segments of older persons who are at four different but not necessarily sequential stages in later life: 'healthy indulgers' (i.e. main focus is on enjoying life rather than 'making it in life'); 'healthy hermits' (i.e. healthy and relatively more socially withdrawn); 'ailing outgoers' (i.e. still active and likely to maintain a high level of self-esteem despite their adverse life condition); and 'frail recluses' (i.e. in isolation and likely to think of themselves as 'old persons'). Such segmentation methods can provide useful insights to help the food sector, service providers and policy makers understand how best to design systems of food delivery and distribution that fit the needs of older people.

In the food sector there has been an increasing recognition that the older population is becoming an important consumer group (e.g. Hollingsworth, 2003). In a study investigating the extent to which older consumers are set in their ways and resistant to change and innovation, Leek *et al.* (1998) found that older consumers were marginally more likely than younger consumers to try, and willing to pay a premium price for, the conceptually new (and healthier) food product, polyunsaturated fatty acid-fed fish. There are examples of food products being targeted specifically at older people. Parry (2004) reports on the re-launch of a wheat biscuit cereal brand in which the manufacturers teamed up with an older people's charity. Other companies prefer to target more broadly and focus on broader age groups with a common interest such as health (Hollingsworth, 2003). The global brand manager of a functional food aimed at lowering cholesterol was quoted as saying: 'I don't see my job as marketing to the over-50s. [. . .] is bought by people who don't take their health for granted and as a specific benefit to a specific need, which is lowering cholesterol' (Lewis, 2005).

Wolfe (1997) considers that marketing to older consumers 'operates against a backdrop of ageing reinforced by gerontology' and 'ignores the brighter side of age: self-realization and human development in later years' (p. 294). To experience empathy with older consumers means to see age as a positive development. Older people generally feel more positive than younger people about their current lives (Cohen, 1989, cited in Wolfe). This lack of understanding has led to high failure rates of new food products designed specifically for older consumers.

Conclusion

Much of the social life of people is focused around food, including shopping, cooking, entertaining and dining out. All of these food-related activities can become of greater importance to older people and yet be more difficult to achieve. Understanding older consumers' behaviour in relation to their choice of food products and services is not only important for marketing, but also is the key to maintaining good health and quality of life. There are still relatively few empirical data regarding the shopping patterns and meal preparation skills of the older community and how these are affected by changes in living circumstances such as the loss of a partner or mobility problems. Many more people, in future, will live alone because of the gender-related differential in survival rates. At the same time the proportion of younger people in the population will decrease, leaving a gap between older people needing help and younger employed workers or relatives able to provide formal and informal support. A more holistic approach to understanding food choice behaviour is needed, which includes the constraints of food procurement if supported independence is to be achieved.

References

American Dietetic Association (2002) Position of the American Dietetic Association: domestic food and nutrition security. *Journal of the American Dietetic Association* 102, 1840–1847.

Anderson, S.A. (1990) Core indicators of nutritional state for difficult-to-sample populations. *Journal of Nutrition* 120, 1557–1600.

Andersson, I. and Sidenvall, B. (2001) Case studies of food shopping, cooking and eating habits in older women with Parkinson's disease. *Journal of Advanced Nursing* 35, 69–78.

Arber, S. and Evandrou, M. (1993) Mapping the territory; ageing, independence and the life course. In: Arber, S. and Evandrou, M. (eds) *Ageing, Independence and the Life Course*. Jessica Kingsley Publishers, London, pp. 9–26.

Arcury, T.A., Quandt, S.A., Bell, R.A., McDonald, J. and Vitolins, M.Z. (1998) Barriers to nutritional well-being for rural elders: community experts' perceptions. *The Gerontologist* 38, 490–498.

Baron, S., Harris, K., Leaver, D. and Oldfield, B. (2001) Beyond convenience: the future for independent food and grocery retailers in the UK. *International Review of Retail, Distribution and Consumer Research* 11, 395–414.

Barrett, J. (1997) The cost and availability of healthy food choices in Southern Derbyshire. *Journal of Human Nutrition and Dietetics* 10, 63–69.

Bartos, R. (1980) Over 49: the invisible consumer market. *Harvard Business Review* 58, 140–148.

Bedell, B.A. and Shackleton, P.A. (1989) The relationship between a nutrition education program and nutrition knowledge and eating behavior of the elderly. *Journal of Nutrition for the Elderly* 8, 35–45.

Bennett, K.M., Hughes, G.M. and Smith, P.T. (2003) 'I think a woman can take it'. Widowed men's views and experiences of gender differences in bereavement. *Ageing International* 28, 408–424.

Bone, P.F. (1991) Identifying mature segments. *Journal of Services Marketing* 5, 47–60.

Borghesani, W.H., de la Cruz, P.L. and Berry, D.B. (1997) Controlling the chain: buyer power, distributive control, and new dynamics in retailing. *Business Horizons* 40, 17–24.

Bowling, A. and Ebrahim, S. (2001) Glossaries in public health: older people. *Journal of Epidemiology and Community Health* 55, 223–226.

Bromley, R.D.F. and Thomas, C.J. (1995) Small town shopping decline: dependence and inconvenience for the disadvantaged. *International Review of Retail, Distribution and Consumer Research* 5, 433–456.

Burt, S.L. (1989) Trends and management issues in European retailing. *International Journal of Retailing* 4, 1–97.

Campion, E.W. (1998) Aging better. *New England Journal of Medicine* 338, 1064–1066.

Caraher, M., Dixon, P., Lang, T. and Carr-Hill, R. (1999) The state of cooking in England: the relationship of cooking skills to food choice. *British Food Journal* 101, 590–609.

Cardello, A.V., Bell, R. and Kramer, F.M. (1996) Attitudes of consumers toward institutional food. *Food Quality and Preference* 7, 7.

Carlson, S.J., Andrews, M.S. and Bickel, G.W. (1999) Measuring food insecurity and hunger in the United States: development of a national benchmark measure and prevalence estimates. *Journal of Nutrition* 129, 510S–516S.

Carrigan, M. and Szmigin, I. (1999) In pursuit of youth: what's wrong with the older market? *Marketing Intelligence and Planning* 17, 222–231.

Caserta, M.S., Lund, D.A. and Obray, S.J. (2004) Promoting self-care and daily living skills among older widows and widowers: evidence from the PATHFINDERS demonstration project. *OMEGA: The Journal of Death and Dying* 49, 217–236.

Charles, N. and Kerr, M. (1988) *Women, Food and Families*. Manchester University Press, Manchester, UK.

Charlton, K E. (1999) Elderly men living alone: are they at high nutritional risk? *Journal of Nutrition, Health & Aging* 3, 42–47.

Cheang, M. (2002) Older adults' frequent visits to a fast-food restaurant. Nonobligatory social interaction and the significance of play in a 'third place'. *Journal of Ageing Studies* 16, 303–321.

Cohen, B.E., Burt, M.R. and Schulte, M.M. (1993) *Hunger and Food Insecurity Among the Elderly*. The Urban Institute, Washington, DC.

Cohen, G.D. (1989) *The Aging Brain*. Springer Publishing, New York, p. 32.

Contento, I.R., Balch, G.I., Bronner, Y.L., Paige, D.M., Gross, S.M., Bisignani, L., Lytle, L.A., Maloney, S.K., White, S.L., Olson, C.M., Swadener, S.S. and Randell, J.S. (1995) The effectiveness of nutrition education and implications for nutrition education policy, programs and research: a review of research. *Journal of Nutrition Education* 27, 277–422.

Contento, I.R., Randell, J.S. and Basch, C.E. (2002) Review and analysis of evaluation measures used in nutrition education intervention research. *Journal of Nutrition Education and Behavior* 34, 2–25.

Cook, J.T. and Brown, J.L. (1992) *Estimating the Number of Hungry Americans*. Center for Hunger, Poverty and Nutrition Policy Working Paper No. he01- 090292. Tufts University, Medford, Massachusetts.

Counihan, C. and van Esterik, P. (1997) *Food and Culture: S Reader*. Routledge, New York.

Crockett, S.J., Heller, K.E., Skauge, L.H. and Merkel, J.M. (1992) Mailed-home nutrition education for rural seniors: a pilot study. *Journal of Nutrition Education* 24, 312–315.

Davidson, K. (2001) Late life widowhood, selfishness and new partnership choices: a gendered perspective. *Ageing and Society* 21, 279–317.

Davis, M.A., Murphy, S.P., Neuhaus, J.M. and Lein, D. (1990) Living arrangements and dietary quality of older US adults. *Journal of the American Dietetic Association* 90, 1667–1672.

de Almeida, M.D., Graca, P., Afonso, C., Kearney, J.M. and Gibney, M.J. (2001) Healthy eating in European elderly: concepts, barriers and benefits. *Journal of Nutrition, Health & Aging* 5, 217–219.

De Castro, J.M. (1994) Family and friends produce greater social facilitation of food intake than other companions. *Physiology & Behavior* 56, 445–450.

De Castro, J.M. (2002) Age-related changes in the social, psychological, and temporal influences on food intake in free-living, healthy, adult humans. *The Journals of Gerontology, Series A, Biological Sciences and Medical Sciences* 57, M368–M377.

Dennison, K.F., Dennison, D. and Ward, J.Y. (1991) Computerized nutrition program: effect on nutrient intake of senior citizens. *Journal of the American Dietetic Association* 91, 1431–1433.

Donkin, A.J.M., Johnson, A.E., Lilley, J.M., Morgan, K., Neale, R.J., Page, R.M. and Silburn, R.L. (1998) Gender and living alone as determinants of fruit and vegetable consumption among the elderly living at home in urban Nottingham. *Appetite* 30, 39–51.

Douglas, M. (1972) Deciphering a meal. *Daedalus* 101, 61–82.

Drewnowski, A., Monsen, E., Birkett, D., Gunther, S., Vendeland, S., Su, J. and Marshall, G. (2003) Health screening and health promotion programs for the elderly. *Disease Management and Health Outcomes* 11, 299–309.

Edstrom, K.M. and Devine, C.M. (2001) Consistency in women's orientations to food and nutrition in midlife and older age: a 10-year qualitative follow-up. *Journal of Nutrition Education and Behavior* 33, 215–223.

Fennell, G., Phillipson, C. and Evers, H. (1994) *The Sociology of Old Age*. Open University Press, Milton Keynes, UK.

Fieldhouse, P. (1995) *Food and Nutrition, Customs and Culture*. Chapman and Hall, London.

Fletcher, A. and Rake, C. (1998) *Effectiveness of Interventions to Promote Healthy Eating in Elderly People Living in the Community: A Review*. Health Promotion Effectiveness Reviews No. 8. Health Education Authority, London.

Frongillo, E.A., Valois, P. and Wolfe, W.S. (2003) Using a concurrent events approach to understand social support and food insecurity among elders. *Family Economics and Nutrition Review* 15, 25–32.

Gibbons, M.D. and Henry, C.J. (2005) Does eating environment have an effect on food intake in the elderly? *Journal of Nutrition, Health & Aging* 9, 25–29.

Goerlich, B. and Stipp, H. (1995) Why youth rules. *American Demographics* 17, 30–31.

Gollub, E.A. and Weddle, D.O. (2004) Improvements in nutritional intake and quality of life among frail homebound older adults receiving home-delivered breakfast and lunch. *Journal of the American Dietetic Association* 104, 1227–1235.

Goodwin, D.R. and McElwee, R.E. (1999) Grocery shopping and an ageing population: research note. *International Review of Retail, Distribution & Consumer Research* 9, 403–409.

Gubrium, J. (1974) Marital desolation and evaluation of everyday life in old age. *Journal of Marriage and the Family* 36, 107–113.

Gustafsson, K., Andersson, I., Andersson, J., Fjellström, C. and Sidenvall, B. (2003) Older women's perceptions of independence versus dependence in food-related work. *Public Health Nursing* 20, 237–247.

Hackman, R.M. and Wagner, E.L. (1990) The senior gardening and nutrition project: development and transport of a dietary behavior change and health promotion program. *Journal of Nutrition Education* 22, 262–270.

Hanson, R.G. (1978) Considering 'social nutrition' in assessing geriatric nutrition. *Geriatrics* 33, 49–51.

Hare, C., Kirk, D. and Lang, T. (1999) Identifying the expectations of older food consumers. More than a 'shopping list' of wants. *Journal of Marketing Practice: Applied Marketing Science* 5, 213–232.

Hare, C., Kirk, D. and Lang, T. (2001) The food shopping experience of older consumers in Scotland. *International Journal of Retail & Distribution Management* 29, 25–40.

Haveman-Nies, A., de Groot, L.P., Burema, J., Cruz, J.A., Osler, M., van Staveren, W.A., for the SENECA Investigators (2002) Dietary quality and lifestyle factors in relation to 10-year mortality in older Europeans: the SENECA study. *American Journal of Epidemiology* 156, 962–968.

Hermann, J.R., Kopel, B.H., McCrory, M.L. and Kulling, F.A. (1990) Effect of a cooperative extension nutrition and exercise program for older adults on nutrition knowledge, dietary intake, anthropometric measures, and serum lipids. *Journal of Nutrition Education* 22, 271–274.

Higgins, M.M. and Clarke Barkley, M. (2003a) Important nutrition education issues and recommendations related to a review of literature on older adults. *Journal of Nutrition for the Elderly* 22(3), 65–78.

Higgins, M.M. and Clarke Barkley, M. (2003b) Evaluating outcomes and impacts of nutrition education programs designed for older adults. *Journal of Nutrition for the Elderly* 22(4), 69–81.

Higgins, M.M. and Clarke Barkley, M. (2003c) Tailoring nutrition education intervention programs to meet needs and interests of older adults. *Journal of Nutrition for the Elderly* 23(1), 59–79.

Higgins, M.M. and Clarke Barkley, M. (2003d) Concepts, theories and design components for nutrition education programs aimed at older adults. *Journal of Nutrition for the Elderly* 23(2), 57–75.

Higgins, M.M. and Clarke Barkley, M. (2004a) Improving effectiveness of nutrition education resources for older adults. *Journal of Nutrition for the Elderly* 23(3), 19–54.

Higgins, M.M. and Clarke Barkley, M. (2004b) Group nutrition education classes for older adults. *Journal of Nutrition for the Elderly* 23(4), 67–98.

Higgins, M.M. and Clarke Barkley, M. (2004c) Barriers to nutrition education for older adults, and nutrition and aging training opportunities for educators, healthcare providers, volunteers and caregivers. *Journal of Nutrition for the Elderly* 23(4), 99–121.

Hockey, J. and James, A. (1993) *Growing Up and Growing Older: Ageing and Dependency in the Life Course*. Sage, London.

Hollingsworth, P. (2003) Food and the aging consumer. *Food Technology* 57, 28–40.

Hughes, G., Bennett, K.M. and Hetherington, M.M. (2004) Old and alone: barriers to healthy eating in older men living on their own. *Appetite* 43, 269–276.

Huijbregts, P., Feskens, E., Räsänen, L., Fidanza, F., Nissinen, A., Menotti, A. and Kromhout, D. (1997) Dietary pattern and 20 year mortality in elderly men in Finland, Italy, and the Netherlands: longitudinal cohort study. *British Medical Journal* 315, 13–17.

Jacobsson, C., Axelsson, K., Österlind, P. and Norberg, A. (2000) How people with stroke and healthy older people experience the eating process. *Journal of Clinical Nursing* 9, 255–264.

Johnson, C.S. (2002) Nutritional considerations for bereavement and coping with grief. *Journal of Nutrition, Health & Aging* 6, 171–176.

Keller, B.K., Morton, J.L., Thomas, V.S. and Potter, J.F. (1999) The effects of visual and hearing impairments on functional status. *Journal of the American Geriatrics Society* 47, 1319–1325.

Keller, H.H., Østbye, T. and Bright-See, E. (1997) Predictors of dietary intake in Ontario seniors. *Canadian Journal of Public Health. Revue Canadienne de Sante Publique* 88, 305–309.

Keller, H.H., Gibbs, A., Wong, S., Vanderkooy, P. and Hedley, M. (2004) Men can cook! Development, implementation, and evaluation of a senior men's cooking group. *Journal of Nutrition for the Elderly* 24, 71–87.

Kerin, R.A., Jain, A. and Howard, D.J. (1992) Store shopping experience and consumer price–quality–value perceptions. *Journal of Retailing* 68, 376–397.

Khaw, K.T. (1997) Healthy ageing. *British Medical Journal* 315, 1090–1096.

Kinsella, K. and Velkoff, V.A. (2001) *Health and Disability. An Aging World: 2001.* US Census Bureau, Series P95/01-1. US Government Printing Office, Washington, DC.

Knoops, K.T., de Groot, L.C., Kromhout, D., Perrin, A.-E., Moreiras-Varela, O., Menotti, A. and van Staveren, W.A. (2004) Mediterranean diet, lifestyle factors, and 10-year mortality in elderly European men and women: the HALE project. *Journal of the American Medical Association* 292, 1433–1439.

Kretser, A.J., Voss, T., Kerr, W.W., Cavadini, C. and Friedmann, J. (2003) Effects of two models of nutritional intervention on homebound older adults at nutritional risk. *Journal of the American Dietetic Association* 103, 329–336.

Laditka, S.B. and Pappas-Rogich, M. (2001) Anticipatory caregiving anxiety among older women and men. *Journal of Women and Aging* 13, 3–18.

Lambert, Z. (1979) An investigation of older consumers' unmet needs and wants at the retail level. *Journal of Retailing* 55, 35–57.

Lang, T. (1994) Feeding the captive stomach: supermarkets, the consumer and competition policy. Paper presented at *XIV International Home Economics and Consumer Research Conference*, Sheffield, UK, 21–22 July.

Lee, J.S. and Frongillo, E.A. (2001a) Factors associated with food insecurity among US elderly: importance of functional impairments. *The Journals of Gerontology. Series B, Psychological Sciences and Social Sciences* 56B, S94–S99.

Lee, J.S. and Frongillo, E.A. (2001b) Nutritional and health consequences are associated with food insecurity among US elderly persons. *Journal of Nutrition* 131, 1503–1509.

Lee, R.A. (1997) The youth bias in advertising. *American Demographics* 19, 46–50.

Leek, S., Maddock, S. and Foxall, G. (1998) Concept testing an unfamiliar fish. *Qualitative Market Research: An International Journal* 1, 77–87.

Leighton, C. and Seaman, C. (1997a) Food retailing: an opportunity for meeting elderly consumers' needs. *Nutrition and Food Science* (4/5), 4i–4vii.

Leighton, C. and Seaman, C. (1997b) The elderly food consumer: disadvantaged? *Journal of Consumer Studies and Home Economics* 21, 363–370.

Lewis, E. (2005) Functional food for thought. *Brand Strategy* 191(April), 50–51.

Locher, J.L., Ritchie, C.S., Roth, D.L., Sawyer Baker, P., Bodner, E.V. and Allman, R.M. (2005) Social isolation, support, and capital and nutritional risk in an older sample: ethnic and gender differences. *Social Science & Medicine* 60, 747–761.

Long, N. (1998) Broken down by age and sex: exploring the ways we approach the elderly consumer. *Journal of the Market Research Society* 40, 73–91.

Lumpkin, J.R., Greenberg, B.A. and Goldstucker, J.L. (1985) Marketplace needs of the elderly: determinant attributes and store choice. *Journal of Retailing* 61, 75–105.

Lyon, P. and Colquhoun, A. (1999) Home, hearth and table: a centennial review of the nutritional circumstances of older people living alone. *Ageing and Society* 19, 53–67.

McAlpine, S.J., Harper, J., McMurdo, M.E., Bolton-Smith, C. and Hetherington, M.M. (2003) Nutritional supplementation in older adults: pleasantness, preference and selection of sip-feeds. *British Journal of Health Psychology* 8, 57–66.

McIntosh, W.A., Shifflett, P.A. and Picou, J.S. (1989) Social support, stressful events, strain, dietary intake, and the elderly. *Medical Care* 27, 140–153.

Mack, R., Salmoni, A., Viverais-Dressler, G., Porter, E. and Garg, R. (1997) Perceived risks to independent living: the view of older, community-dwelling adults. *The Gerontologist* 37, 729–736.

McKie, L. (1999) Older people and food: independence, locality and diet. *British Food Journal* 101, 528–536.

Maddison, D. and Walker, W.L. (1967) Factors effecting the outcome of conjugal bereavement. *American Journal of Psychology* 113, 1057–1067.

Mason, J.B. and Bearden, W.O. (1979) Satisfaction/dissatisfaction with food shopping among elderly consumers. *Journal of Consumer Affairs* 13, 359–369.

Mazis, M.B., Ringold, D.J., Elgin, S.P. and Denman, D.W. (1992) Perceived age and attractiveness of models in cigarette advertisements. *Journal of Marketing* 56, 22–37.

Meiselman, H.L. (1992a) Methodology and theory in human eating research. *Appetite* 19, 49–55.

Meiselman, H.L. (1992b) Obstacles to studying real people eating real meals in real situations. *Appetite* 19, 84–86.

Meiselman, H.L. (2000) *Dimensions of The Meal. The Science, Culture, Business and Art of Eating*. Aspen Publishers, Inc., Gaithersburg, Maryland.

Meiselman, H.L., Hirsch, E.S. and Popper, R.D. (1989) Sensory, hedonic and situational factors in food acceptance and consumption. In: Thomson, D.M.H. (ed.) *Food Acceptability*. Elsevier, London, pp. 77–87.

Meiselman, H.L., Hedderley, D., Staddon, S.L., Pierson, B.J. and Symonds, C.R. (1994) Effect of effort on meal selection and meal acceptability in a student cafeteria. *Appetite* 23, 43–55.

Meiselman, H.L., Johnson, J.L., Reeve, W. and Crouch, J.E. (2000) Demonstration of the influence of the eating environment on food acceptance. *Appetite* 35, 231–237.

Morley, J.E. and Silver, A.J. (1988) Anorexia in the elderly. *Neurobiological Ageing* 9, 9–16.

Moschis, G.P. (1996) *Gerontographics: Life Stage Segmentation for Marketing Strategy Development*. Quorum, Westport, Connecticut.

Moschis, G.P. (2003) Marketing to older adults: an updated overview of present knowledge and practice. *Journal of Consumer Marketing* 20, 516–525.

Moschis, G., Euehun, L. and Mathur, A. (1997) Targeting the mature market: opportunities and challenges. *Journal of Consumer Marketing* 14, 282–294.

Mozaffarian, D., Kumanyika, S.K., Lemaitre, R.N., Olson, J.L., Burke, G.L. and Siscovick, D.S. (2003) Cereal, fruit, and vegetable fiber intake and the risk of cardiovascular disease in elderly individuals. *Journal of the American Medical Association* 289, 1659–1666.

Murcott, A. (1982) On the social significance of cooked dinner in South Wales. *Social Science Information* 21, 677–696.

Murphy, S.P., Davis, M.A., Neuhaus, J.M. and Lein, D. (1990) Factors influencing the dietary adequacy and energy intake of older Americans. *Journal of Nutrition Education* 22, 284–291.

Nijhof, G. (1995) Parkinson's disease as a problem of shame in public appearance. *Sociology of Health and Illness* 17, 193–204.

Oldenburg, R. (1999) *The Great Good Place: Cafes, Coffee Shops, Bookstores, Bars, Hair Salons, and Other Hangouts at the Heart of a Community*. Marlowe and Company, New York.

Parry, C. (2004) Sunny Bisk relaunches and targets older people. *Marketing Week (UK)* 27(26 February), 8.

Payette, H. and Shatenstein, B. (2005) Determinants of healthy eating in community-dwelling elderly people. *Canadian Journal of Public Health. Revue Canadienne de Sante Publique* 96, S27–S31.

Pearson, A., Fitzgerald, M. and Nay, R. (2003) Mealtime in nursing homes: the role of the nursing staff. *Journal of Gerontological Nursing* 29, 40–47.

Piacentini, M., Hibbert, S. and Al-Dajanie, H. (2001) Diversity in deprivation: exploring the shopping behaviour of disadvantaged consumers. *International Review of Retail, Distribution and Consumer Research* 11, 141–158.

Ponza, M., Ohls, J.C. and Millen, B.E. (1996) Serving Elders at Risk: *The Older Americans Act Nutrition Programs, National Evaluation of the Elderly Nutrition Program 1996: 1993–1995*. Mathematica Policy Research, Inc., Princeton, New Jersey.

Population Division of the Department of Economic and Social Affairs of the United Nations Secretariat (2005) *World Population Prospects: The 2004 Revision. Highlights*. United Nations, New York.

Pörn, L. (1993) Health and adaptness. *Theoretical Medicinc* 14, 295–303.

Pound, P. and Gompertz, P. (1998) A patient-centered study of the consequences of stroke. *Clinical Rehabilitation* 12, 338–347.

Prinsley, D.M. and Sandstead, H.H. (1990) *Nutrition and Aging*. Alan R. Liss Inc., New York.

Prothro, J.W. and Rosenbloom, C.A. (1999) Description of a mixed ethnic, elderly population. II. Food group behavior and related nonfood characteristics. *The Journals of Gerontology. Series A, Biological Sciences and Medical Sciences* 54A, M325–M328.

Quandt, S. and Rao, P. (1999) Hunger and food security among older adults in a rural community. *Human Organization* 58, 28–35.

Quandt, S.A., Vitolins, M.Z., DeWalt, K.M. and Roos, G.M. (1997) Meal patterns of older adults in rural communities: life course analysis and implications for undernutrition. *Journal of Applied Gerontology* 16, 152–171.

Quandt, S.A., McDonald, J., Arcury, T.A., Bell, R.A. and Vitolins, M.Z. (2000) Nutritional self-management of elderly widows in rural communities. *The Gerontologist* 40, 86–96.

Quandt, S.A., Arcury, T.A., McDonald, J., Bell, R.A. and Vitolins, M.Z. (2001a) Meaning and management of food security among rural elders. *Journal of Applied Gerontology* 20, 356–376.

Quandt, S.A., Arcury, T.A., Bell, R.A., McDonald, J. and Vitolins, M.A. (2001b) The social meaning of food sharing among older rural adults. *Journal of Ageing Studies* 15, 145–162.

Revenson, T.A. and Johnson, J.L. (1984) Social and demographic correlates of loneliness in later life. *American Journal of Community Psychology* 12, 71–85.

Rolls, B.J. (1999) Do chemosensory changes influence food intake in the elderly? *Physiology & Behavior* 66, 193–197.

Rosenbloom, C.A. and Whittington, F.J. (1993) The effects of bereavement on eating behaviors and nutrient intakes in elderly widowed persons. *Journal of Gerontology* 48, S223–S229.

Rothenberg, E., Bosaeus, I. and Steen, B. (1993) Intake of energy, nutrients and food items in an urban elderly population. *Ageing (Milano)* 5, 105–116.

Rovner, B.W. and Ganguli, M. (1998) Depression and disability associated with impaired vision: the MoVIES Project. *Journal of the American Geriatrics Society* 46, 617–619.

Rowe, J.W. and Kahn, R.L. (1998) *Successful Aging*. Pantheon, New York.

Sahyoun, N.R. and Zhang, X.L. (2005) Dietary quality and social contact among a nationally representative sample of the older adult population in the United States. *Journal of Nutrition, Health & Aging* 9, 177–183.

Sahyoun, N.R., Pratt, C.A. and Anderson, A. (2004) Evaluation of nutrition education interventions for older adults: a proposed framework. *Journal of the American Dietetic Association* 104, 58–69.

Sawchuck, K.A. (1995) From gloom to boom: age, identity and target marketing. In: Featherstone, M. and Wernick, A. (eds) *Images of Ageing: Cultural Representations of Later Life*. Routledge, London, pp. 173–187.

Shahar, D.R., Schultz, R., Shahar, A. and Wing, R.R. (2001) The effect of widowhood on weight change, dietary intake, and eating behavior in the elderly population. *Journal of Aging and Health* 13, 189–199.

Sharkey, J.R. and Schoenberg, N.E. (2005) Prospective study of black–white differences in food insufficiency among homebound elders. *Journal of Aging and Health* 17, 507–527.

Shatenstein, B., Nadon, S. and Ferland, G. (2004) Determinants of diet quality among Quebecers aged 55–74. *Journal of Nutrition, Health & Aging* 8, 83–91.

Short, F. (2003) Domestic cooking practices and cooking skills. *Food Service Technology* 3, 177–185.

Sidenvall, B., Fjellström, C. and Ek, A.-C. (1994) The meal situation in geriatric care – intentions and experiences. *Journal of Advanced Nursing* 20, 613–621.

Sidenvall, B., Lennernäs, M.A.-C. and Ek, A.-C. (1996) Elderly patient's meal patterns – a retrospective study. *Journal of Nutrition and Dietetics* 9, 263–272.

Sidenvall, B., Nydahl, M. and Fjellström, C. (2000) The meal as a gift – the meaning of cooking among retired women. *Journal of Applied Gerontology* 19, 405–423.

Sidenvall, B., Nydahl, M. and Fjellström, C. (2001) Managing food shopping and cooking: the experiences of Swedish women. *Ageing and Society* 21, 151–168.

Smedley, B.D. and Syme, L.S. (eds) (2000) *Promoting Health: Intervention Strategies from Social and Behavioral Research*. National Academy Press, Washington, DC.

Sobal, J. (2000) Sociability and meals facilitation, commensality, and interaction. In: Meiselman, H.L. (ed.) *Dimensions of the Meal: The Science, Culture, Business and Art of Eating*. Aspen Publishers Inc., Gaithersburg, Maryland, pp. 119–133.

Song, Y., Manson, J.E., Buring, J.E. and Liu, S. (2004) A prospective study of red meat consumption and type 2 diabetes in middle-aged and elderly women: The Women's Health Study. *Diabetes Care* 27, 2108–2115.

Spalding, D. (1999) 'Not because they are old'. An independent inquiry into the care of older people on acute wards in general hospitals. *Journal of Human Nutrition and Dietetics* 12, 473–474.

Stitt, S., O'Connell, C. and Grant, D. (1995) Old, poor and malnourished. *Nutrition and Health* 10, 135–154.

Stroebele, N. and de Castro, J.M. (2004) Effect of ambience on food intake and food choice. *Nutrition* 20, 821–838.

Suda, Y., Marske, C.E., Flaherty, J.H., Zdrodowski, K. and Morley, J.E. (2001) Examining the effect of intervention to nutritional problems of the elderly living in an inner city area: a pilot project. *Journal of Nutrition, Health & Aging* 5, 118–123.

Sundström, G. (1994) *Care by Families: An Overview of Trends In Caring for Frail Elderly People: New Directions in Care*. Social Policy Studies No. 14. OECD, Paris.

Swoboda, B. and Morschett, D. (2001) Convenience-oriented shopping: a model from the perspective of consumers research. In: Frewer, L., Risvik, E. and Schifferstein, H. (eds) *Food, People and Society. A European Perspective of Consumers' Food Choices*. Springer-Verlag, Berlin/Heidelberg, Germany, pp. 177–195.

Sydner, Y.M. and Fjellström, C. (2005) Food provision and the meal situation in elderly care – outcomes in different social contexts. *Journal of Human Nutrition and Dietetics* 18, 45–52.

Szmigin, I. and Carrigan, M. (2001) Learning to love the older consumer. *Journal of Consumer Behaviour* 1, 22–34.

Tantiwong, D. and Wilton, P.C. (1985) Understanding food preferences among the elderly using hybrid conjoint measurement models. *Journal of Retailing* 61, 35–64.

Thomas, V. and Wolfe, D.B. (1995) Why won't television grow up? *American Demographics* 17, 24.

Toner, H.M. and Morris, J.D. (1992) A social–psychological perspective of dietary quality in later adulthood. *Journal of Nutrition for the Elderly* 11, 35–53.

Trichopoulou, A. and Critselis, E. (2004) Mediterranean diet and longevity. *European Journal of Cancer Prevention* 13, 453–456.

Trichopoulou, A., Kouris-Blazos, A., Wahlqvist, M.L., Gnardellis, C., Lagiou, P., Polychronopoulos, E., Vassilakou, T., Lipworth, L. and Trichopoulos, D. (1995) Diet and overall survival in elderly people. *British Medical Journal* 311, 1457–1460.

Trichopoulou, A., Costacou, T., Bamia, C. and Trichopoulos, D. (2000) Cancer and Mediterranean dietary traditions. *Cancer Epidemiology, Biomarkers & Prevention* 9, 869–873.

Trichopoulou, A., Costacou, T., Bamia, C. and Trichopoulos, D. (2003) Adherence to a Mediterranean diet and survival in a Greek population. *New England Journal Medicine* 348, 2599–2608.

United Nations Department of Economic and Social Affairs Population Division (2002) *World Population Ageing 1950–2050*. United Nations, New York.

Verbrugge, L.M. and Jette, A.M. (1994) The disablement process. *Social Science & Medicine* 38, 1–14.

Wahlqvist, M.L., Kouris-Blazos, A. and Hsa-Hage, B.H. (1997) Aging, food, culture and health. *Southeast Asian Journal of Tropical Medicine and Public Health* 28(Suppl. 2), 100–112.

Wahlqvist, M.L., Kouris-Blazos, A. and Wattanapenpaiboon, N. (1999) The significance of eating patterns: an elderly Greek case study. *Appetite* 32, 23–32.

Wahlqvist, M.L., Darmadi-Blackberry, I., Kouris-Blazos, A., Jolley, D., Steen, B., Lukito, W. and Horie, Y. (2005) Does diet matter for survival in long-lived cultures? *Asia Pacific Journal of Clinical Nutrition* 14, 2–6.

Walker, D. and Beauchene, R.E. (1991) The relationship of loneliness, social isolation, and physical health to dietary adequacy of independently living elderly. *Journal of the American Dietetic Association* 91, 300–304.

Warde, A. (1997) *Consumption, Food and Taste*. Sage Publications, London.

Wilson, L.C., Alexander, A. and Lumbers, M. (2004) Food access and dietary variety among older people. *International Journal of Retail & Distribution Management* 32, 109–122.

Winter Falk, L., Bisogni, C.A. and Sobal, J. (1996) Food choice processes of older adults: a qualitative investigation. *Journal of Nutrition Education* 28, 257–265.

Wolfe, D.B. (1997) Older markets and the new marketing paradigm. *Journal of Consumer Marketing* 14, 294–302.

Wolfe, W.S., Olson, C.M., Kendall, A. and Frongillo, E.A. (1996) Understanding food insecurity in the elderly: a conceptual framework. *Journal of Nutrition Education* 28, 92–100.

Wolfe, W.S., Olson, C.M., Kendall, A. and Frongillo, E.A. (1998) Hunger and food insecurity in the elderly: its nature and measurement. *Journal of Aging and Health* 10, 327–350.

Wolfe, W.S., Frongillo, E.A. and Valois, P. (2003) Understanding the experience of food insecurity by elders suggests ways to improve its measurement. *Journal of Nutrition* 133, 2762–2769.

World Health Organization (2002) *Active Ageing: A Policy Framework*. Document WHO/NMH/NPH/02.8. World Health Organization, Geneva, Switzerland.

Wylie, C., Copeman, J. and Kirk, S. (1999) Health and social factors affecting food choice and nutritional intake of elderly people with restricted mobility. *Journal of Human Nutrition and Dietetics* 12, 375–380.

16 The Impact of Optimistic Bias on Dietary Behaviour

VICKY SCAIFE,[1] SUSAN MILES[2] AND PETER HARRIS[3]

[1]School of Social Work and Psychosocial Sciences, University of East Anglia, Norwich NR4 7TJ, UK; [2]School of Medicine, Health Policy and Practice, University of East Anglia, Norwich NR4 7TJ, UK; [3]Centre for Research in Social Attitudes, Psychology Department, University of Sheffield, Sheffield S10 2TP, UK

Introduction

Human dietary behaviour is as interesting to members of the public as it is to policy makers and researchers. The mass media presents information on aspects of human dietary behaviour to large audiences, and policy initiatives (e.g. health promotion activities) seek to encourage healthier dietary behaviours amongst members of the public. Concomitantly, a growing research portfolio examines the antecedents, correlates and consequences of human dietary behaviour. The purpose of this chapter is to review one aspect of this portfolio, namely research conducted from a social–psychological perspective examining the impact of 'optimistic bias' (or unrealistic optimism) on human dietary behaviour.

Optimistic bias is the name given to a specific form of optimistic expectation. Optimistic expectations are those expectations that express hopefulness and confidence that favourable outcomes will prevail over unfavourable ones. For example, we may say that an individual who expects to be offered a job after an interview has an optimistic expectation about his/her personal likelihood of obtaining that job. Having optimistic expectations can have both positive and negative effects (Taylor and Brown, 1988; Schwarzer, 1994; Armor and Taylor, 1998). It could represent a functional orientation where an optimistic appraisal of the situation and one's coping abilities assist in the attainment of various favourable outcomes. For example, it has been found that dispositional optimism (stable, generalized expectancies that good things, rather than bad things, will happen), health condition-specific optimism (optimism specifically about future health) and positive efficacy expectations (a belief in ability to cope in demanding situations) have positive effects on physical and psychological well-being in both healthy and unhealthy individuals (Taylor et al., 1992; Leedham et al., 1995; Fournier et al., 2002; Carver et al., 2003; Stiegelis et al., 2003; de Ridder et al., 2004).

It is possible that optimistic bias may be adaptive. Optimistic bias could represent a defensive orientation where unrealistically optimistic predictions about the future lead to risky behaviours being sustained, and the likelihood of undertaking precautionary action being reduced. People's tendency to optimistically believe that others are more likely to experience negative future outcomes than themselves could leave them vulnerable to disappointment or even actual harm (Armor and Taylor, 1998). This optimism becomes problematic first when it is inaccurate, and second if it reduces the likelihood of performing self-protective behaviour. The tendency to erroneously believe that other people are more at risk from a hazard than the self is known as optimistic bias.

There are various ways to measure whether or not expectancies about future outcomes are optimistically biased. The best way is to compare a person's beliefs with the actual likelihood of harm. However, this requires a statistic that is accurate for the particular individual under investigation, which can be problematic to obtain (Weinstein and Klein, 1996). As a result, optimistic bias is more commonly investigated using comparative risk estimates. In such studies, people compare the likelihood of themselves experiencing a negative outcome with the likelihood for other people, with optimistic bias being exhibited when these likelihoods are significantly different, such that the majority of people believe that they are less likely to be at risk than others (this is influenced by, for example, the choice of comparison target and the sample involved; see Weinstein and Klein, 1996 for consideration of these issues).

It must be noted that people are not optimistically biased about anything and everything. For health and safety-related hazards, research on optimistic bias has sought to: (i) identify the specific hazards for which it occurs; (ii) identify the conditions under which it occurs; (iii) consider the nature of its impact upon actual behaviour; and (iv) establish methods for reducing/eliminating it. The interest in optimistic bias arises from concern that optimistic bias may have predominantly negative, rather than positive, effects. Consequently, the remainder of this chapter focuses upon the relationship between optimistic bias and human dietary behaviour. The following sections of this chapter review optimistic bias research in relation to food related hazards and human dietary behaviour. The sections which follow seek to: (i) identify the dietary-related hazards for which optimistic bias occurs; (ii) identify the conditions under which it occurs; (iii) consider the nature of its impact upon dietary behaviour; and (iv) outline methods for reducing/eliminating it. The relevance of optimistic bias research with dietary-related hazards is illustrated within the context of a rise in obesity. This work is then considered in the light of methodological issues.

Optimistic Bias for Dietary-related Hazards

There is much work investigating the extent to which optimistic bias operates in dietary-related domains. Some of this work has investigated the extent to which individuals are optimistically biased about their chances of experiencing negative health events as an outcome of some aspect of diet (e.g. heart disease as an outcome of a diet high in saturated fat; salmonellosis as an outcome of eating eggs).

Other work has investigated the extent to which individuals are optimistically biased about their chances of experiencing negative events associated with aspects of food production and food processing (e.g. food irradiation, food additives). Finally, further work has investigated the extent to which individuals are optimistically biased about their standing, in relation to others, on various diet-related risk factors (e.g. their sodium intake, their fat intake). Each section of this work is now described in turn (for a fuller review of research in this area, see Miles and Scaife, 2003).

Work investigating the extent to which individuals are optimistically biased about their likelihood of experiencing negative events emergent (in part or whole) from aspects of diet has indicated that evidence of optimistic bias has been found for: experiencing a heart attack, heart disease or 'heart trouble' (Hoorens and Buunk, 1993; Harris and Middleton, 1994; Peterson and de Avila, 1995; Raats *et al.*, 1999); experiencing dental problems (e.g. gum disease, tooth decay; Myers and Brewin, 1996; Astrom *et al.*, 1999); developing an alcohol problem (Regan *et al.*, 1995; Klein, 1996); contracting food poisoning (Frewer *et al.*, 1994; Peterson and de Avila, 1995); getting a stomach ulcer (Weinstein, 1983; Harris and Middleton, 1994); having high blood pressure (Weinstein, 1987; Harris and Middleton, 1994); gaining weight or becoming obese (Harris and Middleton, 1994; Sparks *et al.*, 1995; Rothman *et al.*, 1996; Raats *et al.*, 1999); having liver trouble/disease (Harris and Middleton, 1994; Rothman *et al.*, 1996); getting gastritis (Lek and Bishop, 1995); getting indigestion (Raats *et al.*, 1999); experiencing gallstones (Weinstein, 1982, 1987); becoming diabetic (Weinstein, 1982, 1984); feeling unwell generally (Sparks *et al.*, 1995; Raats *et al.*, 1999); developing bovine spongiform encephalopathy (Sparks and Shepherd, 1994); developing vitamin deficiency (Weinstein, 1982; Sparks and Shepherd, 1994); and having a stroke (Harris and Middleton, 1994; Peterson and de Avila, 1995).

Work investigating the extent to which individuals are optimistically biased about their likelihood of experiencing negative events associated with aspects of food production and food processing has indicated that optimistic bias operates for the following potential hazards: microwaves, food irradiation (Frewer *et al.*, 1994; Sparks and Shepherd, 1994), pesticides, genetic modification (Frewer *et al.*, 1994), food additives, food colourings and artificial sweeteners (Sparks and Shepherd, 1994).

Additional findings indicate that individuals are optimistically biased about their standing on a number of dietary-related risk factors including: fat intake (Frewer *et al.*, 1994; Paisley and Sparks, 1998), alcohol, caffeine, energy and sugar intake (Sparks and Shepherd, 1994) and intake of 'unhealthy' food (Whalen *et al.*, 1994).

Taken together, these findings are impressive, and it can be seen from the sample of studies reported here that optimistic bias operates across a wide range of different dietary-related hazards. However, it is not found for all hazards within this domain. For example, optimistic bias does not operate for a number of potential hazards associated with food production and food processing, including: environmental contamination, veterinary drug residues, natural toxicants, hormone residues and packaging materials (Sparks and Shepherd, 1994).

The fact that optimistic bias is found for some hazards and not for others as assessed by the same respondents, at the same time and using the same measurement technique provides some reassurance that optimistic bias is a real phenomenon and not merely an artefact of the measurement procedures employed. It should also be noted that optimistic bias is not always found to the same degree for the same hazard across studies. In particular, research findings regarding whether or not optimistic bias operates for cancer and high blood pressure are inconclusive. Some studies find optimistic bias for high blood pressure (Weinstein, 1984), but others do not (Weinstein, 1983). Generally people are optimistically biased for specific cancers (colon cancer, Rothman *et al.*, 1996; cervical cancer, Eiser and Cole, 2002), but for non-specified cancers some researchers find optimistic bias (Raats *et al.*, 1999) but others do not (Dolinski *et al.*, 1987). It is possible that these inconsistencies are due to different respondents thinking about different types of cancer. However, it is also important to consider the possibility that differences in measurement procedures used across studies may lead respondents in different studies to use different information processing strategies in order to generate risk judgements. Pertinent measurement issues are discussed later.

Negative Effects of Optimistic Bias

As previously stated, one reason for the interest in optimistic biases in personal risk perception is that they may hinder efforts to promote self-protective behaviours (Weinstein, 1989; Weinstein and Klein, 1996; Shepherd, 1999). Most models of health-protective behaviour (e.g. protection motivation theory, Rogers, 1975; the health belief model, Janz and Becker, 1984; the precaution adoption process, Weinstein, 1988) include the individual's perception of personal risk status (or personal vulnerability/susceptibility to a hazard) as a pre-condition for adopting behaviours that reduce risk. In these models, anticipation of a negative health outcome, in combination with the desire to avoid this outcome or reduce its impact, creates motivation for self-protection (Weinstein, 1993). Thus, if people believe that they are not susceptible to an adverse health effect, or less susceptible than others, then it may be more difficult to encourage them to implement sensible precautions.

This could have an effect on the impact of health promotion activities aimed at increasing self-protective behaviour since the vast majority of individuals may consider that the communication is directed at other people who are more vulnerable than themselves. Eiser and Gentle (1989) found that people who smoked, exercised less and had less healthy diets were significantly more likely to dismiss health campaigns as 'irrelevant' (although for drinking alcohol this effect was reversed). This suggests that 'health campaigns are received most favourably by those who "need" them least, as far as the "healthiness" of their own habits are concerned' (p. 118). It has been argued that public health campaigns are ineffective because they fail to change perceptions of personal invulnerability (Tyler and Cook, 1984; McKenna and Myers, 1997). Thus, whilst people may rate a hazard as more risky generally following a campaign, they may not change their rating of personal susceptibility. Weinstein (1988) notes that messages from the mass media and acquaintances provide information allowing people to first become aware of a hazard (i.e. that it exists), and secondly to acknowledge that there is a significant risk associated with the hazard. However, such messages rarely establish who is likely to be affected. Faced with such ambiguity, it is 'relatively easy for people to conclude that it is not their problem' (Weinstein, 1988, p. 362). This is seen when people acknowledge that a hazard poses a threat, but deny that they personally are at risk. However, too often in the literature on optimistic bias the relationship between optimistic bias and the perceived personal relevance of health communications is presumed, not tested.

There is some evidence suggesting that optimistic bias does inhibit performance of self-protective or precautionary behaviours. Burger and Burns (1988) demonstrated that individuals who were optimistically biased were less likely to use effective contraception. Larwood (1978, cited in Helweg-Larsen and Shepperd, 2001) demonstrated that individuals who were optimistically biased were less likely to obtain influenza vaccinations; while Sheer and Cline (1994, cited in Helweg-Larsen and Shepperd, 2001) demonstrated that individuals who were optimistically biased were more likely to engage in high-risk sex. Weinstein and Lyon (1999) found that optimistic bias about personal risk acted as a barrier to health-protective action within the context of testing the home for radon. Helweg-Larsen and Shepperd (2001) cite preliminary experimental evidence suggesting that perceiving the self to be at greater risk than others increases the likelihood of engagement in precautionary behaviour (see e.g. McKenna et al., 1991; Klein, 1997). A review of the literature found no studies examining the relationship between optimistic bias for a dietary-related negative outcome and actual dietary (eating) behaviour. It has been argued that more effort needs to be spent on understanding the behavioural consequences of optimistic biases (van der Pligt, 1994), and this is still the case.

Factors Associated with Optimistic Bias

There has been considerable work focusing on identifying factors which may be correlated with optimistic bias. Although correlation does not imply causality, this work provides insight into the conditions under which optimistic bias typically occurs. This may provide useful information in the future if we wish to predict whether or not optimistic bias may occur for a given health promotion target. A substantial body of literature has indicated that the degree of optimism obtained for a given hazard is related to the perceived controllability of that hazard; individuals are most optimistically biased about hazards which they believe they can personally control (Weinstein, 1980, 1982, 1987; Kulik and Mahler, 1987; van der Velde et al., 1992; Hoorens and Buunk, 1993; Lek and Bishop, 1995; Harris, 1996; Welkenhuysen et al., 1996; c.f. Harris and Middleton, 1994). A number of studies have indicated that individuals are least optimistically biased about their comparative likelihood of experiencing problems considered more likely to occur

(Weinstein, 1987; Eiser et al., 1993), and problems to which more thought has been given (Eiser et al., 1993). Optimistic bias is found for problems associated with a perception that if it has not been encountered in the past it is unlikely to be encountered in the future (Weinstein, 1982, 1987), and problems associated with a stereotype of a 'typical victim' (Lek and Bishop, 1995). In their review, Helweg-Larsen and Shepperd (2001) indicated that individuals also tend to exhibit less optimistic bias following a negative mood induction procedure than they do following a positive mood induction procedure.

Our understanding of the phenomenon has been further clarified by studies demonstrating that optimistic bias is unrelated to perceived severity (van der Velde et al., 1992; Welkenhuysen et al., 1996) and to level of knowledge regarding the risk (Welkenhuysen et al., 1996). There is also some evidence that people exhibit no optimistic bias when faced with a realistic threat (in the sense of having recently occurred or being ongoing, as opposed to a hypothetical threat); Klar et al. (2002) assessed absolute and comparative risk of being the victim of a terrorist attack in a Jewish Israeli population in Israel, and found both a lack of optimistic bias and evidence of precautionary behaviour change. They suggested that optimism (both comparative and absolute) may mainly occur 'when people are asked about future negative outcomes, for which *they are currently not experiencing any behavioral warning or indications*' (p. 216, emphasis in original). There is evidence that experience with a negative event, even if it is not personal experience, creates feelings of vulnerability and reduces optimistic bias (Dolinski et al., 1987; Helweg-Larsen, 1999; Weinstein et al., 2000; Parry et al., 2004). Although Dolinski et al. (1987) found no optimistic bias for threats to health due to radiation in Polish women following the explosion at the Chernobyl atomic power plant, optimistic bias for other threats, including other health threats, was still present. This suggests that the impact of experience with a negative effect on personal vulnerability is specific to the experienced hazard. Thus, it may be that people are more open to health promotion activities after they have experienced a hazard. For example, people who have suffered from food poisoning may be more willing to listen to advice about safe food handing presented by their physician or environmental health officer following this illness.

Attempts to Reduce Optimistic Bias

Work seeking to identify means of reducing or eliminating the bias, in the hope of ultimately facilitating healthful behavioural change, has been driven by findings such as those in the above section and other research describing and discussing the possible causes of the effect. Various methods have been used in these attempts, with varying degrees of success. Both providing conditional base rate statistics (e.g. the chance of developing skin cancer is 15% given low exposure to ultraviolet radiation and 25% given high exposure; Chandler et al., 1999) and reducing perceived social distance between the self and target other (Harris et al., 2000) made respondents' ratings less comparatively optimistic. McKenna and Myers (1997) found that respondents were less likely to report all their skills as better than average when they were informed that they would be taken out and tested on those skills. Making respondents more aware of the relevant risk factors associated with a hazard, and encouraging respondents to consider the risk status of the target other, have also been successful at reducing optimistic bias (Weinstein, 1980; Weinstein and Lachendro, 1982). However, other research has found that merely supplying respondents with information about risk factors can increase optimistic bias (Weinstein, 1983; Weinstein and Klein, 1995); optimistic bias was reduced only when information was provided about the target other's standing on these factors. Other research in this area has been successful at influencing ratings of personal risk judgements by providing self-relevant information (Stapel and Velthuijsen, 1996; Rothman *et al.*, 1999). There is some evidence that people will actually try to maintain their optimistic biases when faced with information about the target other's risk (Rothman *et al.*, 1996). It is apparent that further work is needed in this area to identify appropriate mechanisms for reducing optimistic bias, in particular relation to causes of this effect.

When considering attempts in the literature to alter optimistic bias it is important to be aware that, as described above, optimistic expectations about the future (including optimistic biases about likelihood of adverse effects) can have positive effects on individuals' mental health status. For example, it has been found optimistic beliefs about personal health have a positive impact on self-protective health behaviours, increase attention to health risk information, and lead to greater recall of that information (Taylor *et al.*, 1992; Aspinwall and Brunhart, 1996). Attempts to reduce optimistic bias may well make individuals more appreciative of their health and safety status in relation to others, but we must consider the possibility that reductions in optimistic bias might lead to reductions in self-esteem and psychological well-being. It is also possible that reductions in optimistic bias might lead to the generation of unnecessarily extreme risk aversions. It is likely that sections of the population might exhibit pessimistic bias for some dietary-related hazards. For example, individuals may develop irrational aversions to specific foods, which may negatively impact on their health status. Similarly, individuals with eating disorders may exhibit pessimistic bias regarding outcomes associated with food consumption. Thus, it may be useful to look at the desirability as well as the feasibility of promoting more realistic views in pessimistically biased individuals using the techniques described above.

Optimistic Bias and Obesity: a Current Example

The increasing prevalence of overweight and obesity in both adults and children is a growing concern; as of 2000, the number of obese adults worldwide stood at over 300 million (World Health Organization, 2003). The UK Government has recently outlined recommendations focusing on diet and activity levels for dealing with the increase in overweight and obesity (House of Commons Health Committee, 2004) and the wider health risks associated with a sedentary life-style (Chief Medical Officer, 2004). Thus, motivating people to change their diets and increase their level of physical activity is going to become increasingly important, with health promotion activities in these areas likely to rise. For this reason, it is necessary that any barriers to undertaking the recommended health-protective behaviours are identified and, where possible, overcome.

There is evidence that people tend to both have a greater actual fat intake than recommended and underestimate their fat intake (perceived versus actual intake); furthermore, motivation to change this behaviour is typically low (Glanz et al., 1997; Raats et al., 1999; Oenema and Brug, 2003). Related to this, optimistic bias effects have been found for comparative judgements about the likelihood of experiencing various short- and long-term health problems related to consuming a high-fat diet including feeling unwell due to consumption of a high-fat diet, weight gain, suffering heart attacks and having high blood pressure (Weinstein, 1987; Frewer et al., 1994; Sparks and Shepherd, 1994; Sparks et al., 1995). Moreover, in line with these optimistic expectations, there is also evidence that people claim to eat less of the foods associated with high fat consumption than others (Perloff and Fetzer, 1986; Klein and Kunda, 1993; Sparks et al., 1995; Weinstein and Klein, 1995; Klein, 1996). This suggests that people may misrepresent the actual content of their diet in line with their optimistic biases about risk. 'If individuals do not feel they need to change, because they feel that their diet is already healthy and they are at less risk than the average person, then they are less likely to implement change' (Shepherd, 1999, p. 810).

Even with all the research conducted on optimistic biases in the food domain, little is known about the occurrence and nature of any interpersonal comparisons that are made regarding food issues such as dietary fat intake. Klein and Weinstein (1997) note that whilst we see that people respond to comparison information when it is made available by researchers, we do not know whether or not people engage in social comparison spontaneously when assessing personal risk. Investigating this issue, Oenema and Brug (2003) asked people for details about any comparisons they made when evaluating their own fat intake. They found that respondents did acknowledge comparing themselves to various target others when evaluating their own fat intake, including their partner, relatives, people in the street/shops and friends or acquaintances. This comparison occurred in a number of ways including: observing what other people eat, buy, have in their cupboards and have in their supermarket trolleys; by observing how other people cook; what they look like; and by listening to what other people say about their food habits.

Increasing prevalence of overweight and obesity in children will likely be mirrored by later trends in adult overweight and obesity, indicating a need to start efforts to prevent obesity in early childhood (Troiano and Flegal, 1998; Reilly et al., 1999; Chinn and Rona, 2001). However, there has been very little research investigating optimistic bias, or its impact on food choice decisions in children. Research suggests that there are a number of influences on children's food choices, but long-term health issues associated with food are not important (Neumark-Sztainer et al., 1999; Hart et al., 2002. Food choice in children and adolescents is addressed in other chapters of this book). Indeed, research with parents indicates that they have a short-term health focus with respect to their children's diet (e.g. healthy hair, skin and teeth, and the influence of food choices on behaviour and mood), with little concern for potential long-term consequences (Hart et al., 2003). One study that did investigate optimistic beliefs about risk in children found that children do believe that they are less likely than their peers to experience various health risks including cancer and heart attacks, eating unhealthy food and taking too little exercise (Whalen *et al.*, 1994). Further research is required to investigate any impact of optimistic bias on healthy food and life-style behaviours recommended in health promotion activities aimed specifically at children.

Aspects of Measurement which may Influence the Degree of Optimistic Bias Obtained in Dietary-related Domains

Direct versus indirect measurement

Optimistic bias may be measured using a direct measurement technique or an indirect measurement technique. Under the direct measurement technique respondents make likelihood judgements for themselves compared with others on a single scale (e.g. 'Compared to the average person of my age and sex, the likelihood of me getting colon cancer is . . .'). Under the indirect measurement technique respondents make judgements about their own likelihood of experiencing a negative event on one item (e.g. 'The likelihood of my getting colon cancer is . . .') and judgements about others' likelihood of experiencing a negative event on another separate item (e.g. 'The likelihood of the typical person of my age and sex getting colon cancer is . . .'). Research investigating whether or not optimistic bias operates for dietary-related hazards has utilized both indirect and direct measurement procedures, although there has been a marginal tendency to favour the latter (Miles and Scaife, 2003).

There is evidence suggesting that the type of measurement procedure used does influence the degree of optimism obtained; but the direction of influence under each technique has varied across studies. For instance, Otten and van der Pligt (1996) reported more optimism under the direct measurement technique, whereas Weinstein *et al.* (2000) reported that more optimism was elicited under the indirect measurement technique. Klar *et al.* (2002) and Sutton (2002) both found that the direct measurement technique resulted in more pessimistic bias than indirect measurement. There is some evidence that such differences may be hazard-dependent; for example, Price *et al.* (2002) found that the perceived frequency of occurrence of the hazard interacts with the measurement method to affect the level of optimistic bias shown (direct comparison and frequent events resulted in less optimistic bias than indirect comparison and frequent events).

There is some evidence that when asked to compare themselves to other people using a direct comparison question, respondents are actually only focusing on themselves, rather than on themselves in relation to others (Klar and Giladi, 1999; Kruger, 1999; Eiser *et al.*, 2001; Covey and Davies, 2004). It has been found that comparative ratings correlate positively with absolute ratings for the self, but there is no relationship with absolute ratings for others. It is only when people are asked to rate other people in comparison to themselves that we see both a positive correlation of comparative ratings to absolute ratings for the self, and a negative correlation of comparative ratings to absolute ratings for others (Eiser *et al.*, 2001). However, the less than perfect correlation between perceived absolute risk and perceived comparative risk suggests that the latter is not simply a proxy for the former (Klein, 2002). For these reasons, Covey and Davies (2004) recommend that the indirect measurement technique should be favoured in future research as this method explicitly requires people to think about the comparison others. It is paradoxical, therefore, that the seemingly explicit comparative scale (i.e. the direct one) may not be comparative at all.

In future work using the direct comparison method, we must ask first, when faced with the request to make a direct comparison, if people are actually forming any representation of the other to whom they are supposed to be comparing themselves; and, second, if not and if people are simply focusing on their self, how are they coming up with this rating? It is necessary to be aware that the measurement technique used may influence the results obtained. There is a real need for future research to use both direct and indirect measurement techniques in the same study, for a range of dietary-related hazards, so that the impact of each on the degree of optimism obtained can be more directly assessed.

Self-other focus versus other-self focus

Optimistic bias may be measured using a self-other focus (when people are asked how similar they are to others using direct comparison, or rating the self before other people using indirect comparison), or an other-self focus format (when people are asked how similar others are to themselves using direct comparison, or rating other people before the self using indirect comparison). There is some evidence to suggest that the degree of optimism obtained may vary as a function of this focus. Otten and van der Pligt (1996, Study 1) found that there was greater optimism for the self with a self-other focus than with an other-self focus (see also Eiser *et al.*, 2001); however, they failed to replicate this in their second study. Whilst not directly investigating the impact of comparison order on optimistic bias, a number of other studies using the indirect method have varied the presentation order of the absolute self and other ratings to control for order effects, and no differences in optimism exhibited under the two presentation orders have been found (e.g. Perloff and Fetzer, 1986; Rothman *et al.*, 1996; Whalen *et al.*, 1994). Other researchers have found this order effect for positive events (Hoorens, 1995; note that Eiser *et al.*, 2001 found a stronger effect for positive than for negative outcomes) and a hazard-dependent effect for negative events (Dolinski *et al.*, 1987; Hoorens and Buunk, 1993).

Miles and Scaife's (2003) review indicated that the majority of work investigating optimistic bias in dietary-related domains utilized a self-other focus. To provide reassurance that the degree of bias obtained has not been unduly influenced by this preference, it is important that future research compares the degree of optimism obtained for each format, using both direct and indirect measurement, for a range of dietary-related hazards. If it is confirmed that more optimism is consistently obtained when a self-other focus is used, then the cognitive structures and processes which may underpin this effect will require more thorough elucidation.

Comparison target

It is possible that the latitude which research participants are permitted in their construal of the target other influences the degree of optimism obtained in research work. Research using various comparison targets indicates that the amount of optimistic bias found, and even whether optimistic bias is exhibited at all, depends on exactly who people are asked to compare themselves to. For example, research has found that when people are asked to compare themselves with friends, optimistic bias is not exhibited. Commonly friends are judged to be equally vulnerable as the self and, like the self, are judged to be less vulnerable than other people. Less optimistic bias is also found when people compare themselves to parents and friends. In contrast, when people compare themselves to average or typical others strong optimistic bias is exhibited (Perloff and Fetzer, 1986; Harris and Middleton, 1994; Regan *et al.*, 1995; Klar *et al.*, 1996; Zakay, 1996; Martz *et al.*, 1998; c.f. Hoorens and Buunk, 1993).

In optimistic bias research, the targets for social comparison are usually supplied by the investigator. Even in situations where people are allowed to choose, for example, 'their closest friend' there is no evidence that people would compare themselves with this target spontaneously when thinking about this hazard. It is likely that the comparison other will be dependent on the hazard under consideration; for example, hereditary risks are more likely to require comparison with family members (Klein, 2002). After establishing whether or not people do indeed engage in social comparison to establish their likelihood of experiencing negative effects associated with dietary-related hazards, future work should seek to examine the impact of target specificity on degree of optimism obtained. There is a real need to establish the nature of individuals' comparison preferences in natural settings, beyond the confines of optimistic bias questionnaires, perhaps through the use of diary studies. Having identified people's usual comparison targets under different situations, then this information can be used in health promotion activities. For example, if individuals' real-life comparison preferences are with 'typical' members of particular reference groups, and if a greater degree of optimism is emergent from such comparisons than from comparison with specific individuals (e.g. close friend), then future health communications need to direct individuals to make social comparisons with specific rather than generalized or prototypical others, in order to reduce optimistic bias with a view to effecting more healthy behaviour. One problem with studies using different comparison targets is that factors such as similarity to, liking of, psychological closeness to, type of relationship with, and type of knowledge about the other are often confounded, so it is unclear exactly what aspect of the comparison other is influencing judgements (Klein and Weinstein, 1997). Thus, future work also needs to distinguish between these aspects.

To summarize, it is certainly important to be aware that aspects of the measurement procedure employed may influence the degree of optimistic bias obtained for particular hazards, including those which are dietary-related. However, it is also important to be aware that optimistic bias has been demonstrated to exist for a large number of different dietary-related hazards, using a wide range of different measurement techniques.

General Conclusions

Research evidence to date suggests that an optimistic bias about one's risk likelihood may have an impact on dietary behaviour. There is a small amount of evidence that people exhibiting optimistic biases about their personal susceptibility to experiencing various negative effects associated with different hazards are less likely to undertake self-protective behaviours. However, the research conducted to investigate the impact of optimistic bias on behaviour both in the food domain and in other areas is still extremely sparse. Furthermore, it is also clear that there are a number of measurement issues that may have differential impacts on the level of optimistic bias exhibited. Thus, further work is necessary to elucidate the conditions under which optimistic bias is exhibited for different dietary-related hazards and behaviours. With this information, it will be far easier to identify both the situations where optimistic expectations need to be dealt with, and the means by which this should be done.

References

Armor, D.A. and Taylor, S.E. (1998) Situated optimism: specific outcome expectancies and self-regulation. *Advances in Experimental Social Psychology* 30, 309–379.

Aspinwall, L.G. and Brunhart, S.M. (1996) Distinguishing optimism from denial: optimistic beliefs predict attention to health threats. *Personality and Social Psychology Bulletin* 22, 993–1003.

Astrom, A.N., Awadia, A.K. and Bjorvatn, K. (1999) Perceptions of susceptibility to oral health hazards: a study of women in different cultures. *Community Dental Oral Epidemiology* 27, 268–274.

Burger, J.M. and Burns, L. (1988) The illusion of unique invulnerability and the use of effective contraception. *Personality and Social Psychology Bulletin* 14, 264–270.

Carver, C.S., Lehman, J.M. and Antoni, M.H. (2003) Dispositional pessimism predicts illness-related disruption of social and recreational activities among breast cancer patients. *Journal of Personality and Social Psychology* 84, 813–821.

Chandler, C.C., Greening, L., Robison, L.J. and Stoppelbein, L. (1999) It can't happen to me . . . or can it? Conditional base rates affect subjective probability judgements. *Journal of Experimental Psychology: Applied* 5, 361–378.

Chief Medical Officer (2004) *At Least Five a Week: Evidence on the Impact of Physical Activity and Its Relationship to Health*. Department of Health, London.

Chinn, S. and Rona, R.J. (2001) Prevalence and trends in overweight and obesity in three cross sectional studies of British children, 1974–94. *British Medical Journal* 322, 24–26.

Covey, J.A. and Davies, A.D.M. (2004) Are people unrealistically optimistic? It depends how you ask them. *British Journal of Health Psychology* 9, 39–49.

De Ridder, D., Fournier, M. and Bensing, J. (2004) Does optimism affect symptom report in chronic disease? What are its consequences for self-care behaviour and physical functioning? *Journal of Psychosomatic Research* 56, 341–350.

Dolinski, D., Gromski, W. and Zawisza, E. (1987) Unrealistic pessimism. *Journal of Social Psychology* 127, 511–516.

Eiser, J.R. and Cole, N. (2002) Participation in cervical screening as a function of perceived risk, barriers and need for cognitive closure. *Journal of Health Psychology* 7, 99–105.

Eiser, J.R. and Gentle, P. (1989) Health behaviour and attitudes to publicity campaigns for health promotion. *Psychology and Health* 3, 111–120.

Eiser, J.R., Eiser, C. and Pauwels, P. (1993) Skin cancer: assessing perceived and behavioural attitudes. *Psychology and Health* 8, 393–404.

Eiser, J.R., Pahl, S. and Prins, Y.R.A. (2001) Optimism, pessimism and the direction of self-other comparisons. *Journal of Experimental Social Psychology* 37, 77–84.

Fournier, M., de Ridder, D. and Bensing, J. (2002) Optimism and adaptation to chronic disease: the role of optimism in relation to self-care option to type 1 diabetes mellitus, rheumatoid arthritis and multiple sclerosis. *British Journal Health Psychology* 7, 409–432.

Frewer, L.J., Shepherd, R. and Sparks, P. (1994) The interrelationship between perceived knowledge, control and risk associated with a range of food hazards targeted at the individual, other people and society. *Journal of Food Safety* 14, 19–40.

Glanz, K., Brug, J. and van Assema, P. (1997) Are awareness of dietary fat intake and actual fat consumption associated? A Dutch–American comparison. *European Journal of Clinical Nutrition* 51, 542–547.

Harris, P. (1996) Sufficient grounds for optimism? The relationship between perceived controllability and optimistic bias. *Journal of Social and Clinical Psychology* 15, 9–52.

Harris, P. and Middleton, W. (1994) The illusion of control and optimism about health: on being less at risk but no more in control than others. *British Journal of Social Psychology* 33, 369–386.

Harris, P., Middleton, W. and Joiner, R. (2000) The typical student as an in-group member: eliminating optimistic bias by reducing social distance. *European Journal of Social Psychology* 30, 235–253.

Hart, K.H., Bishop, J.A. and Truby, H. (2002) An investigation into school children's knowledge and awareness of food and nutrition. *Journal of Human Nutrition and Dietetics* 15, 129–140.

Hart, K.H., Herriot, A., Bishop, J.A. and Truby, H. (2003) Promoting healthy diet and exercise patterns amongst primary school children: a qualitative investigation of parental perspectives. *Journal of Human Nutrition and Dietetics* 16, 89–96.

Helweg-Larsen, M. (1999) (The lack of) optimistic biases in response to the 1994 Northridge earthquake: the role of personal experience. *Basic and Applied Social Psychology* 21, 119–129.

Helweg-Larsen, M. and Shepperd, J.A. (2001) Do moderators of the optimistic bias affect personal or target risk estimates: a review of the literature. *Personality and Social Psychology Review* 5, 74–95.

Hoorens, V. (1995) Self-favoring biases, self-presentation, and the self-other asymmetry in social comparison. *Journal of Personality* 63, 793–817.

Hoorens, V. and Buunk, B.P. (1993) Social comparison of health risks: locus of control, the person positivity bias, and unrealistic optimism. *Journal of Applied Social Psychology* 23, 291–302.

House of Commons Health Committee (2004) *Obesity. Third Report of Session 2003–04*, Vol. 1. Available at: http://www.publications.parliament.uk/pa/cm200304/cmselect/cmhealth/cmhealth.htm (accessed 31 October 2005).

Janz, N. and Becker, M.H. (1984) The health belief model: a decade later. *Health Education Quarterly* 11, 1–47.

Klar, Y. and Giladi, E.E. (1999) Are most people happier than their peers, or are they just happy? *Personality and Social Psychology Bulletin* 25, 585–594.

Klar, Y., Medding, A. and Sarel, D. (1996) Nonunique invulnerability: singular versus distributional probabilities and unrealistic optimism in comparative risk judgement. *Organizational Behavior and Human Decision Processes* 67, 229–245.

Klar, Y., Zakay, D. and Sharvit, K. (2002) 'If I don't get blown up . . .': realism in face of terrorism in an Israeli nationwide sample. *Risk Decision and Policy* 7, 203–219.

Klein, W.M. (1996) Maintaining self-serving social comparisons: attenuating the perceived significance of risk-increasing behaviours. *Journal of Social and Clinical Psychology* 15, 120–142.

Klein, W.M. (1997) Objective standards are not enough: affective, self-evaluative and behavioural responses to social comparison information. *Journal of Personality and Social Psychology* 72, 763–774.

Klein, W.M.P. (2002) Comparative risk estimates relative to the average peer predict behavioural intentions and concern about absolute risk. *Risk Decision and Policy* 7, 193–202.

Klein, W.M. and Kunda, Z. (1993) Maintaining self-serving social comparisons: biased reconstruction of one's past behaviors. *Personality and Social Psychology Bulletin* 19, 732–739.

Klein, W.M. and Weinstein, N.D. (1997) Social comparison and unrealistic optimism about personal risk. In: Buunk, B.P. and Gibbons, F.X. (eds) *Health, Coping and Well-being: Perspectives from Social Comparison Theory*. Lawrence Erlbaum Associates, London, pp. 25–61.

Kruger, J. (1999) Lake Wobegon be gone! The 'below-average effect' and the egocentric nature of comparative ability judgements. *Journal of Personality and Social Psychology* 77, 221–232.

Kulik, J.A. and Mahler, H.I. (1987) Health status, perceptions of risk, and prevention interest for health and non-health problems. *Health Psychology* 6, 15–27.

Leedham, B., Meyerowitz, B.E., Muirhead, J. and Frist, W.H. (1995) Positive expectations predict health after heart transplantation. *Health Psychology* 14, 74–79.

Lek, Y. and Bishop, G.D. (1995) Perceived vulnerability to illness threats: the role of disease type, risk factor perception and attributions. *Psychological Health* 10, 205–217.

McKenna, F.P. and Myers, L.B. (1997) Illusory self-assessments – can they be reduced? *British Journal of Psychology* 88, 39–51.

McKenna, F.P., Stainer, R.A. and Lewis C. (1991) Factors underlying illusory self-assessment of driving skill in males and females. *Accident Analysis and Prevention* 23, 45–52.

Martz, J.M., Verette, J., Arriaga, X.B., Slovik, L.F., Cox, C.L. and Rusbult, C.E. (1998) Positive illusion in close relationships. *Personal Relationships* 5, 159–181.

Miles, S. and Scaife, V. (2003) Optimistic bias and food. *Nutrition Research Reviews* 16, 3–19.

Myers, L.B. and Brewin, C.R. (1996) Illusions of well-being and the repressive coping style. *British Journal of Social Psychology* 35, 443–457.

Neumark-Sztainer, D., Story, M., Perry, C. and Casey, M.A. (1999) Factors influencing food choices of adolescents: findings from focus-group discussions with adolescents. *Journal of the American Dietetic Association* 99, 929–934.

Oenema, A. and Brug, J. (2003) Exploring the occurrence and nature of comparison of one's own perceived dietary fat intake to that of self-selected others. *Appetite* 41, 259–264.

Otten, W. and van der Pligt, J. (1996) Context effects in the measurement of comparative optimism probability judgements. *Journal of Social and Clinical Psychology* 15, 80–101.

Paisley, C.M. and Sparks, P. (1998) Expectations of reducing fat intake: the role of perceived need within the theory of planned behaviour. *Psychology and Health* 13, 341–353.

Parry, S.M., Miles, S., Tridente, A., Palmer, S.R. and South and East Wales Infectious Disease Group (2004) Differences in perception of risk between people who have and have not experienced *Salmonella* food poisoning. *Risk Analysis* 24, 289–299.

Perloff, L.S. and Fetzer, B.K. (1986) Self other judgements and perceived vulnerability to victimization. *Journal of Personality and Social Psychology* 50, 502–510.

Peterson, C. and de Avila, M.E. (1995) Optimistic explanatory style and perception of health problems. *Journal of Clinical Psychology* 51, 128–132.

Price, P.C., Pentecost, H.C. and Voth, R.D. (2002) Perceived event frequency and the optimistic bias: evidence for a two-process model of personal risk judgments. *Journal of Experimental Social Psychology* 38, 242–252.

Raats, M.M., Sparks, P., Geekie, M.A. and Shepherd, R. (1999) The effects of providing personalized dietary feedback: a semi-computerized approach. *Patient Education and Counselling* 37, 177–189.

Regan, P.C., Snyder, M. and Kassin, S.M. (1995) Unrealistic optimism: self-enhancement or person positivity? *Personality and Social Psychology Bulletin* 21, 1073–1082.

Reilly, J.J., Dorosty, A.R. and Emmett, P.M. (1999) Prevalence of overweight and obesity in British children: cohort study. *British Medical Journal* 319, 1039.

Rogers, R.W. (1975) A protection motivation theory of fear appeals and attitude change. *Journal of Psychology* 91, 93–114.

Rothman, A.J., Kelly, K.M., Weinstein, N.D. and O'Leary, A. (1999) Increasing the salience of risky sexual behavior: promoting interest in HIV-antibody testing among heterosexually active young adults. *Journal of Applied Social Psychology* 29, 531–551.

Rothman, A.J., Klein, W.M. and Weinstein, N.D. (1996) Absolute and relative biases in estimations of personal risk. *Journal of Applied Social Psychology* 26, 1213–1236.

Schwarzer, R. (1994) Optimism, vulnerability, and self-beliefs as health-related cognitions: a systematic overview. *Psychology and Health* 9, 161–180.

Shepherd, R. (1999) Social determinants of food choice. *Proceedings of the Nutrition Society* 58, 807–812.

Sparks, P. and Shepherd, R. (1994) Public perceptions of the potential hazards associated with food production and food consumption: an empirical study. *Risk Analysis* 14, 799–806.

Sparks, P., Shepherd, R., Wieringa, N. and Zimmermans, N. (1995) Perceived behavioural control, unrealistic optimism and dietary change: an exploratory study. *Appetite* 24, 243–255.

Stapel, D.A. and Velthuijsen, A.S. (1996) 'Just as if it happened to me': the impact of vivid and self-relevant information on risk judgements. *Journal of Social and Clinical Psychology* 15, 102–119.

Stiegelis, H.E., Hagerdoorn, M., Sanderman, R., van der Zee, K.I., Buunk, B.P. and van den Bergh, A.C.M. (2003) Cognitive adaptation: a comparison of cancer patients and healthy references. *British Journal of Health Psychology* 7, 409–432.

Sutton, S. (2002) Influencing optimism in smokers by giving information about the average smoker. *Risk Decision and Policy* 7, 165–174.

Taylor, S.E. and Brown, J.D. (1988) Illusion and well-being: a social psychological perspective on mental health. *Psychological Bulletin* 103, 193–210.

Taylor, S.E., Kemeny, M.E., Aspinwall, L.G., Schneider, S.G., Rodriguez, R. and Herbert, M. (1992) Optimism, coping, psychological distress, and high-risk sexual behavior among men at risk for acquired immunodeficiency syndrome (AIDS). *Journal of Personality and Social Psychology* 63, 460–473.

Troiano, R.P. and Flegal, K.M. (1998) Overweight children and adolescents: description, epidemiology, and demographics. *Pediatrics* 101, 497–504.

Tyler, T.R. and Cook, F.L. (1984) The mass media and judgements of risk: distinguishing impact on personal and societal level judgements. *Journal of Personality and Social Psychology* 47, 693–708.

Van der Pligt, J. (1994) Healthy thoughts about unhealthy behaviour. *Psychology and Health* 9, 187–190.

Van der Velde, F.W., Hookyas, C. and van der Pligt, J. (1992) Risk perception and behaviour: pessimism, realism and optimism about AIDS-related health behaviour. *Psychology and Health* 6, 23–38.

Weinstein, N.D. (1980) Unrealistic optimism about future life events. *Journal of Personality and Social Psychology* 39, 806–820.

Weinstein, N.D. (1982) Unrealistic optimism about susceptibility to health problems. *Journal of Behavioral Medicine* 5, 441–460.

Weinstein, N.D. (1983) Reducing unrealistic optimism about illness susceptibility. *Health Psychology* 2, 11–20.

Weinstein, N.D. (1984) Why it won't happen to me: perceptions of risk factors and susceptibility. *Health Psychology* 3, 431–457.

Weinstein, N.D. (1987) Unrealistic optimism about susceptibility to health problems: conclusions from a community-wide sample. *Journal of Behavioural Medicine* 10, 481–499.

Weinstein, N.D. (1988) The precaution adoption process. *Health Psychology* 7, 355–386.

Weinstein, N.D. (1989) Optimistic biases about personal risks. *Science* 246, 1232–1233.

Weinstein, N.D. (1993) Testing four competing theories of health-protective behavior. *Health Psychology* 12, 324–333.

Weinstein, N.D. and Klein, W. (1995) Resistance of personal risk perceptions to debiasing interventions. *Health Psychology* 14, 132–140.

Weinstein, N.D. and Klein, W.M. (1996) Unrealistic optimism: present and future. *Journal of Social and Clinical Psychology* 15, 1–8.

Weinstein, N.D. and Lachendro, E. (1982) Egocentrism as a source of unrealistic optimism. *Personality and Social Psychology Bulletin* 8, 195–200.

Weinstein, N.D. and Lyon, J.E. (1999) Mindset, optimistic bias about personal risk and health-protective behaviour. *British Journal of Health Psychology* 4, 289–300.

Weinstein, N.D., Lyon, J.E., Rothman, A.J. and Cuite, C.L. (2000) Changes in perceived vulnerability following natural disaster. *Journal of Social and Clinical Psychology* 19, 372–395.

Welkenhuysen, M., Evers-Kiebooms, G., Decruyenaere, M. and van den Berghe, H. (1996) Unrealistic optimism and genetic risk. *Psychology and Health* 11, 479–492.

Whalen, C.K., Henker, B., O'Neil, R., Hollingshead, J., Holman, A. and Moore, B. (1994) Optimism in children's judgements of health and environmental risks. *Health Psychology* 13, 319–325.

World Health Organization (2003) *Controlling the Global Obesity Epidemic*. Available at: http://www.who.int/nutrition/topics/obesity/er (accessed 31 October 2005).

Zakay, D. (1996) The relativity of unrealistic optimism. *Acta Psychologica* 93, 121–131.

Further Reading

Armor, D.A. and Taylor, S.E. (1998) Situated optimism: specific outcome expectancies and self-regulation. *Advances in Experimental Social Psychology* 30, 309–379.

Buunk, B.P. and Gibbons, F.X. (eds) (1997) *Health, Coping and Well-being: Perspectives from Social Comparison Theory*. Lawrence Erlbaum Associates, London.

Helweg-Larsen, M. and Shepperd, J.A. (2001) Do moderators of the optimistic bias affect personal or target risk estimates: a review of the literature. *Personality and Social Psychology Review* 5, 74–95.

Miles, S. and Scaife, V. (2003) Optimistic bias and food. *Nutrition Research Reviews* 16, 3–19.

Weinstein, N.D. and Klein, W.M. (eds) (1996) Special issue: Unrealistic optimism about personal risks. *Journal of Social and Clinical Psychology* 15.

Weinstein, N.D. and Nicolich, M. (1993) Correct and incorrect interpretations of correlations between risk perceptions and risk behaviours. *Health Psychology* 12, 235–245.

This page intentionally left blank

17 Implementation Intentions: Strategic Automatization of Food Choice

THOMAS L. WEBB,[1] PASCHAL SHEERAN[2] AND
CHRISTOPHER J. ARMITAGE[2]

[1]School of Psychological Sciences, The University of Manchester,
Manchester, M13 9PL, UK; [2]Department of Psychology, University of
Sheffield, Sheffield S10 2TP, UK

Introduction

Substantial discrepancies often exist between the decisions that people make about what to eat and their actual consumption of foodstuffs. That is, positive intentions are not necessarily translated into behaviour (see Sheeran, 2002 for a review). For example, Gummeson et al. (1997) found that intentions to eat a healthy breakfast were only moderately related to actual food choices as assessed by a self-report diary. Sheeran et al. (2005a) analysed people's failure to act on their intentions in terms of three processes: intention viability, intention activation and intention elaboration. Intention viability refers to the idea that people may not have the ability, resources or opportunities to act on their intentions. Intention activation is important because alternative goal pursuits (e.g. short-term hedonistic motives) may take precedence over efforts to eat healthily, leading the person to forget their original intention (prospective memory failure) or to prioritize other intentions (goal reprioritization). Finally, intentions may not be translated into behaviour because people fail to engage in, or elaborate in sufficient detail, the particular actions and contextual opportunities that would permit realization of their intention. In short, interventions to change dietary behaviour may need to supplement motivational messages (designed to change intentions) with volitional strategies (designed to ensure intentions are implemented) to ensure dietary change.

Implementation Intentions: Theoretical Overview

Peter Gollwitzer's concept of implementation intentions (Gollwitzer, 1993, 1996, 1999) is arguably one of the most important advances in recent self-regulation research. Implementation intentions are a volitional strategy involving precise behavioural plans that specify when, where and how one will perform

behaviour(s) that lead to goal attainment. Implementation intentions are specified in the form of an if–then plan that creates a mental link between a specified
future situation and a particular goal-directed behaviour. Thus, whereas goal
intentions have the format 'I intend to reach Z!', implementation intentions have
the format 'If situation X arises, then I will perform goal-directed behaviour Y!'
Thus, a person who intends to increase their consumption of fruit and vegetables
might plan when and where to buy their fruit and vegetables and how to
integrate this produce into their diet (cf. Kellar and Abraham, unpublished) by
forming the plans 'When I am next in the supermarket, I will buy at least five
different types of fruit and vegetables!' and 'If I have a midmorning snack, then
I will have a piece of fruit!'

Implementation intentions are important because if–then planning represents a relatively simple, quick and effective strategy to engender behaviour
change. For example, interventions based on implementation intentions have
been used to promote completion of personal projects (Gollwitzer and
Brandstätter, 1997; Oettingen et al., 2002), attendance at cervical cancer
screening (Sheeran and Orbell, 2000), workplace safety training (Sheeran
and Silverman, 2003) and public transport use (Bamberg, 2000). In the
largest review of studies to date, Gollwitzer and Sheeran (2006) found that,
based on 92 studies and a sample size of 8283 participants, implementation
intentions had a medium-to-large effect on goal attainment ($d_+ = 0.65$, where
d_+ refers to the sample-weighted average of d, the unbiased standardized
mean difference between conditions; Hedges and Olkin, 1985). Furthermore,
implementation intentions proved effective across published and unpublished reports, student and non-student samples, self-report and objective
measures of behaviour, and for a wide variety of different goals. Evidence
also indicates that implementation intentions can be effective in promoting
healthy food choice.

Applications of Implementation Intentions in the Domain of Food Choice: a Review

Eating a low-fat diet

Armitage (2004) evaluated the effectiveness of an intervention based on
implementation intentions for reducing dietary fat intake. Two hundred and
sixty-four workers in a medium-sized company were sent a questionnaire
about their dietary behaviours via the internal mail system. In addition, one-
half of the participants received written instructions to form a plan specifying
how they would eat a low-fat diet in the next month ('We want you to plan to
eat a low-fat diet during the next month. You are free to choose how you will
do this, but we want you to formulate your plans in as much detail as possible.
Please pay particular attention to the situations in which you will implement
these plans.'). Fat consumption was assessed one month later by means of a
validated food frequency questionnaire (Margetts et al., 1989). As expected,

participants who supplemented their intention to eat a low-fat diet with a plan specifying how to do so consumed less fat (mean 74 g fat/day) than did participants who had not formed a plan (mean 85 g fat/day).

In a follow-up study, Armitage (2006) categorized the dietary behaviours of a further company-based sample ($n = 554$) into the five stages of change delineated by the transtheoretical model (Prochaska and DiClemente, 1983, 1984). At baseline, 31% of the participants did not eat a low-fat diet and were not thinking about starting (pre-contemplation stage), 25% were thinking about starting (contemplation stage), 22% ate a low-fat diet but not on a regular basis (preparation stage), 7% had begun eating a low-fat diet in the last 6 months (action stage), and 15% had eaten a low-fat diet for more than 6 months (maintenance stage). The key question for Armitage's (2006) study was whether implementation intentions could promote progression through these stages 1 month later.

In short, they could. Participants who formed plans were more likely to progress from their initial stage of change (27% progressed) than were participants who had not formed plans (13% progressed). Furthermore, consistent with the idea that implementation intentions help people to act on their intentions, the intervention was most effective in helping people progress from the pre-contemplation stage (36% versus 15%, for experimental and control groups, respectively) and from the contemplation stage (35% versus 18%, respectively). Armitage (2006) also tested whether implementation intentions prevented regression to earlier stages of change. Contrary to expectations, however, the same proportion of participants in each condition regressed back though the stages. It seems that, in this study at least, different implementation intentions are needed to avoid relapse back into the consumption of fatty foods than are required to promote healthy eating in the first instance.

Instead of asking participants to plan how to avoid eating fatty foods, P. Sheeran and S. Milne (unpublished data) asked participants to plan to consume a particular snack food only on particular occasions. The idea was that participants would probably be unwilling to try to eliminate the foodstuff from their diet and, therefore, a realistic implementation intention would need to respect participants' pre-commitment to indulgence. Participants completed a questionnaire based on the theory of planned behaviour (TPB; Ajzen, 1991) concerning their beliefs about reducing their consumption of a nominated snack food over the following week and a subset formed implementation intentions only to eat the food on specific occasions. Findings from two studies indicated that forming if–then plans to engage in moderate indulgence significantly reduced self-reported snack food consumption over a 1-week period.

Increasing fruit and vegetable consumption

Kellar and Abraham (unpublished) investigated whether forming implementation intentions with respect to acquiring and preparing fruit and vegetables promoted consumption of the recommended daily intake of five portions of fruit and vegetables (RDIFV). Two hundred and eighteen students completed a questionnaire about their dietary behaviour and one-half of the participants were asked to plan when and where they would buy fruit and vegetables during the following week. These participants were also asked to plan both lunchtime and evening meals that incorporated fruit and vegetables. One week later, $n = 146$ of the original sample reported their fruit and vegetable consumption. As expected, participants who formed implementation intentions consumed the RDIFV on more days (mean 3.03) than did participants who did not form a plan (mean 2.28). It is important to note that, although Kellar and Abraham's (unpublished) planning intervention was combined with a motivational message and post-intervention differences were observed between planning and control conditions on measures of intention and anticipated regret, the effect of the planning intervention remained significant after controlling for these differences. Thus, the impact of implementation intentions on behaviour cannot be attributed to changes in motivation or beliefs about eating fruit and vegetables.

The efficacy of implementation intentions for promoting consumption of the RDIFV among a clinical population was tested by Jackson *et al.* (2003). One hundred and nineteen patients with cardiovascular illness were randomly allocated to one of three conditions: participants in the control group were simply asked to eat two extra portions of fruit and vegetables per day over the next 3 months; participants in the TPB group also completed a questionnaire concerning their beliefs about eating two extra portions of fruit and vegetables; finally, participants in the implementation intention group completed the TPB questionnaire and were asked to specify (in conjunction with the researcher) when and where they would eat two extra portions of fruit and vegetables a day over the next 3 months and what they would eat at these times. Participants reported their fruit and vegetable consumption 7 days later, 28 days later and 90 days later. Although all three groups increased their consumption of fruit and vegetables at all three time points, there was no evidence to suggest that participants who formed an implementation intention ate any more fruit and vegetables than did participants in the control and TPB conditions. Furthermore, 90 days later participants who formed plans actually ate less fruit and vegetables than did participants in the other two conditions. Jackson *et al.* (2003) attributed this surprising finding to a lack of flexibility in participants' plans. For example, acting on one's plan to eat a banana for breakfast in the kitchen is impossible if one has run out of bananas. However, an alternative explanation is that forming implementation intentions in conjunction with the researcher led to experimenter demand in the form of unrealistically optimistic intentions and/or extrinsically based motivation. Consistent with this idea, Koestner *et al.* (2002) found that the effectiveness of implementation intentions was undermined when the underlying goal intention was not self-concordant.

Healthy eating (general)

Verplanken and Faes (1999) compared the impact of unhealthy eating habits and an implementation intention manipulation on six aspects of participants' diet recorded over 5 days: variety, fat avoidance, regularity of meals and the amount of vegetables, fruit, and dairy products. Each aspect was rated by a professional dietician as bad (0), reasonable (1) or good (2), and responses across the six aspects were summed to give an overall 'healthy eating' score. Prior to recording their food intake, unhealthy eating habits were measured by asking participants to check which foods they had consumed over the past week from a list of 67 unhealthy foods. In addition, one-half of the sample were asked to form implementation intentions to eat healthily on one of the next 5 days by specifying exactly what they would eat and drink during their chosen day. Regression analyses with the healthy eating score as the dependent variable revealed that both unhealthy eating habits and the manipulation of implementation intentions influenced participants' food choices. Participants who formed implementation intentions were judged to eat more healthily (mean score 6.63) than were participants who did not form implementation intentions (mean score 5.45) Moreover, there was no interaction between the effects of habit and the experimental manipulation – implementation intentions were equally effective for participants with both weak and strong tendencies to eat unhealthy foods.

Two aspects of Verplanken and Faes's (1999) analyses warrant comment. First, the measure of healthy eating was summed across the 5 days, whereas participants only formed an implementation intention with respect to one of these days. It seems possible, therefore, that Verplanken and Faes (1999) underestimated the effect of implementation intentions because the plan was not designed to influence behaviour on 4 out of 5 of these days. It would be interesting to compute a healthy eating score for each day separately and treat the effect of implementation intentions as a within-participants factor in order to further elucidate the impact of the intervention. Second, Verplanken and Faes (1999) also examined whether the effect of implementation intentions could be attributed to participants' desire to appear consistent or to respond in a socially desirable manner. Independent raters compared participants' eating plans with their actual food choices on the specified day. Verplanken and Faes (1999) argued that there was little reason to suspect the operation of consistency or social desirability motives because very few perfect matches occurred between participants' planned foodstuff and the actual foods consumed. However, this finding runs counter to previous work on implementation intentions, which finds a very high correspondence between the specified plan and actual behaviour. For example, in a study of breast self-examination, Orbell *et al.* (1997) found a perfect correspondence between the time and the place that participants specified they would perform breast self-examination and the actual time and place of performance at follow up. One explanation of Verplanken and Faes's (1999) finding is that their results attest to the flexibility of action control under implementation intentions; participants who formed plans did eat more healthily on the specified day, but they flexibly substituted the specified foods with alternatives. As Verplanken and Faes (1999) noted, 'the planned chicken turned out to be beef, and eating an apple became eating an orange' (p. 600). However, this flexibility contrasts with Jackson *et al.*'s (2003) explanation of their findings in terms of a lack of flexibility in planning. Although Sheeran *et al.* (2005b) showed that implementation intentions were flexible to the extent that they were sensitive to changes in the underlying goal intention (i.e. implementation intentions do not influence behaviour if the plan is not supported by a strong, activated goal intention), additional research is warranted to determine whether implementation intentions permit flexible substitution of alternative behaviours if the specified behaviour cannot be enacted.

Consumer behaviour

Bamberg (2002) investigated the effects of forming implementation intentions (with and without a monetary incentive) on purchasing a sample of organic food. Three hundred and twenty students who had seldom bought organic food were given a voucher to buy at least one product in the next 7 days from a local organic food shop. The level of monetary incentive was manipulated by varying the value of the voucher (5 versus 15 German marks) and implementation intentions were manipulated by asking one-half of the participants to decide exactly when they would visit the shop. As expected, for participants with little monetary incentive, forming an implementation intention promoted the purchase of organic food (50% used the coupon) compared with participants who did not form a plan (34%). However, providing a monetary incentive was as effective as forming an implementation intention (54%) and combining the monetary incentive with the implementation intention did not benefit goal achievement over either strategy in isolation (61%). These findings suggest that increased motivation (in the form of a monetary incentive) can sometimes be sufficient to promote healthy food choice; implementation intentions can confer little additional benefit in performance if almost all participants act on their intentions.

Increasing vitamin supplement intake

Finally, implementation intentions have been used successfully to promote the intake of dietary supplements. Sheeran and Orbell (1999, Study 1) provided a bottle containing 50 vitamin C tablets to 136 college students and asked one-half of the sample to specify when and where they would take the tablets. The number of pills remaining in the bottle was counted 10 days later and 3 weeks later. Contrary to expectations, 10 days later there was no difference in the number of pills remaining between implementation intention and control conditions. However, 3 weeks after the intervention, participants who formed implementation intentions had missed significantly fewer pills (mean 1.57) than had participants who did not form implementation intentions (mean 3.53). Sheeran and Orbell (1999) suggested that, in the short term (10 days), simply being motivated to take the supplements was sufficient to ensure consumption and thus implementation intentions conferred no additional benefit. However, in the long term (3 weeks) the volitional demands of remembering to take the pills became much greater and the person was better able to benefit from implementation intention formation. This interpretation (and the discussion of Bamberg's, 2002 results) speaks to the idea that the presence of a self-regulatory problem is an important moderator of implementation intention effects (see Sheeran *et al.*, 2005a).

Mechanisms Underlying Implementation Intention Effects

Implementation intentions are thought to be effective in promoting goal achievement because of psychological processes that relate to both the anticipated situation and the specified goal-directed response (Gollwitzer *et al.*, 2005). First, considerable evidence attests to the idea that the mental representation of the anticipated situation (specified in the if-component of the plan) becomes highly accessible when implementation intentions are formed. Furthermore, this heightened accessibility leads to fast and accurate detection of good opportunities in which to act because people are 'perceptually ready' to encounter these opportunities. For example, Webb and Sheeran (2004) found that, even when the situational cue was embedded in a visual illusion that typically impairs cue detection, forming an implementation intention that specified the cue as a good opportunity to act improved task performance. In sum, people who form implementation intentions are in a good position to identify and attend to the cue specified in the if-component of their plan.

The second process hypothesized to underlie the beneficial effects of implementation intentions relates to the strong link that is formed between the critical situation and the intended response. The mental act of if–then planning forges strong associations between mental representations of opportunities (cues) and actions that promote goal attainment (responses). The consequence is that the person does not have to deliberate about how to act when the specified situation is encountered; instead, the cue triggers the intended behaviour automatically (Gollwitzer, 1999). In other words, there is evidence that action control by implementation intentions is immediate, efficient and does not require conscious intent (Gollwitzer *et al.*, 2005).

The immediacy of action initiation by implementation intentions was demonstrated by Gollwitzer and Brandstätter (1997, Study 3) in a study concerned with counteracting racial prejudice. Participants were asked to take a convincing counter position toward xenophobic remarks presented on a videotape. In addition, one group of participants was asked to form an implementation intention to commit themselves to counter-argue at preselected suitable opportunities. The results suggested that participants who formed an implementation intention seized suitable opportunities to express themselves more immediately (i.e. closer to the specified time) than did participants who had familiarized themselves with these favourable opportunities (see also Brandstätter *et al.*, 2001, Studies 2 and 3). Several experiments have also considered the efficiency of action initiation as a function of implementation intentions. Unlike the performance of participants who only formed goal intentions, manipulations of cognitive load have no deleterious effects on the performance of participants who formed implementation intentions (Brandstätter *et al.*, 2001). Extending this idea, Webb and Sheeran (2003) investigated the relationship between implementation intentions and ego-depletion. Ego-depletion refers to the temporary depletion of self-regulatory capacity by an initial act of self-control (Baumeister *et al.*, 1998; Muraven *et al.*, 1998). Webb and Sheeran (2003) used this idea to test if implementation intentions required self-control resources to be effective. Participants completed a balance-and-maths dual task under ego-depletion versus control conditions and subsequently completed a Stroop colour-naming task (Stroop, 1935). As expected, ego-depleted participants performed worse on the Stroop task. However, ego-depleted participants who formed implementation intentions in relation to the Stroop task performed as well as non-depleted controls. In other words, implementation intention formation means that the intended behaviour can be performed well (or executed appropriately) even when people's self-regulatory resources are diminished.

The final criterion for classifying a response as automatic is to demonstrate that it can operate in the absence of conscious intent. In an illustrative study, Sheeran *et al.* (2005b, Experiment 2) asked participants to complete a series of puzzles as accurately as possible. One-half of the participants were asked to form an implementation intention designed to speed up completion of the puzzles ('As soon as I think I have the answer, I will not deliberate, but press the corresponding number key as quickly as possible!'). In addition, a priming procedure was used to activate the goal of responding quickly outside awareness; a control group did not get this goal activated. The findings revealed that implementation intentions influenced the speed with which puzzles were completed even when the relevant goal was activated through the priming procedure. These findings support the idea that implementation intentions are successful in promoting goal attainment even if participants are not aware that this goal has been activated (see also Bayer *et al.*, 2002, cited in Gollwitzer *et al.*, 2005).

The evidence reviewed so far suggests that implementation intentions enhance: (i) the accessibility of the specified situational cues; (ii) the strength of association between the cue and the intended response; and (iii) goal attainment. However, only two studies to date (Aarts, *et al.*, 1999; Webb and Sheeran, 2004) have provided evidence that the effect of implementation intentions on goal attainment is mediated by cue accessibility and cue–response association strength. Tests of mediation are important in order to rule out the possibility that cue accessibility and strengthened cue–response associations are simply by-products of forming implementation intentions but are not responsible for their success. Aarts *et al.* (1999) investigated whether the behavioural effects of implementation intentions were mediated by enhanced accessibility of the specified environmental features. Participants were asked to form an implementation intention specifying when, where and how they would collect a food coupon (or did not). Next, in an ostensibly unrelated experiment, participants all completed a lexical decision task designed to measure the accessibility of situational cues related to coupon collection (i.e. words related to the location where the coupon should be collected). Finally, Aarts *et al.* (1999) observed whether or not participants collected the coupon. Findings showed that participants who formed an implementation intention were faster to recognize words describing the anticipated situational cues (e.g. left, corridor, swingdoor) and were more likely to collect the coupon than were control participants. Crucially, however, the accessibility of the anticipated situational cues was found to mediate the effect of implementation intentions on behaviour. Thus, this experiment provides good evidence that heightened cue accessibility is one mechanism responsible for the effect of implementation intentions on behaviour.

Webb and Sheeran (2004) replicated and extended the work of Aarts *et al.* (1999) to consider the mediating role of cue–response association strength in addition to cue accessibility. The strength of association between the specified cues and the intended response was assessed using a sequential priming paradigm similar to that used by Bargh *et al.* (1995). Participants were asked to decide (as quickly as possible) if a series of target words were verbs or not. However, prior to some of these targets, words relating to the specified cues were presented subliminally. Cue–response association strength was indexed by examining participants' response latencies to the target behaviour word when it was preceded by words relating to the specified cues. As expected, participants who formed implementation intentions specifying when, where and how they would complete a language task were more likely to act on their intentions than were participants who did not form a plan. Moreover, participants who formed implementation intentions responded faster to words representing the anticipated situational cues and faster to the target behaviour word following subliminal presentation of the situational cues. Finally, mediation analyses revealed that both cue accessibility and the strength of the link between cue and response mediated the impact of implementation intentions on goal attainment. In sum, there is good evidence that implementation intentions promote strategic automatization of goal pursuit; anticipated opportunities are detected easily and these cues elicit the intended response automatically.

Suggestions for Future Research on Implementation Intentions and Food Choice

This section describes several areas of research that we feel warrant further investigation. The majority of studies of implementation intentions in the domain of food choice focus on the behaviour itself (e.g. the number of portions of vegetables eaten each day) rather than the antecedents of behaviour, namely food-related thoughts/cravings and the environmental cues that can trigger consumption. Furthermore, previous research has also tended to neglect cognitive biases that may have an impact on food choice. Accumulating evidence attests to the idea that implementation intentions may be a useful way of modifying these beliefs. Finally, implementation intention research on food choice has, so far, failed to consider the highly social nature of eating.

Modifying thoughts about food and cravings

Dieting individuals face considerable conflict between physiology and cognition; the more weight one loses, the more one's thoughts turn to food and to eating (Keesey and Corbett, 1984; Schlundt and Johnson, 1990). Thus, one of the more important tasks for the dieter is to inhibit these thoughts about food. However, simply being motivated to do so ('I must not think about food') can, ironically, lead to more thoughts about food (Williamson, 1990; Wegner, 1994) or to post-suppression rebound (as soon as the person stops trying to suppress their thoughts about food, they experience more food-related thoughts than they would do normally; Herman and Polivy, 1993). However, there is evidence that implementation intentions can help to avoid ironic processes and rebound effects. Gollwitzer *et al.* (2002, cited in Gollwitzer *et al.*, 2005) adapted a paradigm used by Macrae *et al.* (1994). Participants were asked to describe a typical day in the life of a homeless person and to actively try to avoid thinking about the target in a stereotypical manner. One-half of the participants furnished their goal to suppress their prejudicial beliefs with an implementation intention ('And if I describe a given homeless person, then I will avoid stereotypical statements!'). The findings revealed that participants asked to suppress their stereotypical beliefs and participants who formed implementation intentions described the homeless person in a less stereotypical manner than did participants not asked to suppress their beliefs. Next, after a short filler task, all participants were asked to evaluate 'homeless people in general' using a semantic differential questionnaire. As expected, participants who had to suppress their beliefs in the first task exhibited a rebound effect such that they rated 'homeless people in general' in a more prejudicial manner than did control participants. Importantly, however, participants who formed implementation intentions did not evidence the stereotype rebound observed in participants without implementation intentions. In sum, future research should investigate whether forming implementation intentions can help dieters to control their unwanted thoughts about food while avoiding the ironic costs associated with this suppression.

Modifying environmental cues to consumption

Food cues are central to understanding hunger and cravings (Schachter, 1968). According to Schachter's externality theory dieters find it difficult to control their eating because they are 'super-vigilant' for food-related cues (see also Mogg *et al.*, 1998; Aarts *et al.*, 2001; Alsene *et al.*, 2004). Therefore, one potential future avenue for implementation intentions might be to modify the way that these food-related cues are perceived in an effort to reduce temptation. Work by Walter Mischel (Mischel and Ayduk, 2004; see also Herman and Polivy, 2004) suggests that reducing the sensory allure of the food stimulus itself may reduce the temptation of fatty foods. For example, Mischel *et al.* (1992) found that construing a chocolate bar as a log (or worse) reduced temptation. This paradigm could be modified so that implementation intentions are used to ensure the automation of the reconstrual. For example, participants could be asked to form a plan: 'If I see a chocolate bar, then I will imagine it is made of mud!' Alternatively, Herman and Polivy (2004) suggest that accepting the sensory appeal of chocolate, while keeping in mind its calorific threat, might also be efficacious ('If I am tempted by a chocolate bar, then I will tell myself that this is perfectly understandable, but it's not good for me!').

Reducing pessimistic biases: the 'what the hell effect'

Another domain in which implementation intentions might prove effective is the paradoxical finding that forced consumption of a rich milkshake actually increased subsequent food intake among a sub-sample of dieting participants (Herman and Mack, 1975). It seemed, for these participants, that there was no point in controlling subsequent eating because their efforts to reduce calorific intake had already been violated. Herman and Mack (1975) termed this disinhibition of self-control after an initial breach the 'what the hell effect' (*see* also Tice *et al.*, 2001). Future research might usefully consider whether implementation intentions can help people to contextualize the initial breach and to re-establish control. For example, participants might be asked to tell themselves 'And if I have slipped, then I will remember that it is only a small mistake and I am not much worse off than before!'

Reducing the negative impact of social context on food choice

Food choice is not solely an individual decision; significant others and the wider social context are likely to influence a person's decisions about what to eat (Polivy *et al.*, 1986; Herman *et al.*, 2003). For example, the prototype willingness model (Gibbons *et al.*, 1998) suggests that although people may not intend to engage in health-risk behaviours such as binge drinking they may be willing to if the circumstances are conducive. Similarly, Aarts and Dijksterhuis (2003) found that environmental norms (e.g. displaying good manners when in an upmarket restaurant) had an automatic effect on participants' behaviour. However, there is evidence to suggest that forming a plan to ignore the unwanted social influence ('If I am offered another drink, then I will ignore what other people want me to do and decide for myself!') may have a beneficial influence on goal attainment. For example, Gollwitzer (1998) asked participants to complete arithmetic problems as quickly as possible and to form a plan to ignore distractions ('If my mind gets sidetracked, then I will respond by concentrating on the task at hand!'). While participants worked on the problems they were interrupted by a confederate who asked a series of predetermined questions about how she could find a particular room. Consistent with the idea that implementation intentions can help people to overcome social influences, participants who formed plans to concentrate on the task were quicker to end the conversation with the confederate than were participants who had not formed a plan. Given the highly social nature of eating, it will be important for future interventions based on implementation intentions to target aspects of the social context that could threaten the person's food choice goals.

Concluding Remarks

The present chapter has reviewed eight studies that applied implementation intentions in the context of food choice. Forming an action plan specifying when,

where and how to perform relevant goal-directed behaviour(s) effectively promoted fruit and vegetable consumption amongst a student population (Kellar
and Abraham, unpublished), but not amongst a sample of cardiac patients
(Jackson *et al.*, 2003), consumption of a low-fat diet (Armitage, 2004, 2006; P.
Sheeran and S. Milne, unpublished data), healthy eating in general (Verplanken
and Faes, 1999), consumer behaviour (Bamberg, 2002) and vitamin supplement intake in the long term (Sheeran and Orbell, 1999). Implementation intentions represent a useful intervention for modifying dietary behaviour not least
because planning interventions are quick and economical to implement, but also
because implementation intentions permit dietary change without requiring that
dramatic changes are made to the self or to the environment (Gollwitzer *et al.*,
2005). This consideration is important because even if interventions succeed in
improving the self *vis-à-vis* dietary change (e.g. by providing the skills needed to
cook balanced meals), these benefits may be fleeting and dependent on transient
self-states. What happens, for instance, if the person's thoughts are preoccupied
with other concerns or the self-control resource is depleted after a hard day
at work? Similarly, interventions to change environments relevant to dietary
change are costly (e.g. making organic food readily available) and depend on
the idiosyncratic ways that people interact with the environment. Implementation intentions, on the other hand, only require that the person is motivated
to change their dietary behaviour. If–then planning delegates control of
the intended behaviour to specified environmental cues and, in doing so, goal
pursuit benefits from the immediacy and efficiency associated with automatic
processes. Thus, volitional difficulties associated with conscious, effortful goal
pursuit are circumvented. Research on food choice to date has not fully
capitalized on the benefits of implementation intentions and there is
considerable scope for further studies in this domain.

Acknowledgement

This chapter was supported by an ESRC Postdoctoral Fellowship to the first
author (award no. PTA-026-07-0002).

References

Aarts, H. and Dijksterhuis, A. (2003) The silence of the library: environment, situational
    norm, and social behaviour. *Journal of Personality and Social Psychology* 84,
    18–28.
Aarts, H., Dijksterhuis, A. and Midden, C. (1999) To plan or not to plan? Goal achieve-
    ment or interrupting the performance of mundane behaviours. *European Journal of
    Social Psychology* 29, 971–979.
Aarts, H., Dijksterhuis, A. and DeVries, P. (2001) On the psychology of drinking: being
    thirsty and perceptually ready. *British Journal of Psychology* 92, 631–642.
Ajzen, I. (1991) The theory of planned behavior. *Organizational Behavior and Human
    Decision Processes* 50, 179–211.

Alsene, K.M., Li, Y., Chaverneff, F. and de Wit, H. (2004) Role of abstinence and visual cues on food and smoking craving. *Behavioural Pharmacology* 14, 145–151.

Armitage, C.J. (2004) Evidence that implementation intentions reduce fat intake: a randomized trial. *Health Psychology* 23, 319–323.

Armitage, C.J. (2006) Evidence that implementation intentions promote transitions between the stages of change. *Journal of Consulting and Clinical Psychology* 74, 141–151.

Bamberg, S. (2000) The promotion of new behaviour by forming an implementation intention. Results of a field experiment in the domain of travel mode choice. *Journal of Applied Social Psychology* 30, 1903–1922.

Bamberg, S. (2002) Implementation intentions versus monetary incentive comparing the effects of interventions to promote the purchase of organically produced food. *Journal of Economic Psychology* 23, 573–587.

Bargh, J.A., Raymond, P., Pryor, J. and Strack, F. (1995) Attractiveness of the underling: an automatic power–sex association and its consequences for sexual harassment and aggression. *Journal of Personality and Social Psychology* 68, 768–781.

Baumeister, R.F., Bratlavsky, E., Muraven, M. and Tice, D.M. (1998) Ego-depletion: is the active self a limited resource? *Journal of Personality and Social Psychology* 74, 1252–1265.

Brandstätter, V., Lengfelder, A. and Gollwitzer, P.M. (2001) Implementation intentions and efficient action initiation. *Journal of Personality and Social Psychology* 81, 946–960.

Gibbons, F.X., Gerrard, M., Blanton, H. and Russell, D.W. (1998) Reasoned action and social reaction: willingness and intention as independent predictors of health risk. *Journal of Personality and Social Psychology* 74, 1164–1180.

Gollwitzer, P.M. (1993) Goal achievement: the role of intentions. In: Stroebe, W. and Hewstone, M. (eds) *European Review of Social Psychology*, Vol. 4. Wiley, Chichester, UK, pp. 141–185.

Gollwitzer, P.M. (1996) The volitional benefits of planning. In: Gollwitzer, P.M. and Bargh, J.A. (eds) *The Psychology of Action: Linking Cognition and Motivation to Behavior*. Guilford, New York, pp. 287–312.

Gollwitzer, P.M. (1998) Implicit and explicit processes in goal pursuit. Paper presented at the *Symposium for Implicit vs. Explicit Processes at the Annual Meeting of the Society of Experimental Social Psychology*, Atlanta, Georgia.

Gollwitzer, P.M. (1999) Implementation intentions: strong effects of simple plans. *American Psychologist* 54, 493–503.

Gollwitzer, P.M. and Brandstätter, V. (1997) Implementation intentions and effective goal pursuit. *Journal of Personality and Social Psychology* 73, 186–199.

Gollwitzer, P.M. and Sheeran, P. (2006) Implementation intentions and goal achievement: a meta-analysis of effects and processes. *Advances in Experimental Social Psychology*, in press.

Gollwitzer, P.M., Bayer, U.C. and McCulloch, K.C. (2005) The control of the unwanted. In: Bargh, J.A., Uleman, J. and Hassin, R. (eds) *Unintended Thought*, Vol. 2. Guilford, New York, pp. 485–515.

Gummeson, L., Jonsson, I. and Conner, M. (1997) Predicting intentions and behaviour of Swedish 10–16 year olds at breakfast. *Food Quality and Preference* 8, 297–306.

Hedges, L. and Olkin, I. (1985) *Statistical Methods for Meta-analysis*. Academic Press, New York.

Herman, C.P. and Mack, D. (1975) Restrained and unrestrained eating. *Journal of Personality* 43, 647–660.

Herman, C.P. and Polivy, J. (1993) Mental control of eating: excitatory and inhibitory food thoughts. In: Wegner, D.M. and Pennebaker, J.W. (eds) *Handbook of Mental Control*. Prentice Hall, Englewood Cliffs, New Jersey, pp. 491–505.

Herman, C.P. and Polivy, J. (2004) The self-regulation of eating: theoretical and practical problems. In: Baumeister, R.F. and Vohs, K.D. (eds) *Handbook of Self-Regulation*. Guilford, New York, pp. 492–508.

Herman, C.P., Roth, D.A. and Polivy, J. (2003) Effects of the presence of others on food intake: a normative interpretation. *Psychological Bulletin* 129, 873–886.

Jackson, C., Lawton, R., Conner, M., Lowe, C., Knapp, P., Raynor, T. and Closs, J. (2003) Can implementation intentions increase fruit and vegetable consumption with cardiac patients? Paper presented at the *BPS Division of Health Psychology Conference*, Staffordshire, UK, September.

Keesey, R.E. and Corbett, S.W. (1984) Metabolic defense of the body weight set point. In: Stunkard, A.J. and Stellar, E. (eds) *Eating and its Disorders*. Raven Press, New York, pp. 87–96.

Kellar, I. and Abraham, C. (unpublished) Randomised controlled trial of a brief research-based intervention promoting fruit and vegetable consumption. Manuscript under review.

Koestner, R., Lekes, N., Powers, T.A. and Chicoine, E. (2002) Attaining personal goals: self-concordance plus implementation intentions equals success. *Journal of Personality and Social Psychology* 83, 231–244.

Macrae, C.N., Bodenhausen, G.V., Milne, A.B. and Jetten, J. (1994) Out of mind but back in sight: stereotypes on the rebound. *Journal of Personality and Social Psychology* 67, 808–817.

Margetts, B.M., Cade, J.E. and Osmond, C. (1989) Comparison of a food frequency questionnaire with a diet record. *International Journal of Epidemiology* 18, 868–873.

Mischel, W. and Ayduk, O. (2004) Willpower in a cognitive–affective processing system: the dynamics of delay of gratification. In: Baumeister, R.F. and Vohs, K.D. (eds) *Handbook of Self-Regulation*. Guilford, New York, pp. 99–129.

Mischel, W., Shoda, Y. and Rodriguez, M.L. (1992) Delay of gratification in children. In: Loewenstein, G. and Elster, L. (eds) *Choice over Time*. Russell Sage Foundation, New York, pp. 147–164.

Mogg, K., Bradley, B.P., Hyare, H. and Lee, S. (1998) Selective attention to food-related stimuli in hunger: are attentional biases specific to emotional and psychopathological states, or are they also found in normal drive states? *Behaviour Research and Therapy* 36, 227–237.

Muraven, M., Tice, D.M. and Baumeister, R.F. (1998) Self-control as a limited resource: regulatory depletion patterns. *Journal of Personality and Social Psychology* 74, 774–789.

Oettingen, G., Hönig, G. and Gollwitzer, P.M. (2002) Effective self-regulation of goal attainment. *International Journal of Educational Research* 33, 705–732.

Orbell, S., Hodgkins, S. and Sheeran, P. (1997) Implementation intentions and the theory of planned behavior. *Personality and Social Psychology Bulletin* 23, 945–954.

Polivy, J., Herman, C.P., Hackett, R. and Kuleshnyk, I. (1986) The effects of self-attention and public attention on eating in restrained and unrestrained subjects. *Journal of Personality and Social Psychology* 50, 1253–1260.

Prochaska, J.O. and DiClemente, C.C. (1983) Stages and processes of self-change in smoking: toward an integrative model of change. *Journal of Consulting and Clinical Psychology* 51, 390–395.

Prochaska, J.O. and DiClemente, C.C. (1984) *The Transtheoretical Approach: Crossing the Traditional Boundaries of Change*. J. Irwin, Homewood, Illinois.

Schachter, S. (1968) Obesity and eating. *Science* 161, 751–756.

Schlundt, D.G. and Johnson, W.G. (1990) *Eating Disorders: Assessment and Treatment*. Allyn and Bacon, Needham Heights, Massachusetts.

Sheeran, P. (2002) Intention–behaviour relations: a conceptual and empirical review. *European Review of Social Psychology* 12, 1–36.

Sheeran, P. and Orbell, S. (1999) Implementation intentions and repeated behaviour: augmenting the predictive validity of the theory of planned behaviour. *European Journal of Social Psychology* 29, 349–369.

Sheeran, P. and Orbell, S. (2000) Using implementation intentions to increase attendance for cervical cancer screening. *Health Psychology* 19, 283–289.

Sheeran, P. and Silverman, M. (2003) Evaluation of three interventions to promote workplace health and safety: evidence for the utility of implementation intentions. *Social Science & Medicine* 56, 2153–2163.

Sheeran, P., Milne, S., Webb, T.L. and Gollwitzer, P.M. (2005a) Implementation intentions and health behaviours. In: Conner, M. and Norman, P. (eds) *Predicting Health Behaviour: Research and Practice with Social Cognition Models*, 2nd edn. Open University Press, Buckingham, UK, pp. 276–323.

Sheeran, P., Webb, T.L. and Gollwitzer, P.M. (2005b) The interplay between goal intentions and implementation intentions. *Personality and Social Psychology Bulletin* 31, 87–98.

Stroop, J.R. (1935) Studies of interference in serial verbal reactions. *Journal of Experimental Psychology* 18, 643–662.

Tice, D.M., Bratlavsky, E. and Baumeister, R.F. (2001) Emotional distress regulation takes precedence over impulse control: if you feel bad, do it! *Journal of Personality and Social Psychology* 80, 33–67.

Verplanken, B. and Faes, S. (1999) Goal intentions, bad habits, and effects of forming implementation intentions on healthy eating. *European Journal of Social Psychology* 29, 591–604.

Webb, T.L. and Sheeran, P. (2003) Can implementation intentions help to overcome ego-depletion? *Journal of Experimental Social Psychology* 39, 279–286.

Webb, T.L. and Sheeran, P. (2004) Identifying good opportunities to act: implementation intentions and cue discrimination. *European Journal of Social Psychology* 34, 407–419.

Webb, T.L. and Sheeran, P. (2006) How do implementation intentions promote goal attaimnent? A test of component processes. *Journal of Experimental Social Psychology* (in press).

Wegner, D.M. (1994) Ironic processes of mental control. *Psychological Review* 101, 34–52.

Williamson, D.A. (1990) *Assessment of Eating Disorders: Obesity, Anorexia, and Bulimia Nervosa*. Pergamon Press, New York.

This page intentionally left blank

18 The Use of the Stages of Change Model with Dietary Behaviours

RICHARD SHEPHERD

Food, Consumer Behaviour and Health Research Centre, Department of Psychology, University of Surrey, Guildford GU2 7XH, UK

Dietary Change

Influencing dietary choices in an effective way is not easy. Given recommendations, for example, to reduce fat in the diet (Committee on Medical Aspects of Food Policy, 1994) or to increase the consumption of fruit and vegetables, it is necessary to understand what determines people's choices of foods and what obstacles there might be to effecting such changes. Official recommendations have been in place in the UK since 1984 (Committee on Medical Aspects of Food Policy, 1984) for a reduction of the energy in the diet derived from fat but changes in fat as a percentage of energy at the population level have been slow.

There are a number of theories from psychology on behaviour change which are potentially relevant for dietary change. For example, models of food choice behaviour derived from social psychology such as the theory of planned behaviour (Ajzen, 1991; see also Chapter 3) potentially have implications for attempts at dietary change. Most such theories are continuum theories which provide a prediction of the position of an individual on a continuous variable such as intention and include the variables that will predict intention and behaviour. While individuals will vary on these predictor variables, it is generally assumed that the rules governing the combination of variables will be the same for all individuals. However, there are also models which place people into a series of stages and which predict that the movement of an individual from one stage to the next will be influenced by a given set of factors, but that movement between other stages will be influenced by different factors. There are a number of such stage models, for example the precaution adoption process model (Weinstein and Sandman, 1992) and the health action process approach (Schwarzer, 1992), but the one most commonly used is the transtheoretical model developed by Prochaska and DiClemente (1992). This is described below, followed by a critical examination of the theory and its application to dietary behaviour.

Transtheoretical Model

Within the transtheoretical model it is proposed that health behaviour change consists of five distinct stages (Prochaska and DiClemente, 1992). Prochaska and DiClemente (1992) defined these five stages as pre-contemplation, contemplation, preparation, action and maintenance. These stages are described briefly below.

Individuals are categorized as being in pre-contemplation if they show no serious desire to change their behaviour within 6 months. Pre-contemplators tend to believe there is no need to change and may be unaware that a problem exists. Any changed behaviour at this point is usually the result of pressure from peers or employers, but once the pressure is removed then the old destructive habits will often resume. The goal therefore is for pre-contemplators to progress to the point where they at least consider changing the behaviour. Contemplation follows pre-contemplation and here a person must be thinking about behaviour change within the next 6 months. Prochaska *et al.* (1992) summarized this as the person knowing they need to make changes but feeling they are not quite ready to go forward yet. Goals in contemplation include increasing awareness of the benefits of change and making a definite commitment to change. In the following stage of preparation, individuals have made a definite commitment to change, usually within a month. They may, however, have also unsuccessfully taken action within the last year. In preparation some behavioural change may take place and some researchers believe it to be the early beginnings of the next stage of action. Action is the first point at which significant behaviour change takes place. However, while behaviour change will have taken place, it will only have taken place recently, usually within the previous 6 months. Prochaska *et al.* (1992) believed a trap that many professional practitioners fall into is to neglect the steps needed to move the individual into the final stage of maintenance. The hallmark of maintenance is the successful adoption of the necessary behavioural criterion for at least 6 months. It is essential not to see this as a static stage but as a point where clients actively work to prevent relapse. Individuals at this point might comment that 'they may need a boost now to maintain changes'.

The pattern outlined above represents an idealized form of the five stages through which an individual adopting a health behaviour will sequentially pass. However, an important aspect of health behaviour change, which is also addressed in the transtheoretical model, is relapse. Acknowledging the concept of relapse, Prochaska and Norcross (1999) commented that this might be the rule rather than the exception. Prochaska *et al.* (1992) concluded that a spiral pattern of change rather than a sequential one might be more representative of the real world, in which relapse from action or maintenance to perhaps preparation or in extreme cases back to pre-contemplation is possible. Thus while linear progression from pre-contemplation to maintenance is the ideal, this may rarely be achieved in reality.

In addition to the stages of change, a second central component of the transtheoretical model is the processes associated with change. Analysis of 24 of the most widely used forms of psychotherapy (Prochaska, 1979) showed ten major processes to play a significant role in behaviour change. These are consciousness-raising, self re-evaluation, self liberation, counter conditioning, stimulus control, reinforcement management, helping relationships, dramatic relief, environmental re-evaluation and social liberation. Prochaska *et al.* (1992) believed it to be crucial for process use to be matched to the appropriate stage if people are to move through the stages effectively. Cognitive and affective processes (consciousness-raising, dramatic relief, environmental re-evaluation, self re-evaluation and self liberation) are considered to be most effective in the pre-action stages and the behavioural processes (reinforcement management, social support, counter conditioning and stimulus control) suited to the post-action stages (Prochaska *et al.*, 1992). There has been some support for the factor structure of these processes, including in the dietary area (Bowen *et al.*, 1994).

In addition to the processes of change, Prochaska and DiClemente (1992) also identified decisional balance and self-efficacy as important components of change. Decisional balance was first examined in the Janis and Mann (1977) decision-making model, where decision making is conceptualized as a conflict model. Velicer *et al.* (1985) found that the two critical constructs in measuring the consequences of a decision were the pros and cons of behaviour change. Prochaska *et al.* (1994) believed that, for pre-contemplators, the pros of the problem behaviour outweigh the cons. With individuals in action and maintenance, however, the cons of the problem behaviour outweigh the pros. Clark *et al.* (1991) found high levels of self-efficacy to be predictive of change in numerous studies of addictive behaviours. Velicer *et al.* (1998) in a study of smoking cessation found that self-efficacy increased monotonically across the stages.

In a cross-sectional study of 872 smokers, Prochaska and DiClemente (1983) found process use to broadly match that outlined in the model. Prochaska and DiClemente (1992) found stage of change to be predictive of success with 570 smokers assigned to home-based treatment programmes. However, these studies were with addictive behaviours and a key question is whether the model will generalize across health behaviours. Prochaska *et al.* (1994) found commonalities with stages of change and decisional balance across groups for a range of different health behaviours: smoking cessation, quitting cocaine, weight management, high-fat diets, adolescent delinquent behaviour, safer sex, condom use, sunscreen use, radon gas exposure, exercise acquisition, mammography screening and physicians' preventive practices with smokers. In all cases except one, pros and cons crossed over at preparation, i.e. for stages before preparation cons outweigh pros but for the later stages pros exceed cons.

General Criticisms of the Model

The transtheoretical model has intuitive appeal (Littell and Girvin, 2002) and has been widely used in many areas. A number of commentators have argued that the model has heuristic value (e.g. Davidson, 1992) even when empirical support is less clear, and the model has found favour in many applied settings and in advice to health professionals (e.g. Hunt and Hillsdon, 1996). However, not all researchers have accepted the validity of the model and several have criticized the general model from a variety of perspectives.

Bandura (1997) and Sutton (1996, 2000, 2001) have criticized the concept of a stage model and its validity in relation to health behaviour change. Bandura claimed that the first two stages of the transtheoretical model were merely differing degrees of intention, while the remaining stages were simply 'gradations of regularity or duration of behavioural adoption rather than differences in kind'. The concept of relapse was also criticized by Bandura, who argued that this would not be possible in a true stage model. For example, in Piaget's theory of cognitive development once someone has reached the formal operational stage it is not possible for them to revert to being pre-operational. Overall Bandura believed that the stage classification in the transtheoretical model reveals little not already known to practitioners.

Sutton (1996) emphasized that it is very artificial to categorize individuals into particular stages and to assume that they will cross thresholds between the stages at certain times and start using different processes. Much of the cross-sectional evidence for stages of change suggests that process use follows a linear pattern across the stages rather than showing discontinuities; this can be interpreted as evidence for pseudo-stages rather than true stages (Sutton, 2000). Sutton (1996) believed it to be more helpful to think in terms of states of change rather than stages, with the states carrying no order of sequencing. Overall Sutton describes the theory as an ideal model which may have some value in designing interventions in treatment and clinical or highly controlled settings.

Weinstein et al. (1998) point to a number of criteria that should be met in order to have a valid stage model. These include the need to have an accurate method for classifying people into the appropriate stage; this can be a particular problem for some dietary behaviours (see below). Second, most people should move through the stages in the specified sequence, although there may be some exceptions to this. People at the same stage should face similar issues and problems; the advantage of such a model is that it allows these issues to be addressed for a group of people identified as being at the same stage. Finally, different factors should be important for different stage transitions. If all stage transitions are dependent on the same factors then there is no advantage in having a stage-based model; the same intervention will be effective regardless of the stage. The advantage of a stage model should be that interventions can be targeted specifically at people seeking to move from one stage to the next and that intervention would not be effective for someone at a different stage. Classifying the people into the different stages allows for stage-matched interventions which are hypothesized to be more effective than an overall general intervention.

The boundaries between stages are not hard and fast and in particular the stage timing appears to be arbitrary (Povey et al., 1999): after 6 months a person moves from action to maintenance simply by virtue of the time spent acting in a particular way but this could be set at 1 month, 3 months or any other time interval. Also given the definition of the preparation stage presented above, with the person having some previous unsuccessful attempts at behaviour change, it is not clear how someone can be in the preparation stage on their first time through the stages (Weinstein *et al.*, 1998). Movement through the stages does not follow the correct pattern in many cases and, while some exceptions would be expected, if many people (and maybe a majority of people) do not follow the standard pattern then this calls into question the utility of a stage model. Processes may occur at more than one stage and therefore the differentiation between stages is not really clear-cut. Even when processes can be shown to be used at a particular stage this might be because they are inhibiting movement to the next stage, rather than being the most useful processes at that stage or the processes that will most likely effect a transition to the next stage.

Specific Problems with Dietary Behaviours

While there have been a number of criticisms of the general model there is an extra set of problems in conceptualization and application when considering dietary behaviours. Glanz *et al.* (1994) point out that dietary behaviour merely requires modification and not elimination as in the case of addictive behaviours such as smoking; thus the target might be 35% of food energy from fat or five portions of fruit and vegetables per day. While elimination of a behaviour is easy to characterize and to measure, this is less straightforward in the case of dietary behaviours. The second problem is that many of the targets are really outcomes rather than behaviours. Thus consuming 35% of energy from fat is not a behaviour, but rather a person eats particular quantities of a set of foods and this nutrient intake is the outcome from performing that set of behaviours. A further consequence is that people do not know when they have reached the target, since they do not know their own nutrient intake either before or after they have made changes. Although this problem is eased in the case of behaviours such as fruit and vegetable consumption, where people can more easily estimate whether they do consume five portions per day, the situation is not so straightforward as smoking where the goal is not to smoke at all. In many dietary studies there are no clear end targets set; the aim might be 'to increase fruit and vegetable consumption', 'to reduce fat intake' or 'to avoid high-fat foods'. In these cases it is difficult, both for the participant and the researcher, to know whether the target has been achieved and in many cases it would be possible to change further; thus if a target of 35% of energy from fat is set then after this is achieved there can be a target of 30% energy from fat. With dietary behaviour, multiple changes are needed; for example, changing the amounts consumed of many different foods rather than changing a single behaviour (as in smoking). Although it could be argued that emphasis should be given to a clear and definable behaviour, since that is how the model is conceptualized, there are problems with this since often practitioners are interested in outcomes (e.g. fat intake) rather than a specific behaviour (e.g. eating chocolate biscuits).

In a study on fat intake, Brug *et al.* (1997a) noted that many participants classified in the action and maintenance stages were still consuming above the recommended levels of fat. Thus it appears likely that individuals who in reality need to change dietary behaviour further may classify themselves in post-action stages. This led Mhurchu *et al.* (1997) to question whether the model itself might be comprehensive enough to completely encompass dietary change.

With addictive behaviours self-classification into a particular stage is straight-forward; an individual knows clearly if they have stopped smoking or not. However, defining low-fat behaviour, for example, is not nearly so clear-cut. For example, only a small percentage of participants will know if their fat intake is less than 35% of their energy intake. Thus even if a definition of the target behaviour is given, few will know if they have achieved it. This has led to debate about stage classification for dietary behaviours. Many researchers simply use the participant's perceptions (Glanz *et al.*, 1994; Lamb and Sissons Joshi, 1996; Nigg *et al.*, 1999) as is done for smoking and other forms of behaviour. However, Brug *et al.* (1994) queried this approach, pointing out the dangers of participants wrongly classifying themselves as maintaining a low-fat diet when 55% of participants in their study proved to be unrealistic about their dietary fat intake. Greene *et al.* (1994) and Greene and Rossi (1998) introduced a five-item behavioural criterion, with classification in a post-action stage being dependent on a positive response to at least four items. On the other hand, Kristal *et al.* (2001) emphasized a person's subjective belief about their engagement with dietary change. For example, should an individual who has reduced fat intake from 50% to 38% and has maintained this change for more than 6 months be classified as a pre-contemplator simply because they have not reached the criterion of less than 35% energy from fat? Kristal *et al.* (2001) therefore argued in favour of a simple five-item staging algorithm as this measures a participant's engagement with the dietary change process and not a cut-off point. This issue is far from settled and remains one of the major problems with simply applying the standard measures from the transtheoretical model to dietary behaviours.

Dietary Applications of the Stages of Change Model

While the transtheoretical model was originally formulated and tested mainly in relation to smoking and other addictive behaviours, more recently it has been applied to a variety of behaviours, including various dietary behaviours. Horwath (1999), in a review of the literature on the application of the model to dietary change, found overall that 30 cross-sectional studies and four longitudinal studies had been conducted up until that time. The cross-sectional studies generally classified people into stages and then related one or more of the transtheoretical model constructs (e.g. processes, decisional balance, self-efficacy) to the stage. Horwath (1999), however, pointed out that very few studies focused on the totality of the model but rather focused on single constructs such as the stages of change and their association with nutrient or food group intake.

Cross-sectional studies have shown more positive dietary habits for those participants in the later stages of action and maintenance than those in the earlier stages for fibre intake (Glanz *et al.*, 1994), fruit and vegetable intake (Brug *et al.*, 1997b) and fat intake (Curry *et al.*, 1992; Greene *et al.*, 1994; Lamb and Sissons Joshi, 1996; Steptoe *et al.*, 1996; Brug *et al.*, 1997a; A. Moore, The application of the transtheoretical model to dietary behaviour, unpublished data, University of Surrey, UK, 2002). Also, other parts of the transtheoretical model have been shown to differ across stages. For example, self-efficacy has been found to be higher for those in action and maintenance than for those in the pre-action stages (Glanz *et al.*, 1994; Brug *et al.*, 1997b; Ounpuu *et al.*, 1999; Ma *et al.*, 2002). In general these relationships have been linear such that the later the stage the better the nutrient intake, although this has not always been the case. Van Duyn *et al.* (1998), for example, found fruit and vegetable consumption to be higher in action and maintenance than the other stages, but also found those in pre-contemplation to have higher consumption than those in contemplation or preparation. Self-efficacy has generally shown an increase over the stages rather than discontinuities (Glanz *et al.*, 1994; Brug *et al.*, 1997b; Ounpuu *et al.*, 1999; Armitage and Arden, 2002; Ma *et al.*, 2002).

In a study on fat intake, Moore (unpublished data) found that, in general, use of the processes of change increased linearly across the stages rather than showing discontinuities between stages. Also there was no real difference in the pattern of process use across the stages. Cognitive and affective processes, such as consciousness-raising, showed linear increases, while such processes would be expected to be used more at earlier stages than at the later stages where behavioural processes would be expected to be more important. Armitage and Arden (2002) investigated the distribution of theory of planned behaviour variables (Ajzen, 1991) across stages for consumption of a low-fat diet and found increases in intention, attitude, perceived behavioural control and subjective norm across the stages, a finding common for fruit and vegetable consumption (Armitage *et al.*, 2003) and for exercise (Courneya, 1995).

Thus there is a great deal of evidence that the stages show linear relationships with nutrient and food consumption and also linear increases in transtheoretical model variables such as process use and self-efficacy and with variables external to the model, rather than the discontinuities that a true stage model should show (Sutton, 2000). There are, however, examples of non-linear relationships between some variables and stage. For example, Armitage *et al.* (2003) found ambivalence was experienced least in pre-contemplation and maintenance but was higher in the intermediate stages. While ambivalence is not part of the original transtheoretical model, this would fit with predictions from the transtheoretical model on, for example, decisional balance.

There have been a number of studies that have examined the effects of interventions on stage movement and dietary behaviour. In a longitudinal study over 18 months, Greene and Rossi (1998) found that a feedback intervention increased movement through the stages and accelerated fat intake reduction. Steptoe *et al.* (1999) found brief behavioural counselling based on the model to be effective in reducing smoking, dietary fat intake and increasing regular physical activity.

Although the transtheoretical model argues that process use, self-efficacy and decisional balance pros and cons should differentially predict stage transitions, there is relatively little evidence for this for either dietary behaviours or other forms of behaviour. In a longitudinal smoking study, Prochaska *et al.* (1985)

found self-efficacy predicted the transition from contemplation to action and from action to maintenance, while decisional balance predicted change for those in pre-contemplation and contemplation. Prochaska et al. (1992) showed that people who stayed in the same stage over a long period showed little change in process use while those moving forward showed an increase in overall process use. Dijkstra et al. (2003) investigated which variables predicted stage transitions in smokers. They found that pros of quitting smoking predicted forward movement from pre-contemplation, while self-efficacy predicted movement from preparation to action. There were also trends for lower pros of smoking and high self-efficacy to predict movement from action to maintenance. However, the results from other studies are not entirely supportive of the model. Herzog et al. (1999) found that baseline process use and pros and cons of smoking failed to predict stage transitions at 1- and 2-year follow up.

Courneya et al. (1997, 2001) found that progression and regression across stages for exercise behaviour could be predicted using variables from the theory of planned behaviour including intention, attitude, perceived behavioural control and also social support. These authors, however, did not test the transtheoretical model variables of processes, self-efficacy and decisional balance pros and cons.

In one of the few studies in the dietary field testing what predicts stage transitions (Moore, unpublished data), Moore combined those in the pre-action stages into one group and examined the differences in process use between those who moved forward over 6 months and those who remained in the same stage. Those who moved forward were found generally to have higher use of processes at baseline, significantly so for consciousness-raising, dramatic relief, self re-evaluation, self liberation and counter conditioning; also self-efficacy was found to be significantly higher in those who moved forward. Low-fat behaviour scores increased significantly in the forward movers but not in those who remained in the same stage.

Horwath (1999) argued that the paucity of dietary behaviour research on the model as a whole, and in particular on the processes of change, is a major failing of research related to the model in relation to dietary behaviour. In order to test whether the model is really effective it is necessary to carry out interventions testing stage-matched interventions against controls of mismatched interventions or general interventions in order to demonstrate that the model offers some advantage over other forms of intervention. Horwath (1999) lists only one study which meets this criterion. Campbell et al. (1994) found that stage-matched messages were more effective in reducing fat intake than either a general message or a no message control. However, there was no effect of stage matching the messages on fruit and vegetable consumption. More recently, Moore (unpublished data) failed to find a significant difference between a stage-matched intervention and a general intervention or control aimed at reducing fat intake in diabetic patients. Likewise for exercise, Naylor et al. (1999) found no advantage of stage-matched interventions over non stage-matched interventions.

Thus the model describes quite well differences between individuals in cross-sectional studies, but since many of the variables are found to be linearly related to stage, it is not clear whether the relationships could not be equally well accounted for by continuous rather than stage models. The evidence for predictors of stage transitions is less clear for both dietary behaviours and other types of behaviour. However, for the model to be useful in interventions it needs to be demonstrated that the predictors of movement between stages depend on the stage, i.e. there are different predictors for transition from, for example, pre-contemplation to contemplation than there are from action to maintenance. Finally, there are very few studies examining the key test of the model involving stage-matched versus stage-mismatched or general interventions. Although the model may have potential for more effectively tailoring information for people seeking to change their diets, it requires more critical testing in this field.

Conclusions

The transtheoretical, or stages of change, model appears to offer one means for improving behaviour change through allowing more tailored and personalized interventions. However, due note needs to be taken of the differences between the addictive behaviours, such as smoking, where this model was originally developed, and the types of behaviours of interest to nutritionists. This might necessitate the development of different constructs or different measures of existing constructs specifically for dietary behaviours. While the model offers a means for classifying people and targeting messages more effectively, it needs to be tested critically in order to determine if it really is a useful addition to dietary intervention strategies.

References

Ajzen, I. (1991) The theory of planned behavior. *Organizational Behavior and Human Decision Processes* 50, 179–211.

Armitage, C.J. and Arden, M.A. (2002) Exploring discontinuity patterns in the transtheorectical model: an application of the theory of planned behaviour. *British Journal of Health Psychology* 7, 89–103.

Armitage, C.J., Povey, R. and Arden, M.A. (2003) Evidence for discontinuity patterns across the stages of change: a role for attitudinal ambivalence. *Psychology and Health* 18, 373–386.

Bandura, A. (1997) The anatomy of stages of change. *American Journal of Health Promotion* 12, 9–10.

Bowen, D.J., Meischke, H. and Tomoyasu, N. (1994) Preliminary evaluation of the processes of changing to a low fat diet. *Health Education Research* 9, 85–94.

Brug, J., Assema, V.P., Kok, G., Lenderink, T. and Glanz, K. (1994) Self rated dietary fat intake: association with objective assessment of fat, psychosocial factors and intention to change. *Journal of Nutrition Education* 26, 218–223.

Brug, J., Hospers, J.H. and Kok, G. (1997a) Differences in psychosocial factors and fat consumption between stages of change for fat reduction. *Psychology and Health* 12, 719–727.

Brug, J., Glanz, K. and Kok, G. (1997b) The relationship between self-efficacy, attitudes, intake compared to others, consumption, and stages of change related to fruit and vegetables. *American Journal of Health Promotion* 12, 25–30.

Campbell, M.K., DeVellis, B.M., Strecher, V.J., Ammerman, A.S., DeVellis, R.F. and Sandler, R.S. (1994) Improving dietary behavior: the effectiveness of tailored messages in primary care settings. *American Journal of Public Health* 84, 783–787.

Clark, M., Abrams, D. and Niaura, R. (1991) Self-efficacy in weight management. *Journal of Consulting and Clinical Psychology* 59, 739–744.

Committee on Medical Aspects of Food Policy (1984) *Diet and Cardiovascular Disease*. HMSO, London.

Committee on Medical Aspects of Food Policy (1994) *Nutritional Aspects of Cardiovascular Disease*. HMSO, London.

Courneya, K.S. (1995) Understanding readiness for regular physical activity in older individuals: an application of the theory of planned behaviour. *Health Psychology* 14, 80–87.

Courneya, K.S., Estabrooks, P.A. and Nigg, C.R. (1997) Predicting change in exercise stage over a three year period: an application of the theory of planned behaviour. *Avante* 3, 1–14.

Courneya, K.S., Plotnikoff, R.C., Hotz, S.B. and Birkett, N.J. (2001) Predicting exercise stage transitions over two consecutive 6-month periods: a test of the theory of planned behaviour in a population-based sample. *British Journal of Health Psychology* 6, 135–150.

Curry, S.J., Kristal, R.A. and Bowen, J.D. (1992) An application of the stage model of behavior change to dietary fat reduction. *Health Education Research* 7, 97–105.

Davidson, R. (1992) Prochaska and DiClemente's model of change: a case study? *British Journal of Addiction* 87, 821–822.

Dijkstra, A., Tromp, D. and Conijn, B. (2003) Stage-specific psychological determinants of stage transition. *British Journal of Health Psychology* 8, 423–437.

Glanz, K., Patterson, R.E., Kristal, A.R., DiClemente, C.C., Heimendinger, J., Linnan, L. and McLerran, D.F. (1994) Stages of change in adopting healthy diets: fat, fiber, and correlates of nutrient intake. *Health Education Quarterly* 21, 499–519.

Greene, W.G. and Rossi, R.S. (1998) Stages of change for reducing dietary fat intake over 18 months. *Journal of the American Dietetic Association* 98, 529–534.

Greene, W.G., Rossi, R.S., Richards, G., Willey, C. and Prochaska, J.O. (1994) Stages of change for reducing dietary fat to 30% of energy or less. *Journal of the American Dietetic Association* 94, 1105–1110.

Herzog, T.A., Abrams, D.B., Emmons, K.M., Linnan, L.A. and Shadel, W.G. (1999) Do processes of change predict smoking stage movements? A prospective analysis of the transtheoretical model. *Health Psychology* 18, 369–375.

Horwath, C. (1999) Applying the transtheoretical model to eating behaviour change: challenges and opportunities. *Nutrition Research Reviews* 12, 281–317.

Hunt, P. and Hillsdon, M. (1996) *Changing Eating and Exercise Behaviour*. Blackwell Science, Oxford, UK.

Janis, I.L. and Mann, L. (1977) *Decision Making: A Psychological Analysis of Conflict, Choice and Commitment*. Free Press, New York.

Kristal, A., Hedderson, M., Patterson, E.R. and Neuhausler, M. (2001) Predictors of self-initiated, healthful dietary change. *Journal of the American Dietetic Association* 101, 762–766.

Lamb, R. and Sissons Joshi, M. (1996) The stage model and processes in dietary fat reduction. *Journal of Human Nutrition and Dietetics* 9, 43–53.

Littell, J.H. and Girvin, H. (2002) Stages of change – a critique. *Behavior Modification* 2, 223–273.

Ma, J., Betts, N.M., Horacek, T., Georgiou, C., White, A. and Nitzke, S. (2002) The importance of decisional balance and self-efficacy in relation to stages of change for fruit and vegetable intakes by young adults. *American Journal of Health Promotion* 16, 157–166.

Mhurchu, N.C., Margetts, M.B. and Speller, M. (1997) Applying the stages of change model to dietary change. *Nutrition Reviews* 55, 10–16.

Naylor, P.J., Simmonds, G., Riddoch, C., Velleman, G. and Turton, P. (1999) Comparison of stage-matched and unmatched interventions to promote exercise behaviour in the primary care setting. *Health Education Research* 14, 653–666.

Nigg, C.R., Burbank, P., Padula, C., Dufresne, R., Rossi, J.S., Velicer, W.F., Laforge, R.G. and Prochaska, J.O. (1999) Stages of change across ten health risk behaviors for older adults. *The Gerontologist* 39, 473–482.

Ounpuu, S., Woolcott, D.M. and Rossi, S.R. (1999) Self-efficacy as an intermediate outcome variable in the transtheoretical model: validation of a measurement model for applications to dietary fat reduction. *Journal of Nutrition Education* 31, 16–22.

Povey, R., Conner, M., Sparks, P., James, R. and Shepherd, R. (1999) A critical examination of the application of the transtheoretical model's stages of change to dietary behaviours. *Health Education Research* 14, 641–651.

Prochaska, J.O. (1979) *Systems of Psychotherapy: A Transtheoretical Analysis.* Dorsey Press, Chicago, Illinois.

Prochaska, J.O. and DiClemente, C.C. (1983) Stages and processes of self change of smoking: toward an integrative model of change. *Journal of Consulting and Clinical Psychology* 51, 390–395.

Prochaska, J.O. and DiClemente, C.C. (1992) The transtheoretical approach. In: Norcross, C.J. and Goldfried, R.M. (eds) *Handbook of Psychotherapy Integration.* Harper Collins, New York, pp. 301–334.

Prochaska, J.O. and Norcross, C.J. (1999) *Systems of Psychotherapy: A Transtheoretical Analysis,* 4th edn. Brooks Cole, Pacific Grove, California.

Prochaska, J.O., DiClemente, C.C., Velicer, W.F., Ginpil, S.E. and Norcross, J.C. (1985) Predicting change in smoking status for self-changes. *Addictive Behaviors* 10, 396–406.

Prochaska, J.O., DiClemente, C.C. and Norcross, C.J. (1992) In search of how people change. *American Psychologist* 47, 1102–1118.

Prochaska, J.O., Velicer, W.F., Rossi, J.S., Goldstein, M.G., Marcus, B. and Rakowski, W. (1994) Stages of change and decisional balance for 12 problem behaviours. *Health Psychology* 13, 39–46.

Schwarzer, R. (1992) Self-efficacy in the adoption and maintenance of health behaviours: theoretical approaches and a new model. In: Schwarzer, R. (ed.) *Self-efficacy: Thought Control of Action.* Hemisphere, Washington, DC, pp. 217–243.

Steptoe, A., Wijetunge, S., Sheelagh, D. and Wardle, J. (1996) Stages of change for dietary fat reduction: associations with food intake, decisional balance and motives for food choice. *Health Education Journal* 55, 108–122.

Steptoe, A., Doherty, S., Rink, E., Kerry, S., Kendrick. T. and Hilton, S. (1999) Behavioural counselling in general practice for the promotion of healthy behaviour among adults at increased risk of coronary heart disease: randomized trial. *British Medical Journal* 319, 943–946.

Sutton, S. (1996) Can 'stages of change' provide guidance in the treatment of the addictions? A critical examination of Prochaska and DiClemente's model. In: Edwards, G. and Dare, C. (eds) *Psychotherapy, Psychological Treatments and the Addictions.* Cambridge University Press, London, pp. 189–205.

Sutton, S. (2000) Interpreting cross sectional data on the stages of change. *Psychology and Health* 15, 163–171.

Sutton, S. (2001) Recovery and relapse: back to the drawing board? A review of the applications of the transtheoretical model to substance use. *Addiction* 96, 175–186.

Van Duyn, M.A.S., Heimendinger, J., Russek-Cohen, E., DiClemente, C.C., Sims, L.S., Subar, A.F., Krebs-Smith, S.M., Pivonka, E. and Kahle, L.R. (1998) Use of the transtheoretical model of change to successfully predict fruit and vegetable consumption. *Journal of Nutrition Education* 30, 371–380.

Velicer, W.F., Prochaska, J.O., DiClemente, C.C. and Brandenburg, N. (1985) Decisional balance measure for assessing and predicting smoking status. *Journal of Personality and Social Psychology* 48, 1279–1289.

Velicer, W.F., Prochaska, J.O., Fava, J.L., Norman, G.J. and Redding, C.A. (1998) Smoking cessation and stress management: applications of the transtheoretical model of behaviour change. *Homeostasis* 38, 216 233.

Weinstein, N.D. and Sandman, P.M. (1992) A model of the precaution adoption process: evidence from home radon testing. *Health Psychology* 11, 170–180.

Weinstein, N.D., Rothman, A.J. and Sutton, S.R. (1998) Stage theories of health behavior: conceptual and methodological issues. *Health Psychology* 17, 290–299.

19   What is a Healthy Diet Community?

DEBORAH J. BOWEN[1,2] AND TRACY HILLIARD[1]

[1]School of Public Health, University of Washington, Seattle, WA 98195-7660, USA; [2]Fred Hutchinson Cancer Research Center, 1100 Fairview Ave N, M3-B232, Seattle, WA 98109-1024, USA

Why Are Dietary Change Opportunities and Interventions Important?

What is the evidence for the need for dietary change?

Multiple lines of evidence point to the relevance of dietary change for reducing premature mortality and morbidity. Several nutrients have been implicated in this regard: dietary fat, daily energy, fruits and vegetables, overall fibre and multiple micronutrients. Despite these data and the accompanying recommendations, there is still room for improvement in most Western countries. In addition, people in many developing countries are reporting increases in obesity and other health issues that indicate nutritional problems and imbalances. Taken together, these international experiences indicate that dietary change is a worldwide priority.

How do we get people to change what they eat?

Healthy dietary change has been slow to come, despite the knowledge base for recommendations to improve dietary behaviours. One issue is that dietary knowledge is multilevel and complicated. Often people know little about the nutrient content of the foods that they eat (Geiger, 2001). The knowledge base of appropriate foods and choices is changing rapidly, but these changes could result in confusion and, ultimately, in people simply giving up and consuming preferred or marketed foods, rather than making healthy choices. Economic issues also play a role, although they are currently poorly understood (Drewnowski, 2000). Current national and international efforts to change dietary habits by policy are slow and often confusing (e.g. the food pyramid changes in the USA are one such confusing example).

Even if we could increase knowledge, we know that improvements in knowledge are not enough to produce long-term dietary behaviour changes. We know that simply convincing people that dietary changes might prevent disease or improve health is not the best strategy for actually motivating and supporting changes in behaviour. People might know that they are supposed to consume certain types of foods and avoid others, but this is hard if not impossible in the face of an environment that actually promotes unhealthy eating habits. A world that actually promotes and supports healthy choices would look quite different indeed from the existing system.

One method of producing long-term population-based change is to imagine and then create the vision of an environment that supports the appropriate choices, in affordable, accessible and even desirable ways. This would of course take planning and consideration of the efficacious interventions and opportunities, combined with the finances and opportunities to implement these interventions. However, imagining it is the first step towards obtaining it. So, here we first propose what a healthy community would be, to support healthy dietary intake. We frame this discussion using multiple sectors of community. Then, we discuss the current evidence that supports interventions at each community sector.

What is the Vision for a Healthy Eating Community?

What would a healthy community, focused on promotion of healthy eating, look like? We propose that such a community would provide its citizens with appropriate and accessible health information about what to eat and how to eat it, encourage healthy eating via key sectors and providers, engage in opportunities and encouragement to consume healthy foods at common gathering points and food portals, and take leadership in setting policy and designing messages about healthy eating at the community level. Each of these will be examined in turn.

Current evidence suggests that human–environment interactions play an important role in the dietary and other health-related choices people make (Emmons, 2000). Although they may be more complex to design and implement, dietary change interventions that account for multiple levels of influence are more likely to result in long-term changes in people's dietary behaviours. Therefore, a social ecological approach to dietary interventions is appropriate. The Institute of Medicine recommends a social ecological model for planning public health interventions that incorporates approaches at the individual, interpersonal, institutional, community and policy levels (Smedley and Syme, 2000). This model provides a useful foundation for the construction of dietary change interventions. Box 19.1 presents such a model (Bowen et al., 2005). As can be seen, the causes of health problems and disparities in health outcomes are complex, and range from larger policy issues to individual choices. Each layer can serve as the setting for a healthy eating opportunity or message. The next several sections highlight approaches for dietary interventions representing various levels of this social ecological model. We move from the inner circle, at the level of individual

> **Box 19.1.** Biopsychosocial determinants of health.*
>
> **A. Political**
>
> Federal, state and local policy and law
> Political/geographical environment
> (public safety, food safety, physical
> environment protection, work site
> environmental protection and safety)
> Agriculture and food production
> Education system
>
> Economy
> Public health system
> Health system
> Law enforcement system
> Institutionalized biases
> (e.g. racism, ageism)
>
> **B. Residential**
>
> Residential environment
> Local community health service
> access
> Local public health prevention/health
> promotion
>
> Community economic development
> and employment access
> Community social service access
> School/educational services
> access
>
> **C. Organizational**
>
> Health care benefits
> Occupational issues
> Work and school issues
>
> Social interaction
> Work- or school-related stress
>
> **D. Sociocultural**
>
> Cultural risk environment
> Cultural SES/educational environment
> Cultural context/language
>
> Community social networks/social
> capital
> Religious affiliations
>
> **E. Familial**
>
> Family coping/cohesion/support
> Shared genetic risk
> Shared exposure
>
> Family norms and guidance
> Family roles
>
> **F. Individual**
>
> Demographic information (e.g. age)
> Individual values/preferences/emotions
> Social/economic resources
>
> Stress and reactivity
> Health behaviour levels
>
> *Adapted from McLeroy *et al.* (1988), Patrick *et al.* (1988) and Welton *et al.* (1997).

knowledge, attitudes, etc., through several layers of environmental influence to consider policy at the national and international level.

Individual interventions

In a community that supports dietary change people should have a basic understanding of what makes a healthy diet, how to obtain healthy ingredients and foods, and how to prepare or modify them to consume meals and snacks that promote health. The knowledge regarding healthy eating does not need to be at an expert level, but needs to guide and support choices within cultural norms and personal taste. This knowledge and skill building should be accessible to all people, as they need it and in settings where they might need to apply it to make choices or prepare foods. If personal food preferences and tastes lead people to choose unhealthy foods, then specific strategies need to be provided and supported that help people follow those tastes only to the limits of overall healthy nutrition.

Randomized trials examining various individual intervention strategies such as nutritional counselling and support groups have produced significant changes in dietary fat consumption among study participants (White *et al.*, 1992; Bowen *et al.*, 1994; Boyd *et al.*, 1997; Gorder *et al.*, 1997; Coates *et al.*, 1999). These findings suggest that individual interventions are a successful means for making large changes among healthy individuals. For such studies, participants are recruited who are both interested and able to make large sustained changes in dietary intake in order to test hypotheses over years of study. Many studies of individual interventions have targeted participants with risk factors for chronic disease (Hjermann *et al.*, 1986; Cupples and McKnight, 1994, 1999; Mhurchu *et al.*, 1998; Ornish *et al.*, 1998; Simkin-Silverman *et al.*, 1998; King and Gibney, 1999; Steptoe *et al.*, 1999; Siero *et al.*, 2000; Toobert *et al.*, 2000). The low-income population has also been targeted in several studies of individual interventions (Cox *et al.*, 1995; Hartman *et al.*, 1997; Howard-Pitney *et al.*, 1997; Anderson *et al.*, 2001). It is important to note that virtually none of these studies attempted to study the dietary behaviour of large segments of the population. Overall, these studies of large dietary change in healthy individuals, and these studies of smaller dietary changes among those with chronic disease or low income, all demonstrate that individual interventions can be relatively successful.

Group interventions

Because of group dynamics, some individuals may respond differently to group interventions than they would to those which target the individual. This could also be due to the fact that group interventions tend to encompass more aspects of the social ecological model than do individual interventions. The structure of group interventions may better allow them to address the role of interpersonal, institutional and community influences on dietary behaviours. Which aspect of the social ecological model has the strongest influence on dietary choices may vary from one person to another. Therefore, which aspect may require most intervention in order to produce lasting dietary change may also vary. However, group interventions seem equally as successful as individual interventions. Perhaps the strongest dietary interventions are those which incorporate both an individual and a group intervention component.

Evidence of dietary change resulting from group interventions is strong. Group intervention sessions were associated with increased consumption of fish and fruits/vegetables in people at risk for cardiovascular disease (Siero *et al.*, 2000) and positive changes in low-fat eating behaviours in participants in the Expanded Food and Nutrition Education Program (Hartman *et al.*, 1997).

Group-targeted interventions were demonstrated to be equally effective as those targeting individuals in a study of weight-loss intervention materials (Kreuter *et al.*, 2000). Recipients of The Special Supplemental Nutrition Program for Women, Infants, and Children (WIC Program) who participated in a study that included both an individual and a group intervention component reported increased fruit and vegetable consumption after a 1-year intervention (Havas *et al.*, 1998).

Tailored interventions

Tailoring intervention information to the specific characteristics of the individual in the intervention is one strategy that can make generic interventions feel personal and relevant. Tailoring often involves asking participants in an intervention about their specific dietary habits, their current changes and their plans for future change. Nutritional advice can them be provided, often in printed form, based on the person's characteristics, habits and desires. This type of information should be readily available and easy to obtain. It could be provided at regular intervals as a check-up on progress or maintenance, and should be easy to use for the people who receive it. Advances in the use of technology for delivering interventions could make this type of personalized and relevant support accessible in a wide variety of public places: workplaces, community centres, shopping malls, educational facilities, and even over the Internet.

Tailored interventions tend to focus on producing small changes in a general group of participants not selected for a particular interest or ability (Bowen and Beresford, 2002). Tailored interventions should be particularly relevant to dietary interventions designed for the promotion of healthy eating in diverse communities. Thus, no one single intervention booklet or brochure will be applied to various populations. Tailoring has the potential to reach many people with personalized messages.

The literature indicates that tailored print materials generally outperform non-tailored information when considering both process and outcome measures (Campbell *et al.*, 2006). In a well-designed study, tailored print feedback to change fat and fruit/vegetable intake was successful compared with non-tailored feedback (Campbell *et al.*, 1994). A study of college students demonstrated how tailored sessions with a nutritionist increased fibre consumption (Brinberg *et al.*, 2000). The effectiveness of computer-tailored nutrition education has been attributed to the intensive cognitive processing as a result of individualization, less redundant information and the self-evaluation properties of this approach (Brug *et al.*, 2003). However, additional research is needed about when, why, where and for whom computer-tailored nutrition education is effective. Research on tailored interventions has recently grown to include the use of new forms of media including the Internet, CD-ROM and automated telephone systems. Still, few studies have evaluated the effectiveness of these interactive media to promote health or dietary behaviour changes (Campbell *et al.*, 2006). Thus, additional research needs to be conducted to elucidate whether tailoring via interactive media is as effective as other media in producing dietary behaviour changes.

Once determined, this information could be of particular relevance regarding ways to build healthy eating communities.

Motivational interviewing

Not everyone is ready to create healthy eating plans and patterns at any given moment. Motivational interviewing is a directive, client-centred counselling style for eliciting behaviour change by helping individuals to explore and resolve ambivalence (Rollnick and Miller, 1995). The examination and resolution of ambivalence is the central purpose of this technique, and the counsellor is intentionally directive in pursuing this goal. Motivational interviewing could be a useful approach to produce dietary change in certain individuals. This strategy was originally developed to address the needs of those with addictive behaviours. It has recently been utilized as tool in public health interventions (Miller and Rollnick, 2002). Therefore, for those whose dietary behaviours are associated with some form of addiction, motivational interviewing should be particularly relevant.

Motivational interviewing has been demonstrated as a successful technique to produce dietary changes. However, additional studies need to be conducted to validate the strength of this approach. It has been shown to work well alone, and also as a complementary strategy for other types of intervention activities. In the Eat for Life trial, participants who received phone calls for motivational interviewing in addition to self-help materials exhibited a greater change in fruit and vegetable consumption compared with only self-help materials or the control group (Resnicow *et al.*, 2001). In the Women's Health Initiative, trained dieticians delivered a dietary intervention programme based on motivational interviewing that was demonstrated as efficacious in lowering dietary fat intake (Bowen *et al.*, 2002). In contrast, a study of patients with hyperlipidaemia demonstrated no significant change in dietary fat intake among those receiving both motivational interviewing and standard nutritional counselling, compared with those undergoing standard counselling alone.

Opportunities for support for healthy eating choices

Physicians and health professionals

The health-care visit and provider discussion and counselling are key places for the delivery of positive health messages about appropriate food choices, as well as other preventive issues. Ideally, we could use the tobacco control model as a guide to healthy eating interventions in provider settings. Involvement of the entire office staff and setting is key, with all patient contact including messages about healthy choices. The primary provider could certainly encourage patients to consider or to engage in dietary change, and provide appropriate written and other support for making changes. Regular monitoring could be accomplished by check-ins on progress at annual visits. Referral to dieticians for individual and group intervention could be a key strategy for patients having difficulty making changes on their own.

The evidence for health-care providers, mainly physicians, as a source of intervention activities and endorsement of dietary change is consistent and strong. A randomized trial of self-help materials delivered through primary care practices found significant decreases in dietary fat-related behaviours and increases in fibre-related behaviours in patients of the practice (Beresford et al., 1997). This study asked physicians to advise patients to change what they eat; then patients were provided with nutrition intervention materials by a nurse in the practice. This model of intervention, with the primary provider 'prescribing' or recommending dietary change and following the advice with key nutrition aids, could use the expertise and influence of the health-care setting without burdening the overtaxed provider by providing nutrition counselling.

Dieticians

Nutritional professionals and counsellors are trained to assist people in making healthy choices, often in clinical and hospital settings. Ideally, all medical practices and public health settings should have dietetic professionals to serve as referral sources for individuals who need special assistance. These services should be financially covered by health insurers, and should be accessible during times of specific dietary need, such as pregnancy and lactation, times of growth and development, illnesses and recovery periods that have dietary needs and issues, and at times when people are trying to improve their dietary habits and make healthy changes.

Currently most major hospital settings employ dieticians, and clinical settings with relevant patient populations, such as diabetes clinics, include dieticians on their staff. However, coverage for dietary counselling in the USA is not ubiquitous, and public health nutritional efforts are under-funded. These gaps indicate a lack of full understanding of the importance of nutrition and diet in general health promotion and disease prevention.

Lay health advisors

An additional vision for healthy eating support is the consideration of lay health advisors. In an ideal community, one could turn to non-medical and nutritional experts for simple advice and support for healthy eating – all community settings engage people in helping professions and influential roles, and these people can be strong supporters of choices and actions that improve the quality of one's diet. These types of people can range from community aides and social workers, who have individual client contact, to professionals in other areas besides health, such as grocery store clerks and natural support leaders in community organizations. All of these people and others could be mobilized to provide healthy eating tips and support. There is virtually no research supporting or refuting the use of lay health professionals to improve dietary intake, but future research could use this idea in multiple community settings.

Existing social structures as support and opportunity for dietary changes

Perhaps, in an ideal world, individual interventions for dietary change should be enough to promote healthy eating communities. Because communities are comprised of individuals, one might be led to believe that using intervention strategies to impact individual characteristics influencing dietary behaviours would be most effective. However, this is not necessarily true. Instead, public health professionals must account for more than just one's individual characteristics when planning to impact dietary behaviours. Recall the social ecological model previously discussed calls to incorporate macro-level approaches to influence dietary change. Individual interventions are only a micro-level strategy that can be used to promote a healthy eating community. No individual intervention should stand alone without some accompanying macro-level strategy by its side.

Families

The family is the place in which many of us learn to eat. Families come with diverse structures and functions, but one key function of a family unit is to provide basic sustenance and living quarters for its members, and eating falls into this requirement. Families could be places where young people learn to purchase and prepare healthy foods, to consider long-term consequences of food consumption, and to influence the other members along a path towards nutritious but tasty choices and meals. In the USA children under the age of 12 years eat the majority of their meals at home, but this varies by socioeconomic status and other demographic variables. Still, this provides great opportunity to increase healthy choices using the family as the source of support and influence.

The evidence for the effectiveness of families as a source of healthy eating opportunities is sparse, however. There is some evidence that family food preparers influence their children's (Hannon *et al.*, 2003) and spouses' eating habits in non-intervention settings. One study found that 12 weekly sessions in families, including both parents and children, produced consistent and significant reductions in dietary fat, but at the 4-year follow-up these changes were no longer apparent (Nader *et al.*, 1992). Spouses of women in intensive intervention trials reduced their dietary fat intake significantly, making changes comparable to other direct intervention trials in men (White *et al.*, 1992). More needs to be done to better understand the influences of family on healthy eating choices and to use these influences to improve the healthy eating choices within families.

Schools

The school is in theory an ideal place to provide encouragement, support and tangible opportunity for healthy eating choices. Most children in the developed world go to school, and many schools serve at least one meal daily to the young people who attend the school. In addition, schools provide a structured opportunity to learn about the components and skills needed to make healthy choices through curriculum development. An ideal school youth programme to encourage healthy eating, then, would include lessons on healthy choices and food preparation, healthy options and encouragements during mealtimes. In addition, schools could place limits on or completely eliminate advertising, promotion or sales of unhealthy products. Similar intervention opportunities exist for young adult and adult learning facilities, such as colleges and universities and community learning programmes.

There is some evidence that interventions provided through schools can influence youth dietary choices and behaviours. Several of the National Cancer Institute-funded 5-A-Day programmes were conducted in school settings (Havas et al., 1995) with some success in changing fruit and vegetable consumption. Considerable research by Perry and colleagues has demonstrated long-term success in producing and maintaining children's dietary behaviours, as well as other behaviours, when community and individual intervention components are combined (Kelder et al., 1995). A recent review by French and Stables (2003) found that environment-only interventions in schools settings have been effective for increasing fruit and vegetable consumption among students, including college age students. Other interventions conducted in adult learning settings have shown some promise as sites for intervention (Kumar et al., 1993; Frack et al., 1997; Finckenor and Byrd-Bredbenner, 2000).

Workplaces

The workplace is in some ways an excellent choice for dietary intervention. Most adults work, and therefore contacting large segments of the population over time can be done through workplaces. Workplaces often have relatively formal communications and contact structure, because people interact, exchange information and, indeed, receive payment for their time. In several countries, the employer is also the source of health insurance and health benefits of other types, providing some financial incentive to the employer for improving the health and well-being of employees. Workplaces can distribute information and motivational messages about healthy eating, can arrange for healthy eating opportunities in cafeterias, vending machines and other food sources, can provide classes and educational opportunities for learning about healthy eating, and can promote policy to encourage healthy behavioural choices.

A number of randomized trials have demonstrated that the workplace is a good place for dietary interventions. The Working Well Trial, targeting decreases in fat and increases in fruit and vegetables, was tested in a randomized trial design in worksite settings across the USA (Sorensen et al., 1996). The intervention was multifaceted and multilevel, and the evaluation methods included employee surveys and key informant interviews to identify any worksite-wide changes as a result of intervention participation. The investigators found consistent changes in all nutritional variables at the individual level, as well as at the level of the worksite. Long-term maintenance of these changes was not found (Patterson et al., 1998), providing support for more research into the maintenance of worksite-wide changes. Several studies to increase fruit and vegetable consumption have been successful in increasing frequency of servings using multiple intervention models, including use of cafeteria changes combined with self-help materials (Beresford *et al.*, 2001), use of peer educators to deliver messages to naturally occurring groups within worksites (Buller *et al.*, 1999) and by combining eating guidelines, classes, point-of-purchase labelling within worksites (Sorensen *et al.*, 1992) and, in a follow-up study, family intervention components (Sorensen *et al.*, 1998). A study of blue-collar women workers in North Carolina (Campbell *et al.*, 2002) used a combination of tailored print materials and lay helpers within the worksite to improve fruit and vegetable consumption, as well as fat consumption. Each of these studies contributes to our vision of the workplace as a key component of community health behaviour change.

Religious organizations

The role of religious organizations in health promotion is just beginning to emerge. Many religious settings consider the spiritual needs of the membership or congregation, but improvements in physical health have perhaps been less promoted. However, religious organizations have a keen interest in the health of the people who worship and therefore could be powerful influences on health behaviour. Both the leadership and the membership could play a role in promoting healthy dietary habits, as well as other health behaviours, by serving as role models, by promoting policies and recommendations for healthy eating, and by making nutrition information and nutritious foods available in the religious organization setting. Simple messages to keep oneself and one's family healthy could be very powerful coming from one of the moral and educational leaders of a community setting. The evidence for dietary interventions in religious organizations is consistent, though small. Most studies have shown positive changes in dietary behaviours using tailored messages and motivational counselling (Campbell *et al.*, 1999; Resnicow *et al.*, 2001) and partnerships with churches that include spiritual messages woven into the fabric of the dietary intervention (Baskin *et al.*, 2001; Ammerman *et al.*, 2002). A more recent study found that tailored print and videotape interventions produced stronger improvements in dietary behaviours compared with lay health advisors (Campbell *et al.*, 2004). A multilevel intervention in collaboration with a multi-faith group of religious organizations produced significant changes in both fat- and fibre-related behaviours (Bowen *et al.*, 2004). Taken together, these studies support the religious organization as a setting for health promotion.

Other organizational settings which seem promising as settings for dietary intervention include public and group housing units, rural organizations such as granges, community halls and cooperative extension services, and other places where people gather and communicate. Part of a community vision for health eating promotion includes inescapable and effective opportunities and messages in all regions and areas of people's dwellings and activities. As we continue to explore other organizational settings we can begin to imagine the collective power of these intervention opportunities formed into a seamless community support system for healthy eating.

General community pushes and pulls to eat healthy foods

Purchasing food in grocery stores

Grocery stores and markets where people purchase food are potentially the ideal setting where interventions can be delivered to promote healthy eating communities. Using such a setting could encourage individuals to purchase fresher, healthier foods. If successful, such an intervention may deter individuals from purchasing fast and/or processed foods that tend to be less healthy. Foods need to be labelled to help consumers make appropriate and informed choices, and information on nutritional content must be available at the point of purchase to help with the selection process.

This relies upon two important assumptions: (i) everyone has equal access to a grocery store or market; and (ii) everyone has the ability to shop for meals there based on affordability, availability and quality of the merchandise. Of course, this is not always the case. Unfortunately, many communities only have access to convenience stores and fast-food restaurants. These communities, which may be the most in need of such an intervention, may not even have a grocery store or market in which it could be delivered to them. So first, we must ensure that communities have access to a grocery store or market.

Grocery stores have been used as the setting for several dietary change intervention studies (Jeffery et al., 1982; Kristal et al., 1997; Connell et al., 2001). Interventions in grocery stores have shown mixed results as a successful way to improve the dietary behaviours in communities. Overall, they have shown little efficacy. More research is needed, with innovative strategies, to enable stores to be used as effective health promotion tools. One study provided regular shoppers in interventions grocery stores with audiotapes containing skill-building information and nutritional knowledge tests to use at home (Connell et al., 2001). The store played public service announcements for the 4-week duration of the intervention which were targeted towards all shoppers. In this study, average intake of fruit and vegetables increased, and so did positive beliefs about fruit and vegetable consumption. However, another educational intervention in supermarkets found no significant changes in behaviours of surveyed shoppers compared with those in control supermarkets (Jeffery et al., 1982).

Eating out, and working with restaurants

Although we strive to encourage healthy eating with freshly prepared meals purchased with ingredients from accessible grocery stores, we also know that most people will likely dine out sometimes. So, we would be remiss if we did not consider opportunities for intervention where people purchase food to eat out, other than grocery stores and markets. Consideration should be given to both traditional and fast-food restaurants, concessions stands and vending machines. Legislation could be passed so that restaurants, concessions and vending machines are required to have a minimum number of healthy food options available. Financial incentives could be provided to the owners of restaurants, concessions and vending machines for providing a certain number of healthy food options, and/or offering such items at reduced prices. These food sources could be required by law to regulate portion size, and to provide nutritional information on the food they distribute.

What do we know thus far about the role of eating out in promoting healthy nutrition? Lowering the prices of low-fat snacks in vending machines is one strategy that has been shown to successfully increase the purchase of such snacks in both a university campus (French et al., 2001b) and worksites (French et al., 2001a). A review of nine unrelated restaurant intervention studies found that most restaurants reported increased sales, despite no consistent pattern of menu items targeted for promotion across studies (Seymour et al., 2004). This finding indicates that providing information in the restaurant setting appears to be associated with increased purchase of targeted items. Perhaps it is not the specific intervention strategies that are most important; but instead, it is simply the act of intervening in the restaurant setting that is of particular salience? The authors of the review noted that only one of nine studies had a strong research design (Seymour et al., 2004). Thus, further research needs to be conducted through methodologically sound studies to illuminate how dietary change might be brought about in restaurant settings.

Food pricing and availability

The field of tobacco control has successfully used policy-level interventions to reduce tobacco consumption in several countries (e.g. the USA, the UK, Norway, Canada). We can consider these interventions as a model when we propose policy focused on pricing and availability that might improve the healthiness of dietary habits and choices. Policies regarding nutritional issues may be more controversial than those for tobacco (Jacobson and Brownell, 2000; Nestle, 2003); however, surveys have shown acceptance of polices that impact cost and choice of foods from the general public (Luepker et al., 1994). Policies that effect food consumption could include the support and promotion of agriculture leading to healthy choices, financial support of industries that improve the health quality of the food supply, taxation of foods that are unhealthy and subsidy of healthy choices, and differential pricing of foods based on nutrient value. Some policies that place taxes on 'bad' foods have been enacted with little success in long-term implementation (Campbell et al., 2006). Reasons for the failure have mainly been a lack of agreement on what is good and what is bad. Defining French fries as needing to be taxed might be easy, but adding lobster bisque to the pool of 'bad' foods might be problematic, although both foods have roughly equal fat content. Even snack foods are relatively diverse, and there is no agreement on inclusion of foods into such a label. In addition, in the case of foods there are no studies indicating that such taxation reduces consumption of that specific food, although the case is clearer for tobacco. Therefore, the future of food taxation as a health promotion strategy remains unclear. Overall pricing changes, such as those that reduce or increase the price of the entire food supply or sections of it (e.g. fruits and vegetables), will likely have dramatic agricultural effects and need to be considered in the context of national and international food policy. However, these large-scale changes are likely to have effects on many consumers, and therefore should be considered for future efforts.

Advertising and promotion of foods

The topic of marketing as a health behaviour change strategy is key to changing culture and buying habits of any consumer good, and therefore must be considered regarding food and eating. An optimal advertising and promotion setting in a community would include only limited promotion of unhealthy foods and clear promotion of both guidelines for improving health and the foods that would help individuals meet those guidelines.

Unfortunately, the reality of the situation in the USA is far from optimal. Currently there is very little regulation of food advertising to children and adults in the USA, and as a result, very little advertising time on television and other print arenas is for healthy nutritious food (Gamble and Cotugna, 1999). Companies advertise foods that have high opportunity for return on investment, and these foods are most often prepared foods that are likely to be preferred by many, due to their high fat and sugar content. Over the years many bans and restrictions have been proposed in the USA to limit children's exposure to foods of poor diet quality. Many of these restrictions were rejected due to their potential to limit free speech and are unlikely to be revisited in the near future.

Future Directions for Research and Practice

Where do we go from here in to begin building healthy diet communities? To begin we most continue to consider the role of social context in the design of future interventions. We can do this using the social ecological model as a foundation for modifying old approaches and creating new ones. It is important to note that the virtually none of these previous studies attempted to study the dietary behaviour of large segments of the population. A population health approach to promoting healthy eating communities should be a priority on the future research agenda.

What are the implications for future research? Places where people purchase food have yet to be demonstrated as successful settings for interventions to improve communities' dietary behaviours. Because this setting could be ideal, additional research needs to be conducted regarding how we can make point-of-purchase interventions an effective mechanism for dietary change. In addition, few studies have evaluated the effectiveness of interactive media to promote health or dietary behaviour changes. With technology evolving rapidly in society, it is essential to address this issue as it has the potential to revolutionize the types of dietary interventions delivered in public health practice. Because society is becoming increasingly diverse it will be important to consider theoretical and cultural issues in research pertaining to mediating mechanisms and dietary behaviour change for all future interventions. Tailored interventions may continue to be a strategy that helps us to address these needs appropriately.

References

Ammerman, A.S., Lindquist, C.H., Lohr, K.N. and Hersey, J. (2002) The efficacy of behavioral interventions to modify dietary fat and fruit and vegetable intake: a review of the evidence. *Preventive Medicine* 35, 25–41.

Anderson, J.V., Bybee, D.I., Brown, R.M., McLean, D.F., Garcia, E.M., Breer, M.L. and Schillo, B.A. (2001) 5 a day fruit and vegetable intervention improves consumption in a low income population. *Journal of American Dietetic Association* 101, 195–202.

Baskin, M.L., Resnicow, K. and Campbell, M.K. (2001) Conducting health interventions in black churches: a model for building effective partnerships. *Ethnicity & Disease* 11, 823–833.

Beresford, S.A., Curry, S.J., Kristal, A.R., Lazovich, D., Feng, Z. and Wagner, E. (1997) A dietary intervention in primary care practice: The Eating Patterns Study. *American Journal of Public Health* 87, 610–616.

Beresford, S.A.A., Thompson, B., Feng, Z., Christianson, A., McLerran, D. and Patrick, D.L. (2001) Seattle 5 A Day worksite program to increase fruit and vegetable consumption. *Preventive Medicine* 32, 230–238.

Bowen, D.J. and Beresford, S.A.A. (2002) Dietary interventions to prevent disease. *Annual Review of Public Health* 23, 255–286.

Bowen, D.J., Henderson, M.M., Iverson, D., Burrows, E., Henry, H. and Foreyt, J. (1994) Reducing dietary fat: understanding the success of the Woman's Health Trial. *Cancer Prevention International* 1, 21–30.

Bowen, D.J., Ehret, C., Pedersen, M., Snetselaar, L., Johnson, M., Tinker, L., Hollinger, D., Lichty, I., Bland, K., Sivertsen, D., Ocken, D., Staats, L. and Beedow, J.W. (2002) Results of an adjunct dietary intervention program in the Women's Health Initiative. *Journal of the American Dietetic Association* 102, 1631–1637.

Bowen, D.J., Beresford, S.A.A., Christensen, C.L., McLerran, D., Feng, Z., Hart, A., Tinker, L.F. and Campbell, M. (2004) *Effects of a Multilevel Dietary Intervention in Religious Organisations*. International Society of Behavioral Nutrition and Physical Activity, Washington, DC.

Bowen, D.J., Beresford, S.A.A. and Diergaarde, B. (2005) Social and psychological aspects of ecogenetics. In: Costa, L.G. and Eaton, D.L. (eds) *Fundamentals of Ecogenetics*. Wiley, New York (in press).

Boyd, N.F., Lockwood, G.A., Greenberg, C.V., Martin, L.J. and Tritchler, D.L. (1997) Effects of a low-fat high-carbohydrate diet on plasma sex hormones in premenopausal women: results from a randomised controlled trial. Canadian Diet and Breast Cancer Prevention Study Group. *British Journal of Cancer* 76, 127–135.

Brinberg, D., Axelson, M.L. and Price, S. (2000) Changing food knowledge, food choice, and dietary fibre consumption by using tailored messages. *Appetite* 35, 35–43.

Brug, J., Oenema, A. and Campbell, M. (2003) Past, present, and future of computer-tailored nutrition education. *American Journal of Clinical Nutrition* 77, 1028S–1034S.

Buller, D.B., Morrill, C., Taren, D., Aickin, M., Sennott-Miller, L., Buller, M.K., Larkey, L., Alatorre, C. and Wentzel, T.M. (1999) Randomised trial testing the effect of peer education at increasing fruit and vegetable intake. *Journal of the National Cancer Institute* 91, 1491–1499.

Campbell, M.K., DeVellis, B., Strecher, V.J., Ammerman, A.S., DeVellis, R.F. and Sandler, R.S. (1994) Improving dietary behavior: the effectiveness of tailored messages in primary care settings. *American Journal of Public Health* 84, 783–787.

Campbell, M., Demark-Wahnefried, W., Symons, M., Kalsbeek, W.D., Dodds, J., Cowan, A., Jackson, B., Motsinger, B., Hoben, K., Lashley, J., Demissie, S. and

McClelland, J. (1999) Fruit and vegetable consumption and prevention of cancer: The Black Churches for Better Health Project. *American Journal of Public Health* 89, 1390–1396.

Campbell, M.K., Tessaro, I., DeVellis, B., Benedict, S., Kelsey, K., Belton, L. and Sanhueza, A. (2002) Effects of a tailored health promotion program for female blue-collar workers: health works for women. *Preventive Medicine* 34, 313–323.

Campbell, M.K., James, A., Hudson, M., Haughton, L., Jackson, E., Farrell, D., Tessaro, I. and Demissie, S. (2004) Improving multiple behaviors for colorectal cancer prevention among rural African American church members. *Health Psychology* 23, 492–502.

Campbell, M.K., Gierisch, J. and Sutherland, L. (2006) Interventions to modify dietary behaviors for cancer prevention and control. In: Miller, S.M., Bowen, D.J., Croyle, R.T. and Rowland, J. (eds) *Handbook of Behavioral Science and Cancer.* APA, Washington, DC (in press).

Coates, R.J., Bowen, D.J., Kristal, A.R., Feng, Z., Oberman, A., Hall, W.D., George, V., Lewis, C.E., Kestin, M., Davis, M., Evans, M., Grizzle, J.E. and Clifford, C.K. (1999) The Women's Health Trial feasibility study in minority populations: changes in dietary intakes. *American Journal of Epidemiology* 149, 1104–1112.

Connell, D., Goldberg, J.P. and Folta, S.C. (2001) An intervention to increase fruit and vegetable consumption using audio communications: in-store public service announcements and audiotapes. *Journal of Health Communication* 6, 31–43.

Cox, R.H., Parker, G.G., Watson, A.C., Robinson, S.H., Simonson, C.J., Elledge, J.C., Diggs, S. and Smith, E. (1995) Dietary cancer risk of low-income women and change with intervention. *Journal of the American Dietetic Association* 95, 1031–1034.

Cupples, M.E. and McKnight, A. (1994) Randomised controlled trial of health promotion in general practice for patients at high cardiovascular risk. *British Medical Journal* 309, 993–996.

Cupples, M.E. and McKnight, A. (1999) Five year follow up of patients at high cardiovascular risk who took part in randomised controlled trial of health promotion. *British Medical Journal* 319, 687–688.

Drewnowski, A. (2000) Nutrition transition and global dietary trends. *Nutrition* 16, 486–487.

Emmons, K.M. (2000) Behavioral and social science contributions to the health of adults in the United States. In: Smedley, B.D. and Syme, L.S. (eds) *Promoting Health: Intervention Strategies from Social and Behavioral Research.* National Academy Press, Washington, DC, pp. 254–321.

Finckenor, M. and Byrd-Bredbenner, C. (2000) Nutrition intervention group program based on preaction-stage-oriented change processes of the transtheoretical model promotes long-term reduction in dietary fat intake. *Journal of the American Dietetic Association* 100, 335–342.

Frack, S.A., Woodruff, S.I., Candelaria, J. and Elder, J.P. (1997) Correlates of compliance with measurement protocols in a Latino nutrition-intervention study. *American Journal of Preventive Medicine* 13, 131–136.

French, S.A. and Stables, G. (2003) Environmental interventions to promote vegetable and fruit consumption among youth in school settings. *Preventive Medicine* 37, 593–610.

French, S.A., Jeffery, R.W., Story, M., Breitlow, K.K., Baxter, J.S., Hannan, P. and Snyder, M.P. (2001a) Pricing and promotion effects on low-fat vending snack purchases: the CHIPS Study. *American Journal of Public Health* 91, 112–117.

French, S.A., Story, M. and Jeffery, R.W. (2001b) Environmental influences on eating and physical activity. *Annual Review of Public Health* 22, 309–335.

Gamble, M. and Cotugna, N. (1999) A quarter century of TV food advertising targeted at children. *American Journal of Health Behavior* 23, 261–268.

Geiger, C.J. (2001) Communicating dietary guidelines for Americans: room for improvement. *Journal of the American Dietetic Association* 101, 793–797.

Gorder, D.D., Bartsch, G.E., Tillotson, J.L., Grandits, G.A. and Stamler, J. (1997) Food group and macronutrient intakes, trial years 1–6, in the special intervention and usual care groups in the Multiple Risk Factor Intervention Trial. *American Journal of Clinical Nutrition* 65, 258S–271S.

Hannon, P.A., Bowen, D.J., Moinpour, C.M. and McLerran, D.F. (2003) Correlations in perceived food use between the family food preparer and their spouses and children. *Appetite* 40, 77–83.

Hartman, T.J., McCarthy, P.R., Park, R.J., Schuster, E. and Kushi, L.H. (1997) Results of a community-based low-literacy nutrition education program. *Journal of Community Health* 22, 325–341.

Havas, S., Heimendinger, J., Damron, D., Nicklas, T.A., Cowan, A., Beresford, S.A., Sorensen, G., Buller, D., Bishop, D., Baranowski, T. and Reynolds, K. (1995) 5 A Day for better health – nine community research projects to increase fruit and vegetable consumption. *Public Health Reports* 110, 68–79.

Havas, S., Anliker, J., Damron, D., Langenberg, P., Ballesteros, M. and Feldman, R. (1998) Final results of the Maryland WIC 5-A-Day Promotion Program. *American Journal of Public Health* 88, 1161–1167.

Hjermann, I., Holme, I. and Leren, P. (1986) Oslo study diet and antismoking trial. *American Journal of Medicine* 80, 7–11.

Howard-Pitney, B., Winkleby, M.A., Albright, C.L., Bruce, B. and Fortmann, S.P. (1997) The Stanford Nutrition Action Program: a dietary fat intervention for low-literacy adults. *American Journal of Public Health* 87, 1971–1975.

Jacobson, M.F. and Brownell, K.D. (2000) Small taxes on soft drinks and snack foods to promote health. *American Journal of Public Health* 90, 854–857.

Jeffery, R.W., Pirie, P.L., Rosenthal, B.S., Gerber, W.M. and Murray, D.M. (1982) Nutrition education in supermarkets: an unsuccessful attempt to influence knowledge and product sales. *Journal of Behavioral Medicine* 5, 189–200.

Kelder, S.H., Perry, C.L., Lytle, L.A. and Klepp, K.I. (1995) Community-wide youth nutrition education: long-term outcomes of the Minnesota Heart Health Program. *Health Education Research* 10, 119–131.

King, S. and Gibney, M. (1999) Dietary advice to reduce fat intake is more successful when it does not restrict habitual eating patterns. *Journal of the American Dietetic Association* 99, 685–689.

Kreuter, M.W., Oswald, D.L., Bull, F.C. and Clark, E.M. (2000) Are tailored health education materials always more effective than non-tailored materials? *Health Education Research* 15, 305–315.

Kristal, A.R., Goldenhar, L., Muldoon, J. and Morton, R.F. (1997) Evaluation of a supermarket intervention to increase consumption of fruits and vegetables. *American Journal of Health Promotion* 11, 422–425.

Kumar, N.B., Bostow, D.E., Schapira, D.V. and Kritch, K.M. (1993) Efficacy of interactive, automated programmed instruction in nutrition education for cancer prevention. *Journal of Cancer Education* 8, 203–211.

Luepker, R.V., Murray, D.M., Jacobs, D.R., Mittelmark, M.B., Bracht, N., Carlaw, R., Crow, R., Elmer, P., Finnegan, J., Folsom, A.R., Grimm, R., Hannan, P.J., Jeffrey, R., Lando, H., McGovern, P., Mullis, R., Perry, C.L., Pechacek, T., Pirie, P., Sprafka, M., Weisbrod, R. and Blackburn, H. (1994) Community education for cardiovascular disease prevention: risk factor changes in the Minnesota Heart Health Program. *American Journal Public Health* 84, 1383–1393.

McLeroy, K.R., Bibeau, D., Steckler, A. and Glanz, K. (1988) An ecological perspective on health promotion programs. *Health Education Quarterly* 15, 351–377.

Mhurchu, C.N., Margetts, B.M. and Speller, V. (1998) Randomised clinical trial comparing the effectiveness of two dietary interventions for patients with hyperlipidaemia. *Clinical Science* 95, 479–487.

Miller, W.R. and Rollnick, S. (2002) *Motivational Interviewing: Preparing People for Change*. The Guilford Press, New York.

Nader, P.R., Sallis, J.F., Abramson, I.S., Broyles, S.L., Patterson, T.L., Senn, K.L., Rupp, J.W. and Nelson, J.A. (1992) Family-based cardiovascular risk reduction education among Mexican- and Anglo-Americans. *Family and Community Health* 15, 57–74.

Nestle, M. (2003) The ironic politics of obesity. *Science* 299, 781.

Ornish, D., Scherwitz, L.W., Billings, J.H., Gould, K.L., Merritt, T.A., Sparler, S., Armstrong, W.T., Ports, T.A., Kirkeeide, R.L., Hogeboom, C. and Brand, R.J. (1998) Intensive lifestyle changes for reversal of coronary heart disease. *Journal of the American Medical Association* 280, 2001–2007.

Patrick, D.L., Danis, M., Southerland, L.I. and Hong, G. (1988) Quality of life following intensive care. *Journal of General Internal Medicine* 3, 218–223.

Patterson, R.E., Kristal, A.R., Biener, L., Varnes, J., Feng, Z., Glanz, K., Stables, G., Chamberlain, R.M. and Probart, C. (1998) Durability and diffusion of the nutrition intervention in the Working Well Trial. *Preventive Medicine* 27, 668–673.

Resnicow, K., Jackson, A., Wang, T., De, A.K., McCarty, F., Dudley, W.N. and Baranowski, T. (2001) A motivational interviewing intervention to increase fruit and vegetable intake through black churches: results of the Eat for Life trial. *American Journal of Public Health* 91, 1686–1693.

Rollnick, S. and Miller, W.R. (1995) What is motivational interviewing? *Behavioral and Cognitive Psychotherapy* 23, 325–334.

Seymour, J.D., Yaroch, A.L., Serdula, M., Blanck, H.M. and Khan, L.K. (2004) Impact of nutrition environmental interventions on point-of-purchase behavior in adults: a review. *Preventive Medicine* 39(Suppl. 2), S108–S136.

Siero, F.W., Broer, J., Bemelmans, W.J.E. and Meyboom-de Jong, B.M. (2000) Impact of group nutrition education and surplus value of Prochaska-based stage-matched information on health-related cognitions and on Mediterranean nutrition behavior. *Health Education Research* 15, 635–647.

Simkin-Silverman, L.R., Wing, R.R., Boraz, M.A., Meilahn, E.N. and Kuller, L.H. (1998) Maintenance of cardiovascular risk factor changes among middle-aged women in a lifestyle intervention trial. *Women's Health* 4, 255–271.

Smedley, B.D. and Syme, L.S. (eds) (2000) *Promoting Health: Intervention Strategies from Social and Behavioral Research*. National Academy Press, Washington, DC.

Sorensen, G., Morris, D.M., Hunt, M.K., Hebert, J.R., Harris, D.R., Stoddard, A. and Ockene, J.K. (1992) Work-site nutrition intervention and employees' dietary habits: the Treatwell program. *American Journal of Public Health* 82, 877–880.

Sorensen, G., Thompson, B., Glanz, K., Feng, Z., Kinne, S., DiClemente, C., Emmons, K., Heimendinger, J., Probart, C. and Lichtenstein, E. (1996) Work site-based cancer prevention: primary results from the Working Well Trial. *American Journal of Public Health* 86, 939–947.

Sorensen, G., Stoddard, A., Hunt, M.K., Hebert, J.R., Ockene, J.K., Avrunin, J.S., Himmelstein, J. and Hammond, S.K. (1998) The effects of a health promotion-health protection intervention on behavior change: the WellWorks Study. *American Journal of Public Health* 88, 1685–1690.

Steptoe, A., Doherty, S., Rink, E., Kerry, S., Kendrick, T. and Hilton, S. (1999) Behavioural counselling in general practice for the promotion of healthy behaviour among adults at increased risk of coronary heart disease: randomised trial. *British Medical Journal* 319, 943–947; discussion 947–948.

Toobert, D.J., Glasgow, R.E. and Radcliffe, J.L. (2000) Physiologic and related behavioral outcomes from the Women's Lifestyle Heart Trial. *Annals of Behavioral Medicine* 22, 1–9.

Welton, W.E., Kantner, T.A. and Katz, S.M. (1997) Developing tomorrow's integrated community health systems: a leadership challenge for public health and primary care. *Milbank Quarterly* 75, 261–288.

White, E., Shattuck, A.L., Kristal, A.R., Urban, N., Prentice, R.L., Henderson, M.M., Insull, W. Jr, Moskowitz, M., Goldman, S. and Woods, M.N. (1992) Maintenance of a low-fat diet: follow-up of the Women's Health Trial. *Cancer Epidemiology, Biomarkers & Prevention* 1, 315–323.

20 Eating Behaviour in Obesity

JANE WARDLE

*Health Behaviour Unit, Department of Epidemiology and Public Health,
University College London, London WC1E 6BT, UK*

Historical Perspective on Eating Behaviour Research

In 1968, Stanley Schachter published an influential paper in *Science* (Schachter, 1968) showing that obese and normal-weight people responded differentially to internal and external cues related to food intake. The 'externality theory', as it became known, suggested that obesity was a consequence of being more reactive to external cues such as food palatability and less responsive to internal cues related to hunger and satiety. A series of imaginative studies from Schachter's group made the case that the combination of low sensitivity to satiety and high responsivity to palatability was the underlying cause of overeating, and thereby obesity (Schachter, 1971).

Before long, this elegant theory was challenged by Richard Nisbett's hypothesis that externality was a consequence of the chronic food deprivation practised by many overweight people in an effort to control their weight (Nisbett *et al.*, 1973). Deliberate efforts at weight control, he argued, kept weight below its biologically determined and defended 'set-point'. In support of this, he showed that the highly obese (presumed to have abandoned restraint) were not hyper-responsive to external cues. According to the set-point hypothesis, it was not the eating behaviour that caused the obesity, but the depression of weight below set-point that caused the abnormalities of eating behaviour.

The next step was taken by Peter Herman and Janet Polivy, who extended the notion of the adverse effects of deliberate weight control right across the weight spectrum but, at the same time, detached it from the concept of set-point (Herman and Polivy, 1975). Their carefully designed studies showed that individuals who attempted deliberate control of food intake, regardless of weight status, showed characteristic abnormalities such as under-responsiveness to internal satiety cues and over-responsiveness to external food cues. Restraint theory hypothesized that bringing intake under cognitive control supplanted the 'natural' control mechanisms, and this in turn impeded the delicate processes that should regulate energy intake. On this model, even normal-weight people who restrict their eating would experience problems of control, which would be reflected in behaviours such as emotional eating and binge eating (Wardle and Beinart, 1981; Herman and Polivy, 1990; Polivy and Herman, 2002). Researchers at the time concluded that restraint was unlikely to be an effective means of weight loss and might even, paradoxically, increase weight, because of the disruption of normal regulatory processes (Wardle, 1987a).

At around this time, a new eating disorder was identified, termed 'bulimia nervosa' (Russell, 1979). It was similar to anorexia in terms of the drive for thinness, but differed in that the defining behaviour was not restriction but frequent episodes of binge eating followed by self-induced vomiting. Epidemiological research at that time identified a virtual epidemic of binge eating (Halmi *et al.*, 1981). The burgeoning literature on the hazards of restrained eating had almost predicted that this would happen. Dieting had become more and more popular as young women tried to achieve the slim body shapes promoted in the fashion media, and in so doing – it was argued – they paradoxically impaired their ability to control their eating, and risked developing bulimia nervosa.

The idea that dieting might both cause eating disorders and exacerbate obesity led to an explosion of research into the causes and consequences of dietary restraint, mostly in samples of normal-weight, white, Euro-American students. Many of the disturbances of eating behaviour that had been hypothesized to be causes of obesity were reattributed to restraint; and restraint, rather than obesity, became the primary focus of psychological research into eating behaviour for the next 20 years.

Restraint and Weight Control

In recent years, restraint's role as villain in relation to eating behaviour and weight has begun to be questioned (Peters *et al.*, 2002; Hill, 2004). It has long been clear that not all restrained eaters develop binge eating, but there is now evidence that binge eating often precedes any dieting behaviour, i.e. restraint is neither a necessary nor a sufficient condition (Brewerton *et al.*, 2000; Grilo and Masheb, 2000). More recently it has been suggested that the observed associations between restraint and binge eating could be because a third variable – body dissatisfaction – is associated with both (Stice, 2001; Johnson and Wardle, 2004). Restraint's much vaunted lack of efficacy in achieving weight control has also begun to be questioned. Data from the National Weight Control Registry in the USA show that people who maintain large weight losses have much more restrained eating habits than those who regain their lost weight (McGuire *et al.*, 1999; Wing and Hill, 2001). Consistency and duration of weight-loss efforts may be the key to effective restraint (French *et al.*, 1999; Gorin *et al.*, 2004), along with consistency in monitoring weight and food intake (Boutelle and Kirschenbaum, 1998; Boutelle *et al.*, 1999).

Results from weight-loss programmes – which typically have a strong emphasis on restraint – have also failed to find any evidence that binge eating is increased (Wadden *et al.*, 2004). In an analysis of the impact of restraint changes over the course of obesity treatment, Wardle *et al.* (2001a) found that increased restraint was associated with reduced binge eating, and the greatest reduction of binge eating was among patients who experienced increased restraint coupled with reduced depression.

Restraint theory has played an important role in illuminating the complexities of the interplay between control and loss of control over eating. It highlighted the fact that the intention to restrict food intake does not always lead to effective and sustained reductions in food intake, and might even cause paradoxical increases. But while the initial reaction was to call for everyone to abandon restraint, this is now being replaced by a more balanced consideration of what kind of restraint, under what conditions, and for which groups, might be effective. Research into the psychology of eating behaviour in obesity could also be seen as a victim of psychologists' enthusiasm for the restraint concept. Perhaps the flame can be rekindled as part of the American Psychological Association's 'Decade of Behavior', which aims to generate new knowledge in the behavioural and social sciences 'to prepare the world for the emerging problems in the 21st century'. Obesity is surely going to be one of the most pressing problems in the health domain (http://www.decadeofbehavior.org/about.html).

Obesity, Adiposity and the Environment

Contrary to expectations, anorexia and bulimia are not proving to be the scourge of women's health in the 21st century; rather it is obesity. The epidemic rise in obesity prevalence has been one of the most striking phenomena in the epidemiology of eating and health (James *et al.*, 2001). In most Western countries obesity rates had been low and stable for decades, but after 1980, they started to increase steadily, first in adults and later in children; doubling, trebling and then almost quadrupling in the USA (Mokdad *et al.*, 1999, 2000; Strauss and Pollack, 2001; Ford *et al.*, 2003; Stein and Colditz, 2004).

There is reasonable consensus on the likely suspects for rising adiposity: environmental changes which have made food more palatable, accessible and plentiful, combined with technological changes that have reduced the need for physical activity. Together, these produce ever-stronger pressures towards positive energy balance (Friedman, 2003; Jeffery and Utter, 2003; Prentice and Jebb, 2003). There is less agreement about how the environment can be modified. Everyone wants the same outcome – a reversal of the obesity trends, but not everyone wants to see the environment changed to increase the demands for activity and reduce the opportunities for eating (Brownell and Horgen, 2004). Consumers, policy makers and industry often favour 'choice' over 'compulsion', so while they sign up to initiatives to increase people's opportunities for recreational activity or access to healthy foods, they demur at fiscal or legislative controls. Unfortunately 'choice' inevitably leaves each individual with the challenge of selecting activities and foods that will limit energy intake.

Individual Differences in Adiposity

Even though population weights have been rising fast, there are still enormous individual differences. In Britain, for example, data from the Health Survey for England 2002 show that the thinnest 10% of the population weigh less than half as much as the fattest 10%, with no significant difference in height. And over the past 20 years, the increase in adiposity has been greatest at the higher end of the body mass index (BMI) distribution (Jolliffe, 2004a,b), suggesting that fatter people are even more susceptible than the rest of the population to 'obesogenic' environments.

Gaining weight is a deceptively simple process: it merely involves taking in more energy than is expended. But behind this lies the much more difficult question of why some people find themselves consistently in this state of positive energy balance while others balance intake against expenditure to maintain a stable weight. The best predictor of obesity in a child is obesity in family members. This could be due to shared genes or shared lives, but family studies reveal that BMI similarities largely parallel genetic relatedness (Grilo and Pogue-Geile, 1991; Allison *et al.*, 1996). Sharing genes, more than sharing homes, is what promotes within-family similarity in adiposity (Stunkard *et al.*, 1990; Sorensen and Stunkard, 1993). Most studies have been carried out with adults, but a large twin study on young children's weights found very similar heritability estimates (Koeppen-Schomerus *et al.*, 2001). The conclusion is that, across all ages, around 70% of the variability in BMI within the population is attributable to heritable genetic differences, and around 30% to environmental differences, of which most appears to be in non-shared environmental factors. Whatever the overall environmentally set level, there are always likely to be thinner and fatter individuals, and this variability is largely explained by genetic differences.

Establishing that genetic factors play a part in determining adiposity is quite different from finding out how they exert their effect. At the earlier stages of the genetic revolution, there were expectations that *the* obesity gene would be discovered. There was great excitement when the gene for leptin deficiency was discovered (Zhang *et al.*, 1994) followed by the identification of massively obese children with a mutation in the homologous gene (Montague *et al.*, 1997). But since that time it has become clear that single-gene causes of obesity are exceptional. Current thinking is that there are many genes – possibly hundreds – each contributing a very small amount to variation in weight (Barsh *et al.*, 2000). This highlights the need to study adiposity as a quantitative trait rather than simply comparing groups who fall above and below the obesity threshold. Many genes and many aspects of environment are likely to contribute to the intake and expenditure behaviours that determine weight gain. Most of the emphasis in genetic research has been on the biological processes related to weight regulation. But given that behaviours – eating and activity – are the fundamental determinants of energy balance, they also could constitute steps on the pathway from genes to adiposity (Faith *et al.*, 1997; Wardle *et al.*, 2001b).

Eating Behaviours and Adiposity

Responsiveness to internal cues

The idea that hypo-responsiveness to internal cues of satiety might be part of the phenotype that facilitates positive energy balance has been a significant theme in eating behaviour research for many years. Among the earliest milestones was Stunkard's observation that stomach contractions were temporally associated with reports of hunger in normal-weight people but showed no association with hunger in obese people (Stunkard and Koch, 1964). Soon after, Schachter reported the first 'preload' study, in which participants were fed either sandwiches or nothing prior to a 'taste test' in which they had to taste and rate – and could also eat – a variety of crackers. The normal-weight group ate fewer crackers in the sandwich preload than the 'no food' condition, but the obese group demonstrated no sensitivity to the prior intake, eating as much following the preload as without it (Schachter *et al.*, 1968).

Over the next few years, research into satiety responsiveness was carried out largely within the framework of the restraint construct. However, a flicker of interest in the association between appetitive responses and obesity persisted in the paediatric setting, perhaps because restraint was assumed to be less pertinent to eating behaviour in obese children. A recent study included a comparison of responsiveness to preloads in overweight and normal-weight 8- to 12-year-olds (Jansen *et al.*, 2003). Intake of a wide variety of highly palatable foods was assessed following either a preload or a control condition without food. Overweight children failed to show a reduction of intake after the preload, and importantly, restraint did not moderate the effect. Satiety responsiveness has also been examined in relation to adiposity rather than the overweight–normal weight dichotomy. Johnson and Birch (1994) examined young children's ability to regulate by giving them either a low- or a high-energy preload and assessing their intake at their subsequent lunchtime meal. Compensation was modestly correlated with adiposity in boys although not in girls. A related paradigm has been called 'eating without hunger'; this involves children being fed to satiety and then offered highly palatable foods. Birch and colleagues used this paradigm with 5- to 7-year-old children and showed significant associations between eating without hunger and adiposity (Fisher and Birch, 2002). None of these studies was entirely successful in determining whether the key feature of the excess intake is lowered responsiveness to satiety or greater responsiveness to food cues, but all three suggest that there are differences in eating behaviour related to the degree of adiposity.

Responsiveness to satiety cues has also been investigated through assessments of the micro-structure of meals. Over an individual meal, the rate of eating tends to follow a decelerating curve; which is assumed to reflect a biologically determined satiation process. Meyer and Pudel (1972) did one of the earliest studies showing that obese people did not show this 'normal' deceleration. This was replicated more recently with children (Barkeling *et al.*, 1992): the obese children ate faster, and fewer of them had a decelerated pattern, than normal-weight children. Similar results were found in another study, with more of the obese children and those with Prader–Willi syndrome being 'non-declerators' than the normal-weight children (Lindgren *et al.*, 2000). However, in a larger and more elaborate study of adults in which intake patterns were recorded over five meals, the effect proved elusive (Barkeling *et al.*, 1995): the 38 obese patients ate no faster, ate no more, and were no less decelerated than the 38 normal-weight controls. These are striking inconsistencies in the literature, but one possibility is that obese adults, who exist in a culture that strongly condemns obesity and where advice to 'eat slowly' is widely disseminated as a strategy for weight loss, could be showing some cognitive overlay on any 'natural' eating tendencies. If this is the case, studies on children provide the best test of the theory.

Laboratory methodologies have predominated in research into satiety responsiveness, and this has made testing of large samples prohibitively expensive. An alternative approach is to use a psychometric measure, which loses the objectivity of the behavioural assessment but has the advantage that it reflects behavioural characteristics over many different situations in contrast to the 'snapshot' provided by a single test meal. We have recently developed a parent-completed psychometric instrument for assessing children's eating behaviour (Children's Eating Behaviour Questionnaire; Wardle *et al.*, 2001c) which includes scales to assess satiety sensitivity (e.g. 'my child easily gets full up') and slowness in eating (e.g. 'my child takes a long time to eat a meal'). Satiety scores were significantly correlated with eating behaviour in a test meal, giving confirmation that the two methods are tapping the same underlying concept (Carnell and Wardle, 2006). Contrary to our predictions, we failed to find differences in satiety sensitivity eating between young children from obese and non-obese families (Wardle *et al.*, 2001b). However, we have recently (unpublished data) examined associations with the child's adiposity in the same sample, and found significant negative correlations between adiposity and satiety responsiveness.

Taken together, these results are modestly supportive of the hypothesis that obesity could be linked with lower responsiveness to internal satiety cues, but the literature is still very limited and the results are not entirely consistent across studies, so any conclusions must be tentative.

Responsiveness to external food cues

The externality hypothesis took some serious hits in the heyday of restraint theory, but nevertheless, the idea that hyper-responsiveness to cues such as sight, smell or taste of food could increase the risk of obesity continues to attract interest.

One simple approach to assessing food cue responsiveness is to measure intake of highly palatable foods under conditions of satiety. As discussed above, significant associations between intake of highly palatable foods and adiposity have been found in 5- to 7-year-old children (Fisher and Birch, 2002), but it is not clear whether this reflects hypersensitivity to food cues or insensitivity to satiety cues. An alternative approach has been to compare food intake after exposure to food cues with intake in a control condition. If obese people are stimulated by food cues, then they should eat more after more intensive exposure. Jansen *et al.* (2003) assessed subjective hunger, physiological responses (salivary flow) and food intake (as part of a taste test) after either a control activity (playing) or exposure to the sight and smell of highly palatable foods in a paediatric sample. There were no differences between obese and normal-weight children either in hunger or salivation responses, but the obese children showed a stronger behavioural reaction to exposure, with a greater difference in intake between control and exposure conditions than the normal-weight children.

Responsiveness to external cues has also been assessed psychometrically. In the Three Factor Eating Questionnaire, also known as the Eating Inventory (Stunkard and Messick, 1985), the Disinhibition scale includes items assessing eating in response to food cues, although they are mixed in with items on eating in response to emotional cues. The Dutch Eating Behaviour Questionnaire (DEBQ) has an External Eating scale that specifically assesses eating in response to food cues (van Strien *et al.*, 1986; Wardle, 1987b). Many studies have shown strong associations between external eating and obesity (van Strien *et al.*, 1985; Hays *et al.*, 2002; Provencher *et al.*, 2003), although this has not been entirely consistent (Lluch *et al.*, 2000). Recently a parent-completed version of the DEBQ has been developed (DEBQ-P) which showed significantly higher external cue responsiveness in a clinical sample of obese children (Braet and van Strien, 1997), but similar data from an Italian community sample showed no association (Caccialanza *et al.*, 2004).

Behavioural choice theory has provided a different kind of framework for evaluating responsiveness to foods. The reinforcing value of foods is assessed from responses in a computer task where participants can choose to work for food versus non-food rewards, or for lower versus higher palatability foods. Saelens and Epstein (1996) compared choices for food rewards versus sedentary activity rewards where the 'cost' of sedentary activities remained the same throughout, but that of foods increased progressively. Obese young adults chose to work for food points at a higher rate than the non-obese participants, indicating the relatively higher reinforcing value of food for the obese. Recent work has linked the reinforcing value of food with dopamine genotypes in the context of weight gain after smoking cessation (Epstein *et al.*, 2004).

Emotional eating

One very different aspect of eating behaviour that has been explored as a possible determinant of obesity is eating in response to emotional cues. The psychosomatic approach to obesity (Kaplan and Kaplan, 1957) held that obesity was a consequence either of misinterpretation of emotions as hunger or a form of 'self-medication' to reduce emotional distress. In the early days this was linked with the idea that obese people had extensive psychopathology, but this appeared to be a consequence of self-selection of obese people with psychological problems into therapy. Once larger-scale community studies were carried out, it became clear that there were no systematic differences in either personality or psychiatric illness between obese and normal-weight people (Goldblatt *et al.*, 1965). With time, the psychosomatic theory became more circumscribed and depended largely on the observation that anxiety was associated with reduced food intake in normal-weight individuals, but increased intake in the obese (Slochower, 1976). Curiously, the psychosomatic theory of obesity is probably the one that is most widely promulgated in the media and most popular with the lay public – including obese people themselves. Perhaps this is because it confers some kind of normality on obesity, at the same time attributing it to something outside the individual – the stress of life for example.

As with other aspects of eating behaviour, restraint theory changed the interpretation of the results, with evidence that restraint, rather than weight, was the primary predictor of emotional overeating (Herman *et al.*, 1987). However, the ideas lived on. The key concept became eating in response to emotional cues and it was enshrined in the Emotional Eating sub-scale of the DEBQ (van Strien *et al.*, 1986; Wardle, 1987b). A number of studies have found emotional eating scores to be higher in obese than non-obese adults (van Strien *et al.*, 1985; Fitzgibbon *et al.*, 1993) and findings with the Eating Inventory could be attributed to emotional eating as well as external eating (e.g. Hays *et al.*, 2002). It has been argued that obese people might over-report emotional eating (Allison and Heshka, 1993), in which case studies that utilize the full range of adiposity rather than comparing obese and normal-weight groups might be more informative. Results in children have been mixed, with emotional eating as assessed with the DEBQ-P being higher in clinically obese than non-obese children in one study (Braet and van Strien, 1997), but not in a community sample (Caccialanza *et al.*, 2004). And among the 9- to 10-year-old participants in the National Heart Lung and Blood Institute Growth and Health Study, emotional eating was negatively correlated with adiposity (Striegel-Moore *et al.*, 1999).

The psychosomatic theory gains some support from the literature on the links between stress and eating, where there is evidence that stress has some relationship both with adiposity and choice of energy-dense foods (Bjorntorp, 1995, 2001; Wardle and Gibson, 2002; Steptoe *et al.*, 2004). There is also evidence that the hormone leptin – known as the satiety hormone – might also be involved with the hypothalamus–pituitary–adrenal (HPA) axis (Harris, 2000). These observations, along with new ideas on the role of 'comfort foods' (Dallman *et al.*, 2003) in terms of moderating HPA processes, suggest that there is likely to be continuing interest in the interrelationships between stress, eating and weight.

Adiposity and Eating Behaviour – Identifying Causal Processes

This chapter began by proposing that there is more work to be done by psychologists in understanding human eating behaviour in relation to obesity. There can be no doubt that obese people overeat relative to their energy needs, and therefore research into the control of food intake must be important. Schachter's theory that lack of internal sensitivity to satiety cues and over-responsiveness to food cues are the key characteristics that raise the risk of obesity, lost favour in the heyday of restraint theory but has persisted in the literature, particularly in relation to children's eating styles. The studies discussed in this chapter give some support to the idea that eating behaviours differ between obese and non-obese people, although the results are far from consistent. Psychometric measures have expanded the opportunities for research outside the laboratory, but the results raise questions about the validity of self-reports in the light of the negative stereotypes of obesity, mirroring concerns about the validity of self-reports of food intake and weight.

Few studies have used designs that can identify the direction of causation. Any eating styles that are identified among the obese might be causes of obesity, but they could – as restraint theory argued – be consequences of the weight-loss efforts that obese people engage in. Evidence for associations between eating behaviour and adiposity across the full range tends to support the view that eating behaviour is a cause, because it seems less plausible to invoke restraint effects across lower levels of adiposity. However, this does not rule out the alternative direction of causation. Longitudinal designs are informative: if eating behaviour characteristics can be shown to be correlated prospectively with weight gain, then it is less likely that the obesity caused the eating behaviours, although there could still be a third variable that causes both the eating behaviour and the obesity. Few longitudinal studies have been reported, although one of the earliest studies in the field showed that externality was related prospectively to weight gain in girls attending a summer camp (Rodin and Slochower, 1976) and this has been strongly supported in a much larger study of adult women (Hays *et al.*, 2002).

There can be little doubt that, in an environment where adiposity is increasing dramatically and where there is huge interest in the mechanisms that underlie obesity risk, there must be a case for investing in research into the mechanisms that control initiation and cessation of eating and that determine the size of meals. The genetic revolution does not mean that eating behaviours are irrelevant: they might be crucial factors on the pathways from genes to body fat stores (Faith *et al.*, 1997, 2004; Wardle *et al.*, 2001b). There is already some evidence that eating behaviours could be heritable. Data from 7-day diary records in adult twins showed reasonable heritability (0.32) for the incremental effect of high palatability on intake (de Castro and Plunkett, 2001; de Castro, 2002). Scores on the Disinhibition sub-scale of the Eating Inventory were shown to have a heritability of around 40%, both in a sample of Amish families (Steinle *et al.*, 2002) and in large group of female twin pairs (Neale *et al.*, 2003). The possibility that dopamine receptor genes might be associated with the reinforcing value of food (Epstein *et al.*, 2004) is one of the first studies to link eating behaviour with a specific genetic makeup.

There are also new biobehavioural methodologies that might illuminate mechanisms. Functional neuroimaging studies have shown distinct brain activation in response to food stimuli, with some suggestions of differences between obese and lean individuals (Tataranni and DelParigi, 2003; Wang *et al.*, 2004a,b).

There are likely to be many aspects of food choice that can influence energy balance. The studies described here emphasize responsiveness to food cues, but hedonic and cognitive factors probably play equally important roles.

The challenge in the modern world is to control food intake in the context of an environment with a plentiful, tempting food supply and few demands for energy expenditure. A better understanding of the eating behaviour phenotype will facilitate behavioural and genetic research and should contribute to developments in the clinical management of obesity (Wardle, 2005).

References

Allison, D.B. and Heshka, S. (1993) Emotion and eating in obesity? A critical analysis. *International Journal of Eating Disorders* 13, 289–295.

Allison, D.B., Kaprio, J., Korkeila, M., Koskenvuo, M., Neale, M.C. and Hayakawa, K. (1996) The heritability of body mass index among an international sample of monozygotic twins reared apart. *International Journal of Obesity and Related Metabolic Disorders* 20, 501–506.

Barkeling, B., Ekman, S. and Rossner, S. (1992) Eating behaviour in obese and normal weight 11-year-old children. *International Journal of Obesity and Related Metabolic Disorders* 16, 355–360.

Barkeling, B., Rossner, S. and Sjoberg, A. (1995) Methodological studies on single meal food intake characteristics in normal weight and obese men and women. *International Journal of Obesity and Related Metabolic Disorders* 19, 284–290.

Barsh, G.S., Farooqi, I.S. and O'Rahilly, S. (2000) Genetics of body-weight regulation. *Nature* 404, 644–651.

Bjorntorp, P. (1995) Neuroendocrine abnormalities in human obesity. *Metabolism* 44, 38–41.

Bjorntorp, P. (2001) Do stress reactions cause abdominal obesity and comorbidities. *Obesity Reviews* 2, 73–86.

Boutelle, K.N. and Kirschenbaum, D.S. (1998) Further support for consistent self-monitoring as a vital component of successful weight control. *Obesity Research* 6, 219–224.

Boutelle, K.N., Kirschenbaum, D.S., Baker, R.C. and Mitchell, M.E. (1999) How can obese weight controllers minimize weight gain during the high risk holiday season? By self-monitoring very consistently. *Health Psychology* 18, 364–368.

Braet, C. and van Strien, T. (1997) Assessment of emotional, externally induced and restrained eating behaviour in nine to twelve-year-old obese and non-obese children. *Behaviour Research and Therapy* 35, 863–873.

Brewerton, T.D., Dansky, B.S., Kilpatrick, D.G. and O'Neil, P.M. (2000) Which comes first in the pathogenesis of bulimia nervosa: dieting or bingeing? *International Journal of Eating Disorders* 28, 259–264.

Brownell, K.D. and Horgen, K.B. (2004) *Food Fight: The Inside Story of the Food Industry, America's Obesity Crisis, and What We Can Do About It.* McGraw-Hill, New York.

Caccialanza, R., Nicholls, D., Cena, H., Maccarini, L., Rezzani, C., Antonioli, L., Dieli, S. and Roggi, C. (2004) Validation of the Dutch Eating Behaviour Questionnaire parent version (DEBQ-P) in the Italian population: a screening tool to detect differences in eating behaviour among obese, overweight and normal-weight preadolescents. *European Journal of Clinical Nutrition* 58, 1217–1222.

Carnell, S. and Wardle, J. (2006) Measuring behavioural susceptibility to obesity: validation of the Child Eating Behaviour Questionnaire. *Appetite* (in press).

Dallman, M.F., Pecoraro, N., Akana, S.F., La Fleur, S.E., Gomez, F., Houshyar, H., Bell, M.E., Bhatnagar, S., Laugero, K.D. and Manalo, S. (2003) Chronic stress and obesity: a new view of 'comfort food'. *Proceedings of the National Academy of Sciences USA* 100, 11696–11701.

De Castro, J.M. (2002) Independence of heritable influences on the food intake of free-living humans. *Nutrition* 18, 11–16; discussion 91–92.

De Castro, J.M. and Plunkett, S.S. (2001) How genes control real world intake: palatability–intake relationships. *Nutrition* 17, 266–268.

Epstein, L.H., Wright, S.M., Paluch, R.A., Leddy, J.J., Hawk, L.W. Jr, Jaroni, J.L., Saad, F.G., Crystal-Mansour, S., Shields, P.G. and Lerman, C. (2004) Relation between food reinforcement and dopamine genotypes and its effect on food intake in smokers. *American Journal of Clinical Nutrition* 80, 82–88.

Faith, M.S., Johnson, S.L. and Allison, D.B. (1997) Putting the behavior into the behavior genetics of obesity. *Behavior Genetics* 27, 423–439.

Faith, M.S., Berkowitz, R.I., Stallings, V.A., Kerns, J., Storey, M. and Stunkard, A.J. (2004) Parental feeding attitudes and styles and child body mass index: prospective analysis of a gene–environment interaction. *Pediatrics* 114, e429–e436.

Fisher, J.O. and Birch, L.L. (2002) Eating in the absence of hunger and overweight in girls from 5 to 7 y of age. *American Journal of Clinical Nutrition* 76, 226–231.

Fitzgibbon, M.L., Stolley, M.R. and Kirschenbaum, D.S. (1993) Obese people who seek treatment have different characteristics than those who do not seek treatment. *Health Psychology* 12, 342–345.

Ford, E.S., Mokdad, A.H. and Giles, W.H. (2003) Trends in waist circumference among US adults. *Obesity Research* 11, 1223–1231.

French, S.A., Jeffery, R.W. and Murray, D. (1999) Is dieting good for you? Prevalence, duration and associated weight and behaviour changes for specific weight loss strategies over four years in US adults. *International Journal of Obesity and Related Metabolic Disorders* 23, 320–327.

Friedman, J.M. (2003) A war on obesity, not the obese. *Science* 299, 856–858.

Goldblatt, P.B., Moore, M.E. and Stunkard, A.J. (1965) Social factors in obesity. *Journal of the American Medical Association* 192, 1039–1044.

Gorin, A.A., Phelan, S., Wing, R.R. and Hill, J.O. (2004) Promoting long-term weight control: does dieting consistency matter? *International Journal of Obesity and Related Metabolic Disorders* 28, 278–281.

Grilo, C.M. and Masheb, R.M. (2000) Onset of dieting vs binge eating in outpatients with binge eating disorder. *International Journal of Obesity and Related Metabolic Disorders* 24, 404–409.

Grilo, C.M. and Pogue-Geile, M.F. (1991) The nature of environmental influences on weight and obesity: a behavior genetic analysis. *Psychological Bulletin* 110, 520–537.

Halmi, K.A., Falk, J.R. and Schwartz, E. (1981) Binge-eating and vomiting: a survey of a college population. *Psychological Medicine* 11, 697–706.

Harris, R.B. (2000) Leptin – much more than a satiety signal. *Annual Review of Nutrition* 20, 45–75.

Hays, N.P., Bathalon, G.P., McCrory, M.A., Roubenoff, R., Lipman, R. and Roberts, S.B. (2002) Eating behavior correlates of adult weight gain and obesity in healthy women aged 55–65 y. *American Journal of Clinical Nutrition* 75, 476–483.

Herman, C.P. and Polivy, J. (1975) Anxiety, restraint, and eating behavior. *Journal of Abnormal Psychology* 84, 66–72.

Herman, C.P. and Polivy, J. (1990) From dietary restraint to binge eating: attaching causes to effects. *Appetite* 14, 123–125; discussion 142–143.

Herman, C.P., Polivy, J., Lank, C.N. and Heatherton, T.F. (1987) Anxiety, hunger, and eating behavior. *Journal of Abnormal Psychology* 96, 264–269.

Hill, A.J. (2004) Does dieting make you fat? *British Journal of Nutrition* 92(Suppl. 1), S15–S18.

James, P.T., Leach, R., Kalamara, E. and Shayeghi, M. (2001) The worldwide obesity epidemic. *Obesity Research* 9(Suppl. 4), 228S–233S.

Jansen, A., Theunissen, N., Slechten, K., Nederkoorn, C., Boon, B., Mulkens, S. and Roefs, A. (2003) Overweight children overeat after exposure to food cues. *Eating Behaviors* 4, 197–209.

Jeffery, R.W. and Utter, J. (2003) The changing environment and population obesity in the United States. *Obesity Research* 11(Suppl.), 12S–22S.

Johnson, F. and Wardle, J. (2004) Dietary restraint, body dissatisfaction and psychological distress: a prospective analysis. *Journal of Abnormal Psychology* 114, 119–125.

Johnson, S.L. and Birch, L.L. (1994) Parents' and children's adiposity and eating style. *Pediatrics* 94, 653–661.

Jolliffe, D. (2004a) Continuous and robust measures of the overweight epidemic: 1971–2000. *Demography* 41, 303–314.

Jolliffe, D. (2004b) Extent of overweight among US children and adolescents from 1971 to 2000. *International Journal of Obesity and Related Metabolic Disorders* 28, 4–9.

Kaplan, H.I. and Kaplan, H.S. (1957) The psychosomatic concept of obesity. *Journal of Nervous and Mental Disease* 125, 181–201.

Koeppen-Schomerus, G., Wardle, J. and Plomin, R. (2001) A genetic analysis of weight and overweight in 4-year-old twin pairs. *International Journal of Obesity and Related Metabolic Disorders* 25, 838–844.

Lindgren, A.C., Barkeling, B., Hagg, A., Ritzen, E.M., Marcus, C. and Rossner, S. (2000) Eating behavior in Prader–Willi syndrome, normal weight, and obese control groups. *Journal of Pediatrics* 137, 50–55.

Lluch, A., Herbeth, B., Mejean, L. and Siest, G. (2000) Dietary intakes, eating style and overweight in the Stanislas Family Study. *International Journal of Obesity and Related Metabolic Disorders* 24, 1493–1499.

McGuire, M.T., Wing, R.R., Klem, M.L., Lang, W. and Hill, J.O. (1999) What predicts weight regain in a group of successful weight losers? *Journal of Consulting and Clinical Psychology* 67, 177–185.

Meyer, J.E. and Pudel, V. (1972) Experimental studies on food-intake in obese and normal weight subjects. *Journal of Psychosomatic Research* 16, 305–308.

Mokdad, A.H., Serdula, M.K., Dietz, W.H., Bowman, B.A., Marks, J.S. and Koplan, J.P. (1999) The spread of the obesity epidemic in the United States, 1991–1998. *Journal of the American Medical Association* 282, 1519–1522.

Mokdad, A.H., Serdula, M.K., Dietz, W.H., Bowman, B.A., Marks, J.S. and Koplan, J.P. (2000) The continuing epidemic of obesity in the United States. *Journal of the American Medical Association* 284, 1650–1651.

Montague, C.T., Farooqi, I.S., Whitehead, J.P., Soos, M.A., Rau, H., Wareham, N.J., Sewter, C.P., Digby, J.E., Mohammed, S.N., Hurst, J.A., Cheetham, C.H., Earley, A.R., Barnett, A.H., Prins, J.B. and O'Rahilly, S. (1997) Congenital leptin deficiency is associated with severe early-onset obesity in humans. *Nature* 387, 903–908.

Neale, B.M., Mazzeo, S.E. and Bulik, C.M. (2003) A twin study of dietary restraint, disinhibition and hunger: an examination of the eating inventory (three factor eating questionnaire). *Twin Research* 6, 471–478.

Nisbett, R.E., Hanson, L.R. Jr, Harris, A. and Stair, A. (1973) Taste responsiveness, weight loss, and the ponderostat. *Physiology & Behavior* 11, 641–645.

Peters, J.C., Wyatt, H.R., Donahoo, W.T. and Hill, J.O. (2002) From instinct to intellect: the challenge of maintaining healthy weight in the modern world. *Obesity Reviews* 3, 69–74.

Polivy, J. and Herman, C.P. (2002) Causes of eating disorders. *Annual Review of Psychology* 53, 187–213.

Prentice, A.M. and Jebb, S.A. (2003) Fast foods, energy density and obesity: a possible mechanistic link. *Obesity Reviews* 4, 187–194.

Provencher, V., Drapeau, V., Tremblay, A., Despres, J.P. and Lemieux, S. (2003) Eating behaviors and indexes of body composition in men and women from the Quebec family study. *Obesity Research* 11, 783–792.

Rodin, J. and Slochower, J. (1976) Externality in the nonobese: effects of environmental responsiveness on weight. *Journal of Personality and Social Psychology* 33, 338–344.

Russell, G. (1979) Bulimia nervosa: an ominous variant of anorexia nervosa. *Psychological Medicine* 9, 429–448.

Saelens, B.E. and Epstein, L.H. (1996) Reinforcing value of food in obese and non-obese women. *Appetite* 27, 41–50.

Schachter, S. (1968) Obesity and eating. Internal and external cues differentially affect the eating behavior of obese and normal subjects. *Science* 161, 751–756.

Schachter, S. (1971) Some extraordinary facts about obese humans and rats. *American Psychologist* 26, 129–144.

Schachter, S., Goldman, R. and Gordon, A. (1968) Effects of fear, food deprivation, and obesity on eating. *Journal of Personality and Social Psychology* 10, 91–97.

Slochower, J. (1976) Emotional labeling and overeating in obese and normal weight individuals. *Psychological Medicine* 38, 131–139.

Sorensen, T.I. and Stunkard, A.J. (1993) Does obesity run in families because of genes? An adoption study using silhouettes as a measure of obesity. *Acta Psychiatrica Scandinavica. Supplementum* 370, 67–72.

Stein, C.J. and Colditz, G.A. (2004) The epidemic of obesity. *Journal of Clinical Endocrinology and Metabolism* 89, 2522–2525.

Steinle, N.I., Hsueh, W.C., Snitker, S., Pollin, T.I., Sakul, H., St Jean, P.L., Bell, C.J., Mitchell, B.D. and Shuldiner, A.R. (2002) Eating behavior in the Old Order Amish: heritability analysis and a genome-wide linkage analysis. *American Journal of Clinical Nutrition* 75, 1098–1106.

Steptoe, A., Kunz-Ebrecht, S.R., Brydon, L. and Wardle, J. (2004) Central adiposity and cortisol responses to waking in middle-aged men and women. *International Journal of Obesity and Related Metabolic Disorders* 28, 1168–1173.

Stice, E. (2001) A prospective test of the dual-pathway model of bulimic pathology: mediating effects of dieting and negative affect. *Journal of Abnormal Psychology* 110, 124–135.

Strauss, R.S. and Pollack, H.A. (2001) Epidemic increase in childhood overweight, 1986–1998. *Journal of the American Medical Association* 286, 2845–2848.

Striegel-Moore, R.H., Morrison, J.A., Schreiber, G., Schumann, B.C., Crawford, P.B. and Obarzanek, E. (1999) Emotion-induced eating and sucrose intake in children: the NHLBI Growth and Health Study. *International Journal of Eating Disorders* 25, 389–398.

Stunkard, A. and Koch, C. (1964) The interpretation of gastric motility. I. Apparent bias in the reports of hunger by obese persons. *Archives of General Psychiatry* 11, 74–82.

Stunkard, A.J. and Messick, S. (1985) The three-factor eating questionnaire to measure dietary restraint, disinhibition and hunger. *Journal of Psychosomatic Research* 29, 71–83.

Stunkard, A.J., Harris, J.R., Pedersen, N.L. and McClearn, G.E. (1990) The body-mass index of twins who have been reared apart. *New England Journal of Medicine* 322, 1483–1487.

Tataranni, P.A. and DelParigi, A. (2003) Functional neuroimaging: a new generation of human brain studies in obesity research. *Obesity Reviews* 4, 229–238.

Van Strien, T., Frijters, J.E., Roosen, R.G., Knuiman-Hijl, W.J. and Defares, P.B. (1985) Eating behavior, personality traits and body mass in women. *Addictive Behaviors* 10, 333–343.

Van Strien, T., Frijters, J.E., van Staveren, W.A. and Defares, P.B. (1986) The predictive validity of the Dutch Restrained Eating Scale. *International Journal of Eating Disorders* 5, 747–755.

Wadden, T.A., Foster, G.D., Sarwer, D.B., Anderson, D.A., Gladis, M., Sanderson, R.S., Letchak, R.V., Berkowitz, R.I. and Phelan, S. (2004) Dieting and the development of eating disorders in obese women: results of a randomized controlled trial. *American Journal of Clinical Nutrition* 80, 560–568.

Wang, G.J., Volkow, N.D., Telang, F., Jayne, M., Ma, J., Rao, M., Zhu, W., Wong, C.T., Pappas, N.R., Geliebter, A. and Fowler, J.S. (2004a) Exposure to appetitive food stimuli markedly activates the human brain. *Neuroimage* 21, 1790–1797.

Wang, G.J., Volkow, N.D., Thanos, P.K. and Fowler, J.S. (2004b) Similarity between obesity and drug addiction as assessed by neurofunctional imaging: a concept review. *Journal of Addictive Diseases* 23, 39–53.

Wardle, J. (1987a) Compulsive eating and dietary restraint. *British Journal of Clinical Psychology* 26, 47–55.

Wardle, J. (1987b) Eating style: a validation study of the Dutch Eating Behaviour Questionnaire in normal subjects and women with eating disorders. *Journal of Psychosomatic Research* 31, 161–169.

Wardle, J. (2005) Understanding the aetiology of childhood obesity: implications for treatment. *Proceedings of the Nutrition Society* 64, 73–79.

Wardle, J. and Beinart, H. (1981) Binge eating: a theoretical review. *British Journal of Clinical Psychology* 20, 97–109.

Wardle, J. and Gibson, E.L. (2002) Impact of stress on diet: processes and implications. In: Stansfeld, S.A. and Marmot, M. (eds) *Stress and the Heart*. BMJ Books, London, pp. 124–149.

Wardle, J., Waller, J. and Rapoport, L. (2001a) Body dissatisfaction and binge eating in obese women: the role of restraint and depression. *Obesity Research* 9, 778–787.

Wardle, J., Guthrie, C., Sanderson, S., Birch, L. and Plomin, R. (2001b) Food and activity preferences in children of lean and obese parents. *International Journal of Obesity and Related Metabolic Disorders* 25, 971–977.

Wardle, J., Guthrie, C.A., Sanderson, S. and Rapoport, L. (2001c) Development of the Children's Eating Behaviour Questionnaire. *Journal of Child Psychology and Psychiatry* 42, 963–970.

Wing, R.R. and Hill, J.O. (2001) Successful weight loss maintenance. *Annual Review of Nutrition* 21, 323–341.

Zhang, Y., Proenca, R., Maffei, M., Barone, M., Leopold, L. and Friedman, J.M. (1994) Positional cloning of the mouse obese gene and its human homologue. *Nature* 372, 425–432.

Index

Page numbers in **bold** refer to figures; those in *italic* refer to tables